COPING
WITH
ARTHRITIS

Trigger-point locations with zones of pain reference: front view.

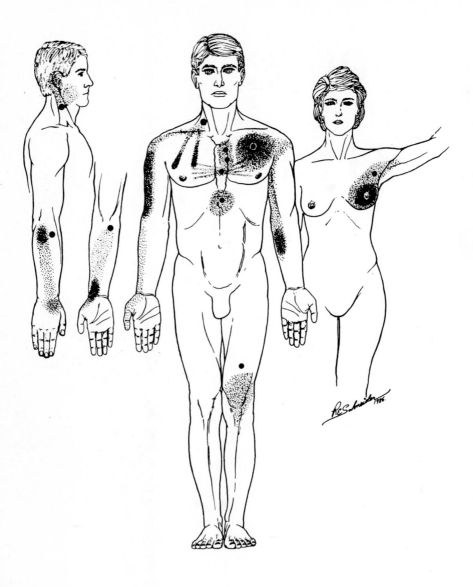

Trigger-point locations with zones of pain reference: back view.

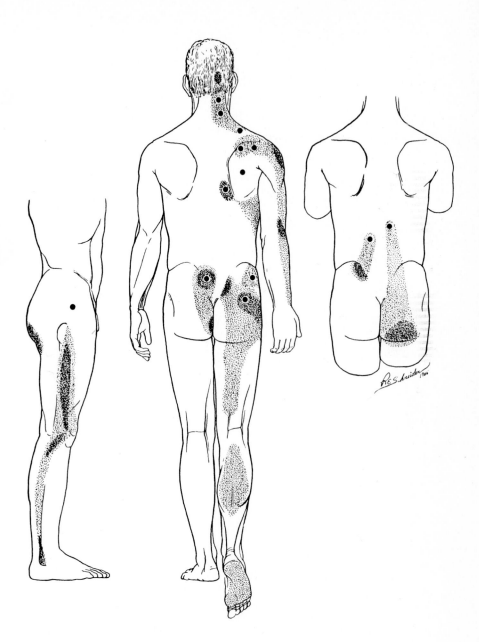

COPING
WITH
ARTHRITIS

MORE MOBILITY, LESS PAIN

Robert P. Sheon, M.D.
Roland W. Moskowitz, M.D.
Victor M. Goldberg, M.D.
with Betty Hueter, M.A.

McGRAW-HILL BOOK COMPANY
New York St. Louis San Francisco Toronto Hamburg Mexico

This book is not intended to replace the services of a physician. Any application of the recommendations set forth in the following pages is at the reader's discretion and sole risk.

1 2 3 4 5 6 7 8 9 D O C D O C 8 9 8 7

ISBN 0-07-056562-7{H.C.}
ISBN 0-07-056561-9{PBK.}

LIBRARY OF CONGRESS CATALOGING-IN-PUBLICATION DATA

Sheon, Robert P.
    Coping with arthritis.

    1. Arthritis—Popular works.   I. Moskowitz, Roland W.
II. Goldberg, Victor M., 1939–   .   III. Title.
[DNLM: 1. Rheumatology—popular works.   2. Self Care—
popular works.   WE 344 S546c]
RC933.S435   1987   616.7'22   87-4043
ISBN 0-07-056562-7
ISBN 0-07-056561-9 (pbk.)

BOOK DESIGN BY PATRICE FODERO
EDITING SUPERVISOR: MARGERY LUHRS

We wish to dedicate this book to our children:

Sarah, Amy, and David Sheon
Josh and Kara Moskowitz
Rebecca, Jonathan, and Eden Goldberg

And to their generation and generations to come
with the hope that they will see the
eradication of these diseases.

And, finally, to Mary, the subject of Chapter 13.
Her life has been a dedication
to the education of future generations:
41 years and 20 summers of happy teaching.

Contents

Acknowledgments

The scientific basis for the medical content of this book may be found in our textbook, *Soft Tissue Rheumatic Pain: Recognition, Management, Prevention*, 2d ed., Lea & Febiger, Philadelphia, 1987. This textbook contains more than 2000 references.

The following illustrations are from our textbook and are reprinted with permission of Lea & Febiger:

Figures:

4-1, 4-3, 4-4, 4-6, 4-7 to 4-10

5-2 to 5-4, 5-6 to 5-8, 5-10

6-2, 6-3, 6-6, 6-10

7-2 to 7-4, 7-6, 7-7, 7-9 to 7-12, 7-14, 7-15

8-1 to 8-4, 8-6

9-2, 9-3, 9-5 to 9-7, 9-9 to 9-12, 9-14, 9-16 to 9-18, 9-21 to 9-23

10-2 to 10-9, 10-11, 10-12

11-2 to 11-8, 11-10, 11-11

The tables, What's Harmful, What's Helpful . . . , are reproduced from R. P. Sheon, "A Joint Protection Guide for Nonarticular Rheumatic Disorders," *Postgraduate Medicine*, 77(5):329–338 (1985), with permission.

Plates 4-1, 4-2, 5-1, 5-2, 6-1, 7-1, 9-1, 9-2, 9-3, 11-1, and 11-2 are reprinted from Henry Gray, *Gray's Anatomy*, 30th ed., Carmine D. Clemente (ed.), Lea & Febiger, Philadelphia, 1985, with permission.

Figures 5-11, 5-12, and 5-13 are reprinted from R.M. Kessler and D. Hertling, *Management of Common Musculoskeletal Disorders*, Harper & Row, Philadelphia, 1983, with permission.

Figure 9-8 is reproduced from S.H. Hochschuler, "Diagnostic Studies in Clinical Practice," *Orthopedic Clinics of North America*, 14:517–526 (1983), with permission.

Figure 12-1 is reprinted from W. S. Wilke and A. H. Mackenzie, "Proposed Pathogenesis of Fibrositis," *Cleveland Clinic Quarterly*, 52:147–152 (1985), with permission.

Figure 14-1 is reprinted from Saul S. Haskell, "Self-examination for Body Alignment," *Orthopedics Today*, 1(4):16 (1981), with permission.

The authors wish to thank our colleagues and patients in Toledo and Cleveland, who taught us much about the art of caring for patients with arthritis and rheumatism.

We wish to thank research secretary Cathy LaCourse and our other assistants and research librarians at Toledo Clinic, University Hospitals/ Case Western Reserve University, Toledo Hospital, and the Arthritis Unit at Flower Hospital; artist and photographer Claire Kirsner; artist Roy Schneider; and photographer Alan Weintraub.

How to Use This Book

Our purpose in writing this book is to help you help yourself. We have tried to anticipate questions patients would like to have answered if they could ask a doctor who would give them all the time they needed. We hope our book will seem that way to you—as if you were sitting down with a doctor who isn't hurried—no, not one doctor, but three. We will help you with workplace or sports injuries, muscle and tendon strains, back pain, nerve entrapment, and arthritis that respond to self-help measures. In many cases these problems can even be prevented. This can be accomplished with the measures detailed in this book.

Many times we will see a patient with a particular joint pain that isn't arthritis at all. Another patient may have a pain that originated in one part of the body and has traveled to the spot that is painful. We show you how to determine the real cause and source of the problem

It is not our aim to put other doctors out of business. We have, however, tried to provide the information you need if you suffer from local aches and pains, strains, or generalized arthritis. First, you need a diagnosis. Then you need to know how to best treat your illness and how to *prevent* or minimize recurrences.

Chapters 1 and 2 provide information about the many disorders that we recognize in our practices. Much can be done for such localized problems as myofascial pain (pain of muscular origin), bursitis, tendinitis, pinched nerves, or osteoarthritis—and often without expensive medical care. We hope you will follow the advice, because it is medically sound. This is a workbook that can provide you with information that will lead to a better, less-stressful, happier life.

We help you sort out your complaints, showing you how to make some self-examination physical findings that either point to a diagnosis or that you can relay to your doctor. We help you evaluate the treatment measures you have tried and suggest what you and your doctor might do. If you are confronted with the possibility of an expensive or invasive test or treatment, we have provided information that will help you decide whether to say "yes" or "no."

If you are working at a job which causes you problems, or if you are thinking of starting a new job, Chapter 3 may help you recognize potentially harmful work positions or hazards. If you can prevent an injury, your health, productivity, and well-being will be enhanced.

If your problem is mostly in one body area, we recommend that you read through Chapter 2 to learn the categories of easily treated soft-tissue rheumatism. Then look through Chapters 4 through 12 and turn to the chapter that relates to that body region. Each of these chapters includes six tables. Among them, a table of danger signs describes symptoms that indicate the need for urgent medical attention. Another table lists symptoms and possible diagnoses. Reading through the chapter, you will learn how to recognize many disorders. Still another table provides self-examination tests and movements that aid in diagnosis. Knowing how to find a trigger point that reproduces your pain can help speed you to the recognition of your problem, treatment, and prevention program.

Once you have a pretty good idea of what is wrong, we help you with some measures you can use for pain relief. In the table of exercises after each chapter, we then indicate exercises you can do to restore strength and muscle tone to that area of your body. If you maintain your respect for pain and don't rush, these exercises should be helpful. But don't just make a dash for these exercises. They will be more beneficial if you read the text that accompanies them. You may even find that you should do only some of the exercises.

But you also will want to consider how you might prevent recurrences, and another table, What's Harmful, What's Helpful . . . , provides a list of aggravating habits or improper body positions that may be causing soft-tissue injury. In addition, the table lists ways to avoid body strain at work, home, or during sports or calisthenic activities. If you are helped by one chapter, we hope you will read through some of the others and learn what is helpful and what is harmful to the other body regions.

But when a condition remains stubborn and you need professional care, each chapter describes what can be done after your doctor's diagnosis—what medications you might find helpful, other measures physicians might consider for your care, and what a referral to a physical therapist or occupational therapist might offer. If you still haven't had success, a table of persistent causes suggests some activities that may be aggravating the problem.

If you hurt all over, turn to Chapters 12 and 13. We have seen many patients with fibrositis or rheumatoid arthritis who do much to help themselves. Many times we are in awe of our patients who, often in severe pain and sometimes severely disabled, continue with a full and meaningful life. In Chapter 12 we say that anyone who is afflicted with arthritis and can still cope is a hero. We really believe that, and we want to help you get the maximum from your life. We point out what measures you can take to improve the quality of your life. With the help of a supportive physician, you can learn what features might lead to a diagnosis more quickly, what tests are most helpful, and some of the treatment measures your doctor might consider.

Sometimes a local problem is aggravating a bigger problem. For example, chest-wall pain syndromes are very common in patients with arthritis and connective-tissue diseases; and they are happy to learn that they don't have a heart problem. Local treatment and exercise can go a long way to ease suffering. We don't have any magic pills or theories. But even if you have rheumatoid arthritis or lupus erythematosus, we probably can help you cope—help you reduce your pain and disability. On those days when it all seems too much to manage, read through the chapter on Mary (Chapter 13). We think she will give you what it takes to manage.

Chapter 14 on sports includes many ways to avoid injuries from conditioning and sport activities. If you have suffered an injury, you'll learn what we think is best for immediate care. Each major sport and conditioning activity has unique problems that are worth your consideration.

Chapter 15 provides information about commonly used drugs, rub-ons, assistive devices, and some not-so-helpful treatment measures. There's no need to be a stoic about arthritis pain. Take advantage of every creature comfort you can find which makes life easier—long-handled nippers to pick up out-of-reach articles on the floor or shelves, zipper pulls and buttoners, or a light-weight electric blanket for cold nights to avoid the weight of heavier blankets. Many catalogs are available that make it easy to find such useful items without even leaving your home to shop for them. Catalogs and books that feature these items are listed in the Appendix.

Terms about arthritis and rheumatism that your doctor might use can be found in the Glossary.

The Index can help you find the condition, body site, or treatment modalities covered in our book.

We doubt, however, that you will read the book cover-to-cover. Rather, you will perhaps be like the boy in high school who was asked whether he had read straight through any books. He said his favorite was the *Sears Catalog*, and he liked to look up things he needed to know.

We hope you will find our ideas not only helpful but also cost-effective. If we can save you a prolonged series of visits to your doctor, if we can speed your recovery, or if we can improve your productivity, then our efforts will have been rewarded.

It is part of the cure to wish to be cured.

—Seneca, *Hippolytus*

CHAPTER 1

Arthritis: Past, Present, Future

Arthritis, in one form or another, affects more men and women than any other disease. It can and does appear from infancy until very advanced ages. The Arthritis Foundation has studies showing that 97 percent of all people over 60 have enough arthritis to be seen on x-rays.

Although we have documented evidence that arthritis existed 3500 years ago, it probably was present many centuries before that. Despite these statistics, and unlike the majority of our diseases, to date there have been no revolutionary cures. However, this book will show that much can be done to alleviate and even prevent arthritic pain and other rheumatic-pain disorders.

The term "arthritis," then, can be applied to maladies of both the bony and the soft-tissue parts of muscles and joints. When we want to be precise, we will refer to the specific type of arthritis by name—that is, osteoarthritis, gout, rheumatoid arthritis, etc. Included in the broad term arthritis are at least 250 different disturbances manifested in everything from pain in joints to pain in membranes, tendons, and even skin! Although joint inflammation with swelling, pain, and stiffness is not uncommon, much of the discomfort and disability may also result from tissue surrounding and connecting the joints. Different tissues do different things. Muscles and tendons move the bones, ligaments tie them together, bursal sacs cushion them, and nerves send the messages that activate the joints. These soft supporting tissues may cause serious trouble, and cause it more often than the joints. Cartilage, ligaments, tendons, bursas, muscles, fascial tissues, fatty tissue, and nerves may also be affected (Figure 1-1). In arthritis there can be almost as many aches and pains as there are movements of our body parts, and the onset can be slow or rapid.

If you now have arthritis, you will want to do everything possible to end your discomfort. If you are without symptoms, you will find measures here that can *prevent* arthritis pain and some of the crippling which often accompanies it. If you think you are immune, don't forget that "97 percent."

A century ago aches and pains and even a limp were taken for granted. Because life was often brief, they were not a concern. Then, following World War II, we became a sedentary society. More of us entered the white-collar work force. We bought overstuffed, unsupportive furniture, and we sat for hours at a time watching tele-

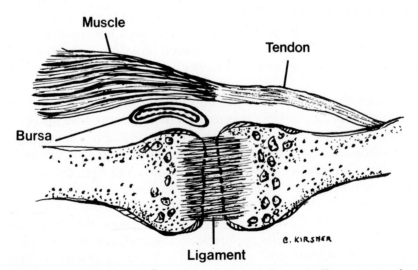

Muscle

Tendon

Bursa

C. KIRSHER

Ligament

Figure 1-1. Diagram of a joint. Note location of muscle, ligament, tendon, tendon sheath, and bursa. The bursa, a moist sac, protects muscle from underlying bone and assists smooth muscle movement across the body surface. Tendons are the stringy ends of muscles that attach to bone. Ligaments are joint hinges.

vision. We gave up dancing, a wonderful exercise. Our muscles grew flabby. Joints sagged, loosening supporting tissues, and postures slumped. Nerves became stretched. If, on occasion, we undertook a strenuous task, our flabby muscles objected and were susceptible to injury.

Now we take our bodies more seriously. Recently health clubs, adult-education programs, and other exercise regimens have become popular. The whole nation has become conscious of body-conditioning activities such as jogging, walking, and cross-country skiing. A recent study of Harvard alumni indicates you do live longer and better if you exercise regularly. People are also into many other activities such as handicrafts and home remodeling. Many minor skeletal deformities result in injuries during these activities, and although we can expect to live a lot longer, we feel threatened when we notice evidence of aging or joint distress. It is pleasing to look forward to more years, but we want them to be comfortable years. As longevity increases and exercise becomes ever more active, arthritis will continue to worsen unless we take preventive action.

Common, everyday, repetitive movements—often unconscious—can be a primary cause of arthritis pain. Many times a day a salesman flings his briefcase over his shoulder as he gets behind the wheel of his car. He retrieves the case each time by reaching backward over the seat. Before too long he develops a painful shoulder. A homemaker who is addicted to romantic novels, often reading two an evening, suffers from pain in her wrists, numbness, and weakness in her hands—all from holding the book and turning pages. Her hands ache badly when she awakens, and she must shake them violently to get rid of the pain. A person prone to talking on the phone cradles the receiver between shoulder and chin, ending up with arthritis neck pain.

Behavior disorders contribute to many musculoskeletal injuries. The compulsive person—the one who says, "I am going to finish this job if it kills me"—is likely to have such a disorder. This is particularly true of someone who enjoys knitting, needlepoint, woodworking, playing a musical instrument, etc. Such individuals are prone to tendinitis, carpal-tunnel syndrome, trigger finger, and other disabilities. The combination of the compulsive personality and a mild structural disorder often produces musculoskeletal disabilities.

It has even been established that most factory accidents involving back injuries occur during the first hour at work. They usually happen to the employee who has driven a given distance to get there—

very likely gripping the steering wheel in a rather desperate fashion. Speaking of work, statistics show that 26.6 million days are lost annually in regular jobs to arthritis and rheumatic-pain disorders, for a total of $6.046 billion in lost wages. To that figure add the annual direct and indirect cost of medical care, and the total economic impact is $13.269 billion. It's quite a tab for one disease!

We often think that medical specialization is a fairly recent concept and lament that doctors are getting ever more limited in the area they will treat. Actually, specialization is ages old, having existed among the Egyptians in 1500 B.C.—and once was even more precise than it is today. Long before medicine was a science, it was an art; long before it was an art, it was a religion. Each part of the body was the province of a different "priest," who could treat only that particular component. Moreover, the treatment had to follow a careful, prescribed-by-law ritual. Any deviation in the administration of the cure meant capital punishment. And what did the remedies consist of? There is no mention in Garrison's *History of Medicine*[1] of the eye of newt used by Macbeth's witches, but many other strange substances found their way into the doctor's little black bag. Equal parts of the fat of the lion, hippopotamus, crocodile, goose, serpent, and ibex were compounded and rubbed on bald pates. Other pharmacopoeias contained blood, excreta, and visceral parts of birds and reptiles. One concoction consisted simply of equal parts of writing ink and cerebrospinal fluid. (Perhaps even the "hair of the dog" was taken.) Small wonder that if there was no improvement in the patient within 4 days, the "doctor" was allowed to try something new. So, although there is no actual record of what was used to treat arthritis, many mummies attest to the fact that there was crippling from joint disease, which the Egyptians labeled "hardening in the limbs." You may use your imagination to visualize the "cures" they concocted.

Through the centuries treatments came and went, but even as late as 1940 doctors were all over the lot searching for ways to deal with arthritis. One popular method involved an electrical machine with a variety of glass wands which produced a violet glow, sparks, and a sizzling sound when they were brought into contact with flesh (Figure 1-2). The device was low in price and quite a phenomenal

---

1. F. H. Garrison, *History of Medicine,* W. B. Saunders, Philadelphia, 1929.

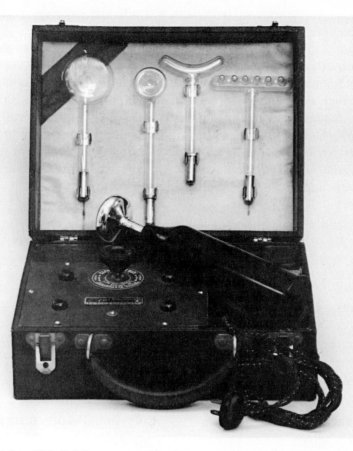

Figure 1-2.   This "violet ray machine" was used to "cure" many types of rheumatism about 50 years ago. Our fascination with electricity for medical purposes has a long history.

value because it could also "cure" acne, abscesses, functional aphonia (psychologic loss of voice), anemia, and asthma. And, that's only the A's. Undoubtedly, too, you have heard of copper bracelets, honey and vinegar, kelp, and a strict fish-and-poultry diet. Before you chortle and feel superior, keep in mind that $1.75 billion a year is *still* spent for quackery to cure arthritis.

    Just 30 years ago most hospitalized arthritis cases were the result of tuberculosis, gout, or rheumatic fever. Today most patients with these three diseases now manage very well on an outpatient basis.

    But still there are more than 100 inflammatory-arthritis conditions, usually associated with pain, warmth, and swelling. Also, there are noninflammatory, degenerative-arthritis diseases that damage the bony joints and cartilage. All of these conditions can now be diagnosed, and attention can now focus on their cause, cure, and maintenance. But there remain hundreds of rheumatic conditions for which no cause is known. Health-care professionals do, however, recognize the significance of bad habits and aggravating activities. Unfortunately, once injured, some tissues have little capacity for recovery or healing. Prevention is vitally important.

Today all of the following are being used in the treatment of arthritis and all are reputable, valuable methods:

Medication	Walking aids
Rest	Surgery
Exercise	Heat
Posture correction	Rehabilitation
Splints	

All of these professionals are involved in some part of the problem:

Dentist	Physical therapist
Osteopath	Occupational therapist
Rheumatologist	Professional sports instructor
Orthopedist	Chiropractor
Physiatrist	Orthotist
Podiatrist	Occupational nurse
Personal physician	

Work strains, poor posture, and slack musculature can be aided by mobilizing and conditioning exercises. Tables and illustrations of exercises are provided in this book. You may, however, have to check with your physician if you have a hiatus hernia (a swallowing disruption) or a heart problem or if you are beyond middle age. A new exercise should be undertaken cautiously and gradually.

Because pain and spasm often cannot be measured, limited research has been undertaken on them. Furthermore, tests that measure spasm, degeneration, or altered function of muscles, tendons, and ligaments are also frequently inadequate. Although some of the advice we provide represents art rather than science, the advice is safe, reliable, and inexpensive. Furthermore, some new measurement tools are becoming available, and we will describe them.

In this book we strive to help you better understand the diverse approaches to rheumatic-pain disorders. Also, we want to provide you with the ability to identify and manage painful or disabling conditions, and to do it without resorting to expensive, invasive procedures. Most important, we aim to help you prevent arthritis in areas of the body where you do not have it.

The book can guide you whether you have an advanced case of arthritis or are still in its early stages and concerned about your future. You may begin with any problem area. As you read the suggestions, a bonus will be your appreciation of proper body mechanics while resting, sleeping, sitting, or performing your job, recreation, or home activity. Simple, sane body mechanics are lost when you develop an aggravating habit; if we can teach you to substitute a good habit for a bad one, much pain and disability will be prevented. If you want to try a new activity and are fearful, this book can show you helpful ways to begin.

The book is not meant to be a substitute for a physician's advice and care. But it is a self-help book, designed to let you work on your own. Do not try to diagnose and treat significant problems of arthritis or bursitis. Please consider the book a guide to understanding your aches and pains, which may be manageable.

In Chapters 4 to 12, we deal with pain in the various parts of the body, from the head to the feet. In addition there are chapters on soft-tissue rheumatic pain in general and also on pains arising from employment. We will examine how well someone with very severe arthritis manages to cope. There is a chapter on preventive measures for sports enthusiasts. Also covered are pain that seems to hit every part of your body, but at different times, and even the pain that hits all these parts at the *same* time. We also devote a chapter to emotionally induced pain and another to the various medications for arthritis.

At the end of Chapters 4 to 12 are a series of tables. The first table in each chapter contains a list of danger signs to alert you to the need for professional advice and treatment. The second table describes self-examination techniques to help you correctly identify your problem. Next are tables to help you pinpoint those habits of everyday life that may be aggravating your problem and a number of corrective measures and habits that may ease the pain. Finally, we have included a table of exercises, with illustrations, to help you prevent or alleviate arthritic discomfort.

CHAPTER 2

Soft-Tissue Rheumatic-Pain Disorders

Diagnosis of many soft-tissue rheumatic-pain disorders has been hampered by the lack of reproducible measurement of the pain and spasm. Also, terminology for occupations or activities (such as "weaver's bottom" or "tennis elbow") and the overlapping of conditions (for example, carpal-tunnel syndrome and trigger finger) confound our ability to study or generate data for these disorders. It was only after World War II when electrical nerve studies provided measurement of pinched-nerve syndromes that these nerve-entrapment disorders gained validity and recognition.

Classification

We have divided the 150 or so common soft-tissue rheumatic-pain disorders into five major groupings, as described in Table 2-1, at the end of this chapter. These will be discussed in detail in the material on each body region. This chapter will acquaint you with these disorders in general and with their treatment. Also, we will present some of the emerging techniques for studying these conditions.

Myofascial Pain

Myofascial pain is often felt in the neck, back, or limbs. It is pain in or around muscles. Because present technology does not provide objective measurement of muscle spasm, the recognition of myofascial pain is an art as well as a science. The term implies deep, aching pain in one body area at a distance from a *trigger point*. Pressure upon that point will reveal a hard, painful area within the tissue. Thus, the trigger points are said to actuate pain in a "target zone of pain reference," which is at some distance from the trigger point. Secondary trigger points lie within this pain zone and are also called *myalgic points, tender points,* or *trigger zones* (Plates 2-1 and 2-2). The trigger points may result from acute trauma or minor injury, from the repeated minor microtrauma of daily living, or from the chronic strain of sedentary living habits. They also occur in systemic inflammatory disorders or infections. Visible swelling is rare.

What causes persistent muscle pain? If broken bones or surgical incisions will heal within 6 weeks, then it just doesn't make sense that bursitis, tendinitis, or muscle injuries should last months, as they often do. The degree of injury to a tissue depends on the state of conditioning of the tissue, degree of overuse, and type and severity of the injury. John Bonica, a physician-researcher in Seattle, has suggested that chronicity often results from a pain-spasm-pain cycle. Once tissue is injured, pain substances in the injured tissues irritate nerve endings. The nerves carry up messages of injury to the brain and carry back messages that actualize in swelling, spasm, and increased blood flow (seen as warmth or redness). The dull ache of injury is a result. Chemical changes in the tissue occur, with increased lactic acid and potassium. These intensify the spasm and pain. The muscle fibers may then choke off their own blood supply! These changes occur more rapidly in sedentary individuals than in athletes.

Injury or trauma must be considered more broadly than direct injury. Most cases of persistent muscle spasm (myofascial pain) result from *microtrauma*—the injury that results from the improper body mechanics of our daily living. The mechanics will be considered throughout these pages.

Tendinitis and Bursitis

Tendinitis is a clinical and pathologic disorder with common features of local pain and dysfunction. Sport and calisthenic activities,

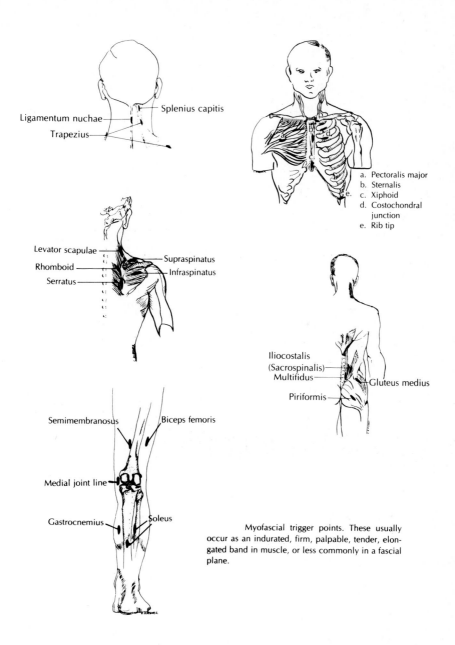

Ligamentum nuchae
Trapezius
Splenius capitis

a. Pectoralis major
b. Sternalis
c. Xiphoid
d. Costochondral junction
e. Rib tip

Levator scapulae
Rhomboid
Serratus
Supraspinatus
Infraspinatus

Iliocostalis (Sacrospinalis)
Multifidus
Piriformis
Gluteus medius

Semimembranosus
Biceps femoris

Medial joint line

Gastrocnemius
Soleus

Myofascial trigger points. These usually occur as an indurated, firm, palpable, tender, elongated band in muscle, or less commonly in a fascial plane.

Plate 2-1. Typical locations for trigger points in injured or strained muscles. (Trigger-point maps based on work of Janet Travell.)

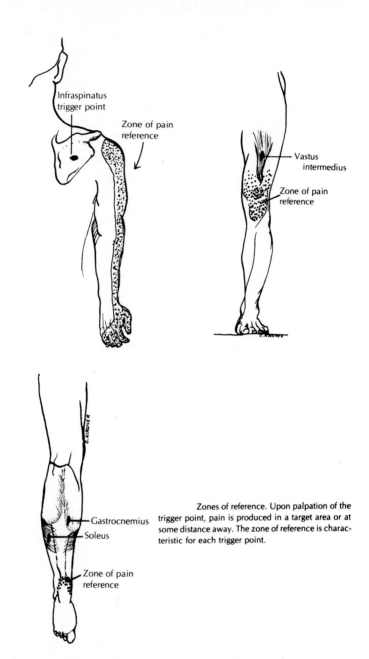

Zones of reference. Upon palpation of the trigger point, pain is produced in a target area or at some distance away. The zone of reference is characteristic for each trigger point.

Plate 2-2.   Typical trigger points with location of pain always at a distance from the trigger point. You probably wouldn't know you had a trigger point unless you knew when and how to press it.

hobbies, and jobs that require repetitive motion may give rise to inflammation and degeneration. *Triggering* is a unique disturbance associated with tendinitis: a finger will suddenly lock and must be pulled passively. A snapping is perceived as the digit "unlocks." Triggering occurs in 20 percent of the cases of tendinitis in upper limbs.

Bursitis is an inflammation of the bursas, the saclike structures that form after birth to protect the soft tissues against underlying bony prominences. Common sites for inflammation of these sacs are behind the elbow, about the knee, in front of the kneecap, and on the side of the hip.

Alexander Monro II of Edinburgh provided the first atlas of some 40 bursas. The term "bursitis" originates from the end of the eighteenth century. In 1788 the society that followed the second bourgeois revolution consisted of princes and their political power; laborers and freemen, who provided the basic work force; and the new middlemen, the purse ("la bourse"), who were the businessmen. The latter class and their banks ensured that lubrication made for a frictionless, easy-running society.[1] Hence the aptly applied term, "bursa"! The word *bursa* also comes from the word for "bag" or "pouch" in medieval Latin and the Greek word for "skin" or "hide."

Structural Disorders

The structural disorders include short leg, scoliosis (curvature of the spine), lateral patellar subluxation (displaced kneecap), and flat feet. We must keep in mind that structural disorders are important in the prevention of soft-tissue injury among athletes and those participating in conditioning activities. In one study of medical students, 69 percent had from one to seven different structural abnormalities. Joint laxity was the most common; next was restricted joint motion. Other common findings were scoliosis, short leg, flat feet, and misalignment of the kneecaps.

Nerve Entrapment

Neurovascular entrapment disorders may occur within the spinal canal (spinal stenosis) or along the course of a peripheral nerve. A sensation of swelling and pain, as well as numbness and tingling away from the site of entrapment, should suggest the condition.

---

1. E. G. L. Bywaters, "Lesions of Bursae, Tendons, and Tendon Sheaths," *Clinics in Rheumatic Diseases,* 5:883–918, 1979.

Generalized Pain Disorders

These are the "I hurt all over!" syndromes. One of these generalized pain disorders is the *fibrositis syndrome,* in which tender points are found. When pressed, these tender zones produce pain in a nearby area. Fibrositis is a disease characterized by pain, stiffness, and tenderness of muscles. Sleep disturbance, constant aching, and fatigue are also part of the disease; in addition, patients are never completely free from pain. *Polymyalgia rheumatica* (pain involving many muscles) is an acute, painful stiffness about the shoulders and hips in older people. In contrast, people with *psychogenic rheumatism* (rheumatism which originates in the mind) may be perfectly fine at times, but then again they may have the "touch-me-not" syndrome, where all parts of the body are painful to the touch. *Chronic benign pain* may result from a trivial injury or surgery; it can lead to widespread, aching pain. *Reflex sympathetic dystrophy* is one of the most painful forms of arthritis. There may be little to see—perhaps whiteness or some redness of the skin in addition to slight swelling—but there is a throbbing, burning, aching pain, usually in an arm or leg. Doctors think of it as a short-circuiting of the nervous system.

Diagnosis

Intra-articular arthritis is arthritis within the joint, and doctors think of it as true arthritis. Although this true arthritis is what most people worry about, the symptoms of joint pain are often the result of soft-tissue disturbances such as bursitis, tendinitis, muscle spasm, and pinched nerves. Here are some helpful ways to distinguish soft-tissue problems from arthritis.

1. The usual physical findings, the tests of inflammation, and the x-ray features of arthritis are normal or as expected for the average healthy individual of that age.
2. Symptoms of soft-tissue problems often are worse after resting. Whereas intra-articular disease (true arthritis) is worse with use and relieved by rest, these conditions of the soft supporting tissues often awaken you from sleep or are accentuated

after sitting and relieved with movement. Of course, overuse may aggravate them as well.

3. Most of these conditions have other aggravating factors that lead to recurrences. These include improper resting positions, prolonged repetitive movements, and a lack of respect for pain.

4. Physical-examination tests and maneuvers can reproduce or exacerbate symptoms. We will teach you many of these, so you can test yourself.

5. Simple management can provide relief, and this response to treatment will support the diagnosis. These five features are summarized in Table 2-2 at the end of this chapter.

Presently great interest lies in using newer technology in the diagnosis of soft-tissue rheumatic-pain problems. These new diagnostic methods include scintigraphy, computed tomography, thermography, magnetic resonance imaging, and further refinement of electrodiagnostic testing.

Scintigraphy, or *radionuclide scanning,* which is performed with a harmless amount of a radioisotope, has proved of value in a number of the soft-tissue rheumatic disorders. These scans use a measuring device similar to a Geiger counter combined with x-ray film. The scan will show such things as tumors, infections, and inflammation before any bone changes appear on ordinary x-ray films. Scans also can show fractures that may not be visible on ordinary x-rays. In addition, their use is valuable in reflex-sympathetic dystrophy and in frozen-shoulder diagnosis for evaluation and assessment of disease, sacroiliac-joint involvement in low-back pain, vascular injury, osteonecrosis (the pathologic death of a cell or group of cells in contact with living cells in a bone), knee pain, and perhaps certain chest-wall pain disorders. Another important use is for detection of rheumatoid arthritis before its appearance.

Computed axial tomography (CT scan or CAT scan) links x-ray with a computer to obtain three-dimensional pictures. It has been used in diagnosing back and neck problems, hip pain, lipomas (fatty growths), cysts, and bursitis, as well as the possibility of stenosis (narrowing) of the carpal canal as a cause for carpal-tunnel syndrome. It is used mostly to detect abscesses and tumor conditions.

Thermography is a diagnostic technique that records infrared radiation that emanates spontaneously from the body's surface and provides a thermogram or mathematical recording of its temperature and local thermal differences. It is of great interest because the technique is gaining refinement through increased quality. Heat emission from the body can be recorded by thermography; and microwave thermography may provide a noninvasive, simple, permanent record of sympathetic-nervous-system abnormality when nerve-root or myofascial disease is present. But the technique is only one example of many diagnostic tools that are being researched at this time.

Magnetic resonance imaging (MRI) is another new and noninvasive technique. It involves the use of very strong magnets in combination with computer technology. Although time-consuming and costly, MRI does provide a three-dimensional view of the body and tissue. It can measure changes in metabolism by using magnetic forces rather than x-rays and holds great promise for measuring changes in muscles and tendons. Presently it is used for identifying cancers, spinal and brain abnormalities, heart disease, and abdominal disorders. This technique may also have diagnostic value in metabolic muscle disturbances and mass lesions near the spine or in the extremities.

Does Treatment Really Help?

Whether treatment really helps has been a tough question because we have no good yardsticks to measure pain, spasm, or the emotional impact of pain and disability. But we can now measure the time an injured worker has been disabled and the time until a sport participant resumes activities. The new electronic exercise devices that print out graphs of a person's strength may allow objective measurement of the effort an individual makes toward gaining strength. Studies at the University of Alabama of strength-training programs found that any exercise program with voluntary maximal effort resulted in muscle strengthening. They could not find one method superior to another. Similarly, aged individuals also respond to treatment if they make the effort.

In 1984 the American Medical Association (AMA) Council on Scientific Affairs published a review of numerous exercises for the elderly and found that older sedentary persons benefit if they begin exercising at a low level and increase gradually, with each exercise session starting with a 3- to 5-minute warm-up. One of our patients, aged 92, got down on the floor every day to perform a back program. She had not walked without assistance in 35 years, but in *just 6 weeks* she had conditioned herself to the point that she could leave the house unassisted. Five years later she went to London and kept up with her group on walking tours!

Back-extension exercises have been advocated by a New Zealand therapist for patients with limited lumbar movement associated with muscle spasm. Results revealed improvement in 2 months in 80 percent of the patients, and most reported they could abort an attack of pain by performing the exercise.

Group exercise has been developed for the YMCA by physiatrists. They reported the results of 12,000 people who had enrolled and completed a 6-week program. Pain diminished and trunk strength improved in 80 percent of the patients, irrespective of past surgery. Success related directly to maintenance of strength.

Back schools that incorporate at-the-workplace education have resulted in significant improvement in the quality of life for participants. Simple education and the use of exercise such as we describe in these chapters allowed twice as many of these patients to return to work compared with those receiving no such education or exercise. Similarly, persons receiving disability benefits who took a group-exercise program (including bending exercises, pool therapy, and the back-school education) had encouraging results. Seventy-two percent of them were employed within 6 months even though half of them had had back surgery previously. Half the patients had had symptoms of longer than 3 months' duration when they entered the program.

Manipulation techniques, some of which are used throughout this book, were rigorously examined in Britain. There, investigators tested such treatment against sham or placebo physical therapy (inappropriate movements or exercise) and found that manipulation alone at first provided relief from symptoms, but that the benefit did not last. By 2 months the effect had worn off. Similarly, manipulation provided relief more quickly than massage, but the benefit was brief. Manipulation, in the long run, does not save money. Several studies have compared the total cost of various treatment methods, including manipulation, and none was less costly or more effective.

In the treatment of tendinitis, a Canadian sports clinic reported results of friction massage and stretching, followed by strengthening. Of 200 patients, mostly between ages 16 and 50, treated once daily for 6 weeks, 87 percent either completely recovered or greatly improved. This was true for those with tennis elbow as well as lower-limb sport injuries to tendons. These experts stress eccentric strengthening, a type of off-center balanced exercise in which muscles lengthen as they strengthen. An example when exercising the elbow muscles would be to slowly lower a weight held with an elbow, first bent and then gradually extended.

Following an initial constriction, using ice for 20 minutes produces dilation of blood vessels. This "milking" effect may remove waste products and edema from injured tissue. In one study, ice treatment of ankle injuries resulted in 17 fewer days of disability.

In up to 90 percent of patients, leg cramp can benefit from the Daniell exercise, as described on page 250. In other education programs investigators report that back education was retained at an 80 percent level 6 to 18 months later. An interesting adjunct to the various treatment programs, another study concluded that people who bought health books had 6 percent fewer doctor visits than patients who didn't try to "keep up" with developments in health.

Table 2-1
Soft-Tissue Rheumatic-Pain Disorders

Myofascial pain: Regional pain with trigger points

Tendinitis and bursitis: Inflammation or degeneration of these anatomically identifiable structures

Structural disorders: Short leg, scoliosis (curvature of the spine), lateral patellar subluxation (displaced kneecap), flat feet

Nerve entrapment: Thoracic-outlet syndrome, carpal-tunnel syndrome, and tarsal-tunnel syndrome (pinched nerve near the inner anklebone)

Generalized pain disorders: Fibrositis (muscular rheumatism), benign pain, reflex sympathetic dystrophy (swollen, painful short-circuiting of the nervous system), and psychogenic rheumatism (rheumatism of mental origin)

Table 2-2

Features of Nonarticular Rheumatism

No signs or tests indicate systemic inflammation.
Pain is often worse with rest and improved with movement.
Aggravating habits are common and cause recurrences.
Physical-examination tests and maneuvers reproduce symptoms.
Treatment provides relief, thus corroborating diagnosis.

CHAPTER 3

The Pains of Work: "My Job Is Killing Me!"

Almost everyone who develops pain or has an accident while working blames the job—"My job is killing me!" However, it isn't necessarily so.

For example, John R. complained to his supervisor that his new job was harming his hands. His task required handling small parts, turning them over, then lifting the tray of parts onto a rack. He wasn't bothered during the workday, but would awaken some mornings with swollen, aching, numb hands. Other workers had no difficulty with the job, so John's supervisor suggested a review of other factors. (In reading the chapter on the hand, you will find the real culprits in John's problem.) John had been drinking a lot of caffeinated beverages and had become a hand clencher. On his way home from work, he unconsciously clutched the steering wheel. At night he also clenched his fists and jaws as he slept. In addition, he had begun working on his car, on a lift, at a local garage. He was working overhead and causing a congestion of the thoracic outlet (nerves and vessels going down the arms). After correcting these aggravating habits, John tolerated his job very well.

Arthritis research in conditions that are work-related has been hampered by difficulties in diagnosis, terminology, measurement, and politics within the workplace. Arthritis, known colloquially by such descriptive terms as "slipped disc," "weaver's bottom," "coal-miner's beat knee," or "golfer's elbow," can result from a number of structural disturbances. These conditions are really a number of different conditions, and each one may involve a different injured tissue.

Many questions must be considered:

> Does the worker have a monotonous and tedious task, one that involves making repetitive movements or remaining in a fixed position a long time? Does he or she lift above or below a mechanically strainful height? How many workers performing the same job have been disabled?

> What is the atmosphere of the workplace? Is the milieu conducive to good work habits? What about safety, lighting, and temperature? Are the tools and machine adaptable to the physical features of the worker?

> Does the worker have a good relationship with coworkers and management? How does the company help the injured worker? How quickly is proper care given?

> What physical characteristics, habits, and attitudes does the worker bring to the workplace? How much time has the worker lost in the past? Are physical characteristics of the worker important in satisfactory job placement?

These and other considerations are under scrutiny by experts in the medical field. Methods that will educate management to consider these and other facets of occupational injury are being studied in the United States, as well as in many other countries.

Until recently health-care costs were accepted without question or scrutiny. Now, in an effort to control runaway expenses, many companies have begun self-insured plans that offer employees incentives for maintaining good work habits and good health. Suddenly back and other soft-tissue injuries have become important. Companies' medical personnel promote this wellness. Their efforts also include preventing injury through improving health and motivating the worker to be more cautious.

As our labor population ages and grows increasingly concerned about health, a change is occurring. For example, we now have exercise physiologists in the sports departments of community hospitals, sport-medicine specialists, increased visiting-nurse services, home-health aids, and health educators—all with the support of industry.

Origins of Disability

In addition to the huge impact musculoskeletal (arthritic and rheumatic) disability has on our economy, studies at Yale University reveal that this condition ranks first among disease groups that adversely affect our quality of life. Of workers who take early retirement, 16 percent do so because of musculoskeletal disorders. Researchers in Denmark, in a 3-year study of disability pensioning due to these disorders, showed that both medical and social factors are involved.

Cumulative trauma may be a factor. Government figures show that in 1982 some 580,000 musculoskeletal injuries were treated in the United States. Cumulative trauma disorders that result from repetitive motion include the carpal-tunnel syndrome, tendinitis, ganglions, bursitis, and tennis elbow. These are often caused or aggravated by repeated twisting or awkward postures, particularly when they are combined with high force. Vibration-associated injuries include degenerative-disc disease and low-back pain. Vibration of one limb or body segment, as caused by a chain saw or jackhammer, is associated with "vibration syndrome," characterized by intermittent numbness, blanching of the fingers, and reduced sensitivity of touch.

Trauma must be defined more broadly than simply as direct blows to muscle. In fact, most cases of persistent myofascial pain result from the so-called microtrauma (tiny injuries) of daily living, including many instances resulting from improper body mechanics. Back pain in Swedish workers was reported to result from:

1. Static work postures, such as prolonged sitting or bending over, or frequent bending and twisting.
2. Forceful or sudden unexpected movements.
3. Repetitive work motions.
4. Vibration, such as from working on trains or buses or riding a tractor.

5. Social problems that include alcoholism, drug dependency, and divorce.

6. Tasks that were less than a match for the worker's strength. ("Heavy" work was only sometimes related.)

In another study of back pain and disability in Swedish workers, the disability was not correlated with diminished work satisfaction, inability to influence the work situation, less demand for concentration, overtime work, or heavy work. But in another study, conducted in the United States, injuries were more common among persons who had boring jobs, jobs in which they had no choice in the tempo of the work, and jobs that required driving a longer distance to work. In other studies, back pain was most common in workers between the ages of 35 and 55, with the duration of the pain increasing with age. Back pain was more likely to occur in persons of lower social class, in those who had drug or alcohol problems, in those who were divorced or had family problems, and in those with less education than the average person. Ruptured discs occurred more often after age 40 in persons who spent more time in a car (particularly without cruise control). Ruptured discs were more likely to occur in those who smoked and had chronic coughs. Lastly, ruptured discs also appeared in persons who either got insufficient physical exercise or who participated in baseball, golf, or bowling.

Feelings about work or tensions in interpersonal relations can cause injuries. British researchers noted that 36 percent of injuries reported as accidental were, in fact, not the result of accidents. Similarly the investigators were suspicious of lifting injuries as a cause of back pain. Their studies revealed that the reported injury was only the *alerting factor,* and that the workers had numerous other reasons for back pain. Also, they noted the high correlation of a worker's back injuries with driving long distances and with the occurrence of the injury in the first hour of work. Was the back really pain-free before the worker came to the workplace? Swedish investigators noted that workers who felt they had little chance of influencing methods or tempo in their jobs were more likely to suffer back pain. Also, workers who had diminished work satisfaction or held jobs that were considered monotonous or boring suffered back pain. In addition to long-distance driving, vibration from riding trains or trucks has similarly been noted as being related to back pain. Similar findings were reported by researchers at Yale. Another British researcher noted that 40 percent of back complaints allegedly resulted from work injuries that had occurred within the first hour of work. The persons with back pain also had driven the farthest.

Personal characteristics and habits can also be factors. Investigators in the United States and Britain recognized that back injury was more likely in persons who had a previous history of low-back pain. Age, weight, and stature were not important. Height, they thought, may be related, but scoliosis and other curvatures of the spine and leg-length discrepancy were not correlated with back pain. Degenerative changes of the intervertebral discs or spinal joints did not correlate with low-back pain, type of work, or absence from work. Currently, lumbar-spine x-rays should be reserved for the elderly or for patients with abnormal physical-examination findings or known diseases, or for those experiencing major trauma or taking drugs that can affect the spine.

Another team of U.S. and British investigators devised a questionnaire to predict the prevalence and nature of back pain. Pain that had developed with a slow onset before age 40, that persisted for 3 months or more, and that was accompanied by morning stiffness, correlated with the presence of ankylosing spondylitis (inflammatory arthritis of the spine). In an industrial complex, they found 16 cases among 1880 persons with back pain. Thus the chance of serious arthritis in workers with back pain was about 1 percent.

Joint laxity (loose joints) is a common musculoskeletal finding and may account for up to 70 percent of back pain in women with no other objective finding. In other studies, smoking and coughing were correlated with back pain. Insufficient exercise or participation in bowling, golf, cross-country skiing, jogging, or baseball may predispose one to back pain.

A researcher at the University of Michigan devised an isometric strength test in which the subject was placed in a stooped position with hands 20 inches above the floor and 20 inches in front of the ankle. The subject then applied a lifting force to a testing device. On average, female workers' strength-test scores were 70 percent of those of their male counterparts. The worker and the job could then be matched, and when they were, the future back-injury rate was reduced significantly. Other studies report similar findings between women and men for grip, arm flexors, and back extensors. Social problems (drinking, divorce, family conflict, antisocial behavior, etc.) are much more common in people who have back pain. Persons with higher education tend to find jobs that are less likely to injure their backs. Studies to determine predictable features that lead to back pain are under way.

Summary

Any person who suffers from disability beyond the expected duration should be considered for psychological interview. Chronic pain (of more than 6 months' duration) no longer serves as nature's warning. A complex adaptation-and-defense protection mechanism may have become operational. Pain then may serve to maintain the individual's psychic equilibrium, and he or she becomes pain-focused. To avoid a psychologically painful circumstance a person may use a pain complaint to avoid facing the real problem. This is called an *adaptation-and-defense pain mechanism*.

Consider these four R's when a person develops increasing disability despite apparently adequate treatment:

Roles: The ability to carry on relationships as parent, spouse, student, or breadwinner. Look for loss of self-esteem.

Reactions: The patient's emotional response to the disorder—anger, hostility, anxiety, discouragement, or defeat. Patient education is needed here.

Relationships: Insurmountable problems at work, in the family, in school, or in friendships. The patient may be beating his head against a wall!

Resources: Has the patient tapped community programs, counselors, minister? Has she used simple joint-protection methods to reduce stress?[1]

In summary, most people work; therefore, most of us will suffer a soft-tissue or bony-arthritis problem. But work alone is seldom the cause of aches and pains. Examine all aspects of your daily life in identifying potential aggravations that affect your work.

---

1.   D. H. Neustadt, "Commentary: Psychosocial Factors in Rheumatic Disease," *Ortho Review,* 13:114–115, 1984.

CHAPTER 4

The Head and Neck

Among the most common complaints bringing people to physicians are aches and pains of the head and neck. Arthritis and rheumatism can cause headaches—particularly in association with numbness and tingling in the back of the scalp; a sensation of a tight band around the head with pain in the eye region; headache that occurs upon awakening in the morning and in association with a tight feeling in the muscles of the back of the neck; or pain in the region of the jaw, side of the face, ear, or throat. Although "arthritis," when it is evident on x-rays of the neck or jaw, is often believed to be the cause of the pain, we now know that in fact the changes which appear on the x-rays are very common in those over 40 and may not relate to symptoms.

It is important that any evidence of arthritis be carefully correlated with your symptoms. More commonly, the symptoms are not due to arthritis of the bones, but rather to disturbances of the muscles, ligaments, or nerves in the head and neck area (Plates 4-1 and 4-2). Not only can many of these problems be corrected, but they can often be prevented if you can learn what habit or strain causes the muscle to become irritated, to tighten up, and to create pressure which results in symptoms. Pain and spasms of the neck muscles can

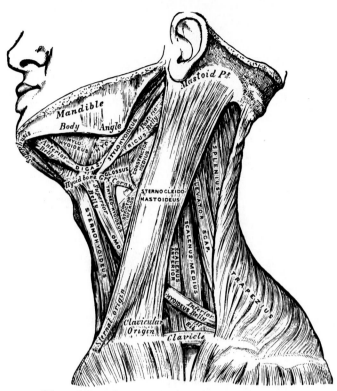

Plate 4-1. Anatomy of the neck, side view.

result in many symptoms throughout the head and neck, even into the arms and chest areas.

There are clusters of inappropriate and improper habits in daily living—including using too much coffee, tea, cola, or chocolate—that can give rise to symptoms in the head and neck area. If you can recognize and correct these habits, you may break up a pain-spasm-pain cycle that leads to muscle spasm, spinal pain, or jaw-joint pressure, and, ultimately, to arthritis damage in the small joints of the region. In fact, there is evidence that arthritis damage in the jaw joint can heal if pressure from jaw clenching is stopped with a plastic bite splint used particularly at night (Figure 4-1). Tables outlining danger signs in the head and neck (Table 4-1), self-examination techniques (Table 4-2), possible causes of persistent head and neck pain (Table 4-3), habits that aggravate or ease the symptoms (Tables 4-4 and 4-5), and helpful exercises designed to alleviate pain (Table 4-6) are located at the end of this chapter. Three cases that illustrate head and neck problems follow.

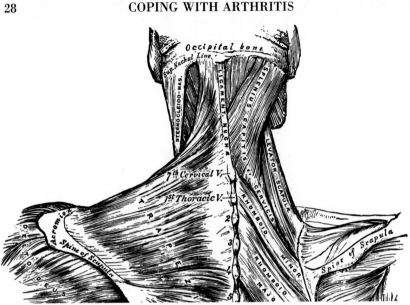

Plate 4-2.   Anatomy of the neck, rear view.

The TMJ Syndrome

If you have neck pain or headache and notice a painful jaw when chewing, particularly at breakfast, you should consider temporomandibular joint (TMJ) syndrome as a cause. First, try the following:

1. Cut out stimulating beverages for 2 weeks.
2. Practice relaxation or listen to quiet music before retiring.
3. Both morning and night, perform the first two jaw exercises detailed in Table 4-6 and Figure 4-2.

If you do not improve in 2 to 3 weeks, consult your dentist for a checkup and possible use of a bite protector or splint. Drugs that are helpful include meprobamate and/or amitriptyline before bedtime. Surgery should be reserved for those who have tried all of these measures.

SALLY M.: TOO ORGANIZED AND TOO HARD-WORKING

Sally M., 26 years old, has always been hard-working, strict, aggressive. She knows she is rough on herself, that she is overly organized, that she is sensitive to criticism. She also doesn't exactly shine in interpersonal relationships, partly because she has difficulty controlling her emotions. Too, she often suffers from morning fatigue and muscle irritability. Like others in her family, she has a short fuse.

When Sally awakens in the morning, she often finds her jaws are tired, chewing is painful, and jaw clicking is common. Upon arising she also finds her hands tightly clenched; while telephoning or driving, she always clutches tightly. Sally is concerned about this tension and would like to remedy it. Personality revision, however, isn't always easy.

During a period when she was undergoing the stress of a new job, she got into an argument with her boyfriend. As if that weren't enough, Sally experienced an uncontrolled pain-spasm-pain cycle in her jaw. Doctors theorize this cycle results when the nervous system is excited by pain impulses, and then certain centers in the brain send nerve messages to muscles that increase their tension.

In Sally's case the original area of stress was the muscles that clamp the jaw tight. Because of her unconscious jaw clenching, these muscles

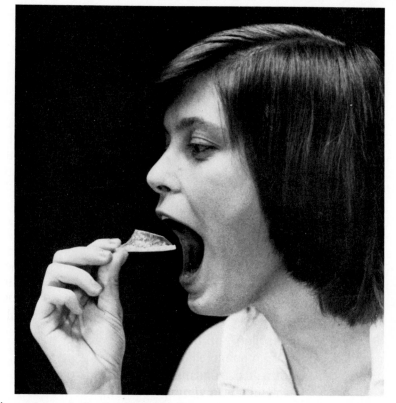

Figure 4-1.   A plastic bite splint for use as a jaw-joint spacer during sleep.

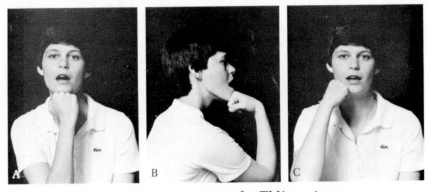

Figure 4-2.   Jaw exercises for TMJ syndrome.

became tired and sent their impulses into the brain, which in turn caused spasm and contraction in the muscles of the back of her neck.

Sally began to notice dull headaches, more pronounced at the back of the head and neck, morning fatigue, restless sleep, painful chewing, and a dull aching in the ears and jaw. At first the symptoms were only occasional, but they grew in both frequency and severity. Sally thought of consulting an ear, nose, and throat doctor or a dentist. If she had, she probably would have been told that nothing was wrong, or she may have been given dental care. (Dentists are becoming increasingly aware of the relationship between jaw clenching and headaches.)

As Sally grew ever more irritable from fatigue, chronic discomfort, and dissatisfaction, her symptoms grew in intensity and severity. She still attempted to maintain her ambitious pace, drinking more coffee or other caffeine products during the day—but this stimulated the nervous system and further accelerated the pain-spasm-pain cycle.

If you identify with Sally, her remedy may help you. Fortunately, she recognized that this was not the first time her nervous system had overreacted. Once, she had had a prolonged gastrointestinal upset that was, after much medical investigation, diagnosed as stress. Sally decided to control her nervous system through relaxation techniques, which included biofeedback (see Chapter 13), and to discontinue colas, chocolate, tea, coffee, and even decaffeinated dark beverages. She also cut down on her activities and tried in every way to reduce stress. Relaxation techniques brought the most relief. Other things she might have tried include selfhypnosis with a trained instructor, yoga, jogging, or meditation. These techniques can provide an individual with the ability to calm the nervous system—particularly the *autonomic* nervous system, which controls spasm, palpitation, sweating, and changes in skin temperature.

Sally also had to examine her goals and interpersonal relationships. With the help of a close friend, she gained insight into how hard she had been on herself and her acquaintances. A *perfectionist* who was never quite satisfied, she often projected this unhappiness onto others, causing strife with close family members, her boyfriend, and other friends. As Sally changed, she became more happy and positive. Her mother said one day, "Well, finally Sally is growing up." Yes, growing up—largely through easing up, on others and especially on herself.

Later, at the suggestion of the psychologist who administered the biofeedback, Sally decided to seek dental assistance. An orthodontist (it isn't only children they see!) fitted her with a plastic bite splint. He also suggested jaw-balancing exercises (Table 4-6). Finally, he advised Sally to use the bite splint long after her symptoms began to disappear. Because jaw clenching is an unconscious habit, only prolonged use of the splint allows the patient to eliminate the habit.

It Really Isn't Whiplash!

Pain in the neck is very prevalent because injuries in this area are very common, and so is arthritis. Accidents do cause whiplash injuries, but they are not all that frequent. Very few people go through life without injuring the head or neck; therefore, it is very difficult to correlate neck pain with neck injury. Even when severe arthritis is evident on x-rays, neck pain may be absent. The individual with evident arthritis may not have had pain until an injury occurs. At that time the x-rays will reveal the arthritis. Obviously the arthritis has taken years to develop. When an x-ray examination following an injury reveals severe spurring, believe it or not, those spurs have taken years to develop; and they may have caused only a little stiffness or slight loss of neck movement. Another truth is that most people with neck pain do get better, regardless of what the x-rays reveal. Exceptions, of course, would include fractures, subluxations (incomplete dislocations), or tears in the spinal ligaments. When an injury has occurred and pain persists despite treatment, you must consider other aggravating factors. The self-examination techniques described in Table 4-2 can help you-pinpoint some abnormalities in the neck.

RUTH D.: NO TIME FOR A BREAK

Ruth and Fred D. had been married only a few years and were struggling to keep up—not so much with the Joneses, but rather with cost-of-living accelerations. So that they might have more of the things they desired,

Ruth began working for her husband, keeping the books of their small business. In her new family job, she spent hours at her desk without rest breaks. One day, while she was returning from an errand, her car was struck in a rear-end collision. Ruth's head was thrown forward and backward; and the result was a moderate flexion-extension injury, often called a whiplash. She did not seek medical attention immediately because she considered the injury slight.

Worried about being behind in her bookkeeping, she started putting in even longer hours. But the later she worked, the more the back of her neck ached. Stiffness and headaches came close behind; her head felt like it weighed a ton, and it drooped forward. Using a thicker pillow seemed to ease the pain; but in the morning, the pain and stiffness were even worse. Finally after she had consulted a series of physicians, a doctor ordered an x-ray examination. At 47, Ruth was told she had spurs on her neck bones; arthritic changes appeared on the x-rays. Her doctor informed Ruth that the auto injury had perhaps aggravated the arthritis. He gave her medication and advised physical therapy, which eventually enabled her to resume her long hours at her desk. But soon the pain returned in even greater severity.

A little later Ruth and Fred went on a vacation during which they golfed and hiked. Sleeping on soft, thin pillows seemed to help her neck; but when she returned home and resumed the harmful, prolonged hours at her desk, the pain returned. Only then did Ruth associate her pain with her work. Now she felt she was on the right track. And she was. Breaking up the prolonged worktime with short rest breaks and getting up and stirring about helped. So did interspersing filing with bookkeeping. And she resumed using a thin, soft pillow. The pain slowly subsided.

Myofascial Neck Pain

The previous example demonstrates the importance of always considering an aggravating habit in cases of persistent neck pain. When chronic pain does result from such a habit, the pain often involves the muscles of the back of the neck and is often worse after one sits or sleeps; but better during body movement and neck movement. The pain may be an isolated complaint or part of a generalized muscle irritation with stiffness and pain in other body areas after rest.

To control local pain, many patients find ice massage helpful. Tender muscles can be massaged with the corner of an ice cube. Hold the cube with a towel; rub the ice directly onto the skin. Press deeply as you slowly rub up and down over the most tender areas. Rub for 1 to 5 minutes. Repeat every few hours. Stretch the neck muscles after each ice treatment.

Ibuprofen, available without prescription, seems particularly helpful for relief of neck muscle pain. The usual dosage is two tablets two to four times daily (with meals and at bedtime).

Pain that awakens you from sleep; numbness and tingling in your shoulder, arm, or hand; or other danger signals described in Table 4-1 demand prompt medical examination.

MALCOLM L.: A HOCKEY PLAYER WHO GOT IT IN THE NECK

One of us (R.S.) had a 22-year-old male patient, Malcolm L., who had sustained a head injury while playing amateur hockey. The following year was very unproductive for him, and he suffered most of the time from an aching discomfort along the side of his neck. Examination from time to time revealed no special findings.

Finally, after a great many consultations, Malcolm spoke of working on his computer. A large portion of his day was spent working on his papers, which he said always lay beside the computer waiting for him. The to-and-fro motion of his head as he typed was causing the problem. It was suggested that he obtain an easel with a flexible elbow to hold the papers at eye level. He clamped it to his desk and was "cured." Malcolm is just fine today. Now you see why the first question physicians usually ask is likely to be, "What repetitive little movements do you make in your work or recreation?"

Feeling worse after rest is the cardinal feature of muscular rheumatism. If muscles have tightened in the neck region, turning the head to either side may be more difficult; as the muscles tighten the joints of the neck, spurs may block side-to-side head movement. But when the muscles are relaxed or stretched, these spurs can be stretched apart somewhat to bring improved neck motion. Table 4-2 will help you perform a self-examination. When you recognize and correct a bad habit, you may still have to use mobilizing exercises to reestablish the integrity of the neck muscles and ligaments. Neck exercises can begin with a simple warm-up: roll the head to the side and downward and then turn the chin to the other side. Now tilt the ear toward the shoulder and repeat on the opposite side. For acute pain, begin with exercise 3 in Table 4-6 and then proceed to exercises 4 through 6; review Figure 4-3. If the neck pain continues after 2 or 3 weeks or if grinding noises occur, try exercise 7.

Sleep Well—And Correctly

Resting positions that help muscular neck pain include the use of a very thin, soft pillow or rolled-up towel under the neck or around

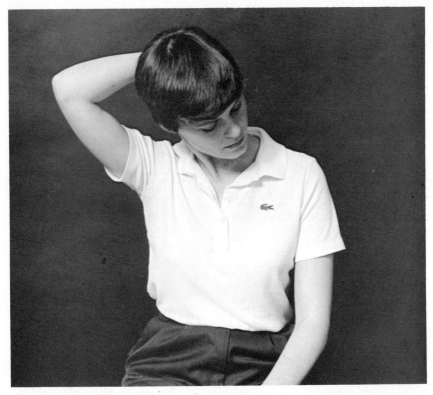

Figure 4-3.   Sternomastoid stretch exercise.

the neck while reclining. To sleep, lie on your back with your legs elevated and use a sofa cushion of 8- to 10-inch elevation under your feet and lower legs, as shown in Figure 4-4. Your arms should lie at the side of the body and not overhead. Later, when acute pain has subsided, you may lie on either side; but keep your arms below breast level. Never sleep on your stomach. If you cannot break the habit of sleeping on your stomach, try this: Roll up a blanket lengthwise and prop it alongside your body. While lying on your side, keep your lower leg bent forward, with the knee beneath the rolled-up blanket. The blanket should keep you from rolling over on your stomach. Sandbags can also be used alongside your body. If all else fails, use two pillows under your belly while you sleep on your stomach. Various neck pillows that open the nerve canals are available, including the Cervipillo and the Wal-Pilo.

If you have muscular neck pain, you should avoid sitting or lying on a sofa. Similarly, avoid a reclining chair that forces the head

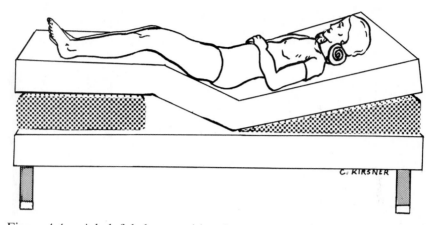

Figure 4-4.   A helpful sleep position for someone suffering from chronic neck or back pain.

forward. A wing chair is ideal for reading. A chair should be tall enough to support the back of the head, have a back that inclines slightly backward from the vertical, allow both feet to touch the floor, and be tall enough for you to rise without gripping the sides of the chair and pushing off.

Also helpful is a 30-inch foam-rubber wedge to prop you up in bed while you read or watch television. If you can't find one, you can improvise, using a plywood base covered with foam rubber.

How effective are these treatments? One study noted that just improving the sleeping position with a neck pillow provided relief from neck pain in 68 percent of patients. On the other hand, it has been reported that three patients have had strokes following chiropractic manipulation of the neck. We strongly advocate that you try self-help exercise and proper neck positioning before you place your neck in the hands of others! Most patients respond to these measures within 2 or 3 weeks.

Cervical Traction

Sometimes your physician or therapist will recommend cervical traction to stretch the soft tissues of the neck, to relieve spasm, and to separate the vertebrae. The variety and methods of neck traction used attest to its safety if employed according to your therapist's instructions. If you are using cervical traction, it is helpful to protect your teeth by using a rubber or foam mouth guard or strips of plastic

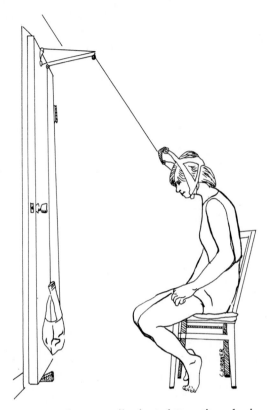

Figure 4-5.   A commonly prescribed neck-traction device for home or office use.

sponge between your teeth. Sometimes cervical traction requires more than 20 pounds to eliminate grinding noises during head rotation. Most patients prefer traction with the head pulled forward, as shown in Figure 4-5.

Arthritis, Bursitis, and Neuralgia

Bursitis and neuralgia can also occur as a result of bad habits involving the head and neck.

SARAH M. AND HER TV NAPS

Sarah M. complained of occasional attacks of sharp, stabbing pain in the back of her head on the right side, which left a tingling and numb sensation that persisted for several hours. These attacks often occurred in the morning when Sarah began to read the mail. Sometimes they would awaken her from sleep in the early hours. One day she awakened with severe pain in the middle of the back of her neck. Sarah was rather obese and had grown somewhat stooped with age (Figure 4-6). Because the hump at the back of her neck was similar to her mother's, Sarah had taken it for granted. But one day Jane, her daughter, remarked that the "dowager's hump" was becoming more evident. Sarah mentioned to Jane the new pain at the back of her neck. An avid reader, Jane was "up" on the latest medical news as presented in the popular magazines. She began questioning her mother to determine possible causes of her neck strain.

Now, Jane realized that for some time Sarah had been falling asleep while watching television. With her head dropping down and forward, almost resting on her chest, she would sleep for half an hour or so without changing her position. Naturally, she felt a little stiff upon awakening. Jane knew that it is bad to remain in one position for even half an hour without moving. Still she was puzzled: why was Sarah experiencing pain in the morning? What Jane didn't realize was that muscle spasm from overstretching takes many hours to develop. Thus the simple act of falling asleep in a chair was causing early-morning muscle spasm high in the neck region at the splenius capitis, a muscle high in the back of the neck (Figure 4-7). This muscle overlies the occipital nerve, and the muscle spasm causes irritation of that nerve; the result is numbness, tingling, and stabbing pains up the back of the skull.

Jane needn't have felt she was slow in figuring out her mother's problem. The relationship between falling asleep in a chair and neuralgic head pain is not often or readily appreciated. To break that habit, Jane suggested

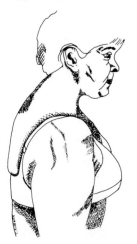

Figure 4-6. Forward drooping of the head, neck, and shoulders caused by long-term poor posture.

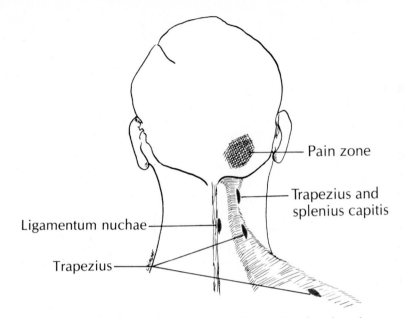

Pain zone

Trapezius and
splenius capitis

Ligamentum nuchae

Trapezius

Figure 4-7.   The trigger-point map for the head and neck.

that if Sarah would use a kitchen stool to watch television, she wouldn't
be likely to fall asleep. Sarah decided against using the stool, but she did
begin changing places several times during each TV session.

And what of the more acute pain in the middle of the dowager's hump?
Several days previously, Sarah had spent a burst of energy cleaning the
upper cabinets in her kitchen. Being somewhat short, she had worked several hours with her head tilted up. This had caused bursitis to develop
between two bones deep in the dowager's hump. The neck-strengthening
exercise (Table 4-6, exercise 4) can actually diminish a dowager's hump
and interspinal bursitis! Obviously, many months of exercise are required
to change the neck-bone alignment; but it can be done, with excellent results (Figure 4-8).

Important Points

This discussion of simple bad habits and the resulting neck and face
pain is meant to prompt your examination of the use of your body
in daily living. If you are suffering from pain and disability or limitation of movement in the head and neck region, you may recognize
bad habits that can be reversed. If so, symptoms should disappear.
However, a word of caution! Table 4-1 lists danger signs that require
urgent medical attention!

Other causes of persistent neck pain and stiffness are profiled in the tables at the end of the chapter. In addition, chronic recurrent complaints of the head and neck may stem from nervous temperament, compulsiveness, a family or personal history of migraine, caffeine sensitivity, and body mechanics that are improper at rest, work, or play. Prolonged sitting or standing in one position is harder work than lifting 40 pounds! If you think of your head as a 12-pound ball balanced on top of a pole and of those little neck muscles doing all the work to hold that ball motionless, you can see how strainful prolonged sitting or standing can be to the neck muscles. Never sit more than half an hour without getting up. Change positions often.

The "birdwatcher's neck" is a common cause of neck strain. Imagine someone looking at birds through binoculars with the neck and head jutted forward. You can do this unconsciously during conversations or when driving. Try to be conscious of your head position.

Also, lying propped up on a sofa or in a bed with the head jutted forward or falling asleep in a chair and allowing your head to drop forward can result in overstretching your neck muscles. This, in

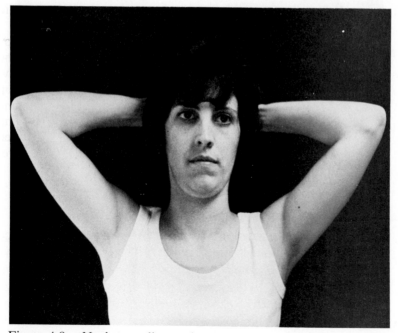

Figure 4-8.   Neck-to-wall exercise to strengthen the neck muscles.

turn, may cause muscle spasm many hours later. You can see that the aggravating habit may be in operation long before neck pain and headache begin.

Neck noises may result from tendons snapping across bony spines or from the small spinal joints under pressure from tense, taut neck muscles. If a "noisy neck" is also painful, the cause is usually very tense, irritated muscles. Heavy, pendulous breasts can tug on the neck. A support brassiere, as shown in Figure 4-9, can help. Trigger points may develop in these neck and upper back muscles. Shoulder strengthening exercises (exercise 5, Table 4-6) are helpful.

GLADYS G., THE GO-GETTER "VOLUNTEER OF THE YEAR"

Almost anyone over 50 who has x-rays taken of the neck will probably be told they have some arthritis. It is a very common finding. Occasionally the condition is painful, but many people have some arthritis of the neck without suffering much discomfort at all. An illustration is Gladys G., a woman in her early sixties who regularly came to her doctor's office com-

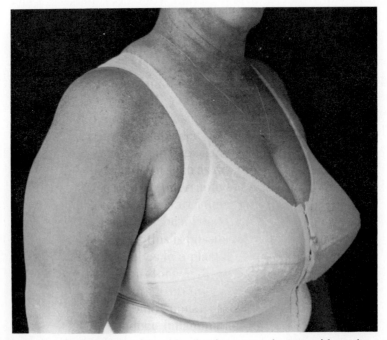

Figure 4-9. A brassiere with wide elastic straps that provides adequate support.

plaining of severe headaches. Because her neck was also stiff much of the time, she thought she had arthritis.

Gladys was a go-getter of the first order. She was number one on the hit list when people needed a chairman for a project—church, Welcome Wagon, and so on. Although her doctor felt arthritis was not the culprit, Gladys continued to insist that it must be. After all, he had said the x-rays showed some. Yes, some, but not enough to cause all her pain.

Actually, Gladys was a workaholic, even though she didn't have a traditional job. Her position as the town's "Volunteer of the Year" was her bugbear. She readily admitted that she rarely stopped once she began her day; and during the evening, after hours on the phone, she would often work until 3 or 4 A.M. In fact, she took great pride in her late hours. The doctor wasn't certain what they represented to her, but suspected they were a perk of some kind.

How did her doctor know her lifestyle was causing her tension headaches (for that's what they were)? The consistency of the headaches was the main clue, but Gladys herself provided the proof when she suddenly changed her lifestyle after meeting an attractive widower. Now she had little time to volunteer. She had her own project; her "excruciating headaches" suddenly stopped. She was a new woman: a relaxed new woman. Moral: there is a cure for almost everything, but it isn't always in the doctor's office, nor on prescription blanks.

Relaxation techniques can "unwind" a tense or high-strung nervous system and provide long-term control of other psychophysiologic disease states such as hypertension, functional diarrhea and spastic colon, chest pain, and tension headaches. There is no such thing as a true muscle relaxant. A new drug called cyclobenzaprine (Flexeril) shows much promise, but no pill will actually lengthen a muscle contracted in spasm. Chronic muscle spasm should be treated mechanically with physical therapy and exercise. Aggravating habits that induce the muscle spasm must be eliminated.

Arthritis of the small joints at the back of the neck will occur in late life in all of us. Wear and tear lead to spur formation on these neck bones. Knobby finger joints are a similar formation. However, only a few of us will develop symptoms from neck arthritis. Most common is stiffness and a little loss of neck movement. Grating noises often occur. All of these complaints will decrease if you avoid the aggravating habits detailed in Tables 4-4 and 4-5 and perform exercises 3 through 6 described in Table 4-6. Aspirin for weather sensitivity and pain (two regular-strength tablets every 4 to 6 hours) is often as good as more expensive medications.

When to Seek Professional Help

If you note any of the danger list items, see your doctor at once. Also, if these measures don't satisfy, the physician should check for a more serious condition such as hypertension, sinus infection, glaucoma, or one of many other medical problems common to the head and neck. Brain tumors are the least likely. For example, out of all the patients admitted to a large referral clinic for a suspected brain tumor in 1 year, 95 percent had other causes for their symptoms—and these were the patients who had specialists worried.

Your physician can prescribe some safe painkillers, a muscle relaxant such as cyclobenzaprine, anti-inflammatories, or tricyclic relaxants to raise your pain threshhold (Chapter 15).

Physical therapists can help provide pain relief by using local heat and stretching devices. They can also guide you in a specific home program of exercise. Occupational therapists will provide advice about muscle and joint strain.

Table 4-1

Danger Signs in the Head and Neck

Fever and chills
Intense headache or spasmodic, stabbing pains
Mental dullness
Visible swelling
Swollen lymph glands
Blood in the ear, eye, nose, or mouth
Disturbed vision, smell, or taste
Numbness or weakness

Table 4-2

Self-Examination of the Head and Neck

1. Sit sideways in front of a full-length mirror; hold a smaller mirror so that you can see your profile. Note alignment of shoulders, neck, and head. Are you allowing your head to drop forward? Are your shoulders rounded forward as in Figure 4-6? Now sit straight, tucking the chin in like a soldier. Throw shoulders back and upward. If it feels clumsy, you nevertheless look more pleasing.

2. Sit in your favorite chair, take a book, and read for several pages. Stop, but don't move your head position. Note the distance between your eye and the center of the book. It should be about 16 inches. If it is much different, you may need an eye examination.
3. Rotate your chin toward each shoulder. You should be able to get your chin almost to the shoulder. Now tilt your head backward, then forward. This motion should be free of pain or grinding. Lastly, tilt your ear toward your shoulder, first to the right, then to the left. This should also be pain-free.
4. To examine tender points, tilt your head forward; poke gently at the back of the neck where it joins the skull (over the splenius capitis as seen in Figure 4-7) about an inch to each side of the midline). Gradually press more deeply. Pain that radiates to the scalp suggests occipital (back part of head) neuralgia from spasm of the muscle. Now tilt the chin down and to the right and gently press the left side of the neck. Note extreme tenderness over the sternomastoid (also called "sternocleidomastoid") about 2 inches below the ear (halfway to your collarbone). This is a muscle of the neck that flexes the head (Plate 4-1). Repeat the procedure to test the right side, tilting chin down and to the left.

   Now, with head straight, poke the muscles between the neck and shoulders, and then the muscles between the shoulder blade and neck. If you can detect painful points, you may want to try the exercises or consult your doctor.

Table 4-3
Possible Causes of Head and Neck Symptoms

Complaint	Possible Cause
Neck pain, headache	Muscle-contraction headache (tension headache); jaw clenching; myofascial neck pain
Headache, tingling scalp	Occipital neuralgia
Pain in the side of the face, jaw, or ear	Jaw clenching (TMJ syndrome)
Pain in the throat or neck	Obesity and hiatus hernia; migraine-headache disorder; anxiety
Neck-grinding noises	Arthritis and tight neck muscles
Neck cannot be turned fully	Arthritis

Table 4-4

Possible Causes of Persistent
Head and Neck Problems

Complaint	Possible Aggravation
Pain in the back of the neck	Lying with the head propped forward, as on the arm of a sofa, or using thick pillows; jutting the head forward instead of holding it upright; lying in a reclining chair with a headrest that thrusts the head forward; improper eye-to-work distance (proper distance is 16 inches); frequent changes in head position because of poor adjustment to wearing bifocals or working in an improper position at a computer terminal
Pain behind upper neck and back of head	Prolonged working overhead such as in painting a ceiling or washing windows (arms should never remain overhead for very long); sleeping on your stomach with arms overhead; falling asleep in your chair and allowing your head to drop forward and down
Pain at one side of neck	Cradling a telephone between your head and shoulder in order to use both hands

Table 4-5

What's Harmful, What's Helpful for the Head and Neck

Harmful	Helpful
Sitting or standing for more than 30 minutes can induce more neck strain than lifting heavy objects.	Alternate tasks in which the body does not move (e.g., knitting) with tasks that allow the body greater movement (e.g., sweeping).
Lying on a sofa with the head propped forward, falling asleep in a chair and allowing the head to drop forward, or lying on more than one thin pillow stretches the muscles at the back of the neck. Hours later, these muscles may go into spasm, resulting in headache, stiff neck, or limited neck movement. Avoid the "birdwatcher's neck."	Align the entire trunk, chest, and head on a slanted wedge or a very large pillow to watch television or read in a reclining position. Anyone with hiatus hernia, sinus trouble, or heart disease who has been told to sleep in a propped-up position should elevate the entire mattress or the head of the bed rather than simply putting two or three pillows under the head.
Sleeping on the stomach can strain the neck.	Sleep on the side or the back, keeping the arms below the level of the chest.
Clenching the jaw can cause muscle spasm in the neck.	Use a bite spacer, relaxation techniques, or muscle relaxants.
Storing items in the kitchen at a level that is too high or too low can strain the neck.	Store items that are used daily no higher than shoulder height or lower than knee level. If storage is a problem, use a step stool to avoid tilting the head excessively.
Working too close to materials can strain the neck.	Maintain the proper hand-to-eye distance of 16 in (about 40 cm). Position work materials in such a way that the neck remains straight. Place a computer screen at eye level.

(continued)

Harmful	Helpful
Incorrectly using the telephone can cause neck pain.	If both hands must be free during phone conversations, use a speaker phone, headphone, or a shoulder holder and make your conversations as brief as possible.

Table 4-6
Jaw and Neck Exercises

These exercises should each be performed twice a day for at least 1 to 2 minutes' duration.

1. *Jaw balancing:* With the mouth open an inch, place your fist in front of your lower jaw and try to jut the jaw forward against the immovable fist. *No motion actually occurs* (Figure 4-2).
2. *Jaw balancing:* Place your fist on one side of the jaw and similarly thrust your lower jaw against the fist. Do this on the other side. Finally place your fist beneath the lower jaw and thrust against it. In each instance hold the thrust for 10 seconds and repeat six times in each direction. Perform the exercise morning and evening (Figure 4-2).
3. *Mobilizing exercises:* These exercises can be done with a rolled towel and performed on the bed. First, lie face down, towel under the forehead; push forehead down firmly for 6 seconds. Repeat three times. Then lie face up, towel under the back of the head, and push down hard for 6 seconds. Repeat three times. Next, lie on one side with your ear on the towel. Press down hard for 6 seconds. Repeat three times. Do the same on the opposite side. Finally, sit upright. Rotate the head and neck with a firm, steady, circular motion for 12 seconds. Lift and lower head during the rotation.
4. *Neck strengthening:* Back up to a wall with your feet 6 inches from the wall. Place your hands behind your head and push your buttocks against the wall; then push your head and shoulders back against the wall. Your hands act as a cushion between your head and the wall. Begin a gradual, forceful thrust of the head backward to the wall, keeping your chin tucked in like a soldier at attention. As you thrust your head backward, your arms are loose, and you allow your hands to act as a cushion behind your head. You should

feel a sensation of muscle tension in the back of the neck. Maintain this thrust for up to 30 seconds, relax it for a second, and then repeat up to 2 minutes (Figure 4-8).

5. *Neck and shoulder strengthening:* Exercise your neck and shoulder muscles with two weights, each 2 to 10 pounds. You can make these from socks lined with a plastic freezer bag and filled with gravel, sand, or dirt. You can hold the weights at the sides of your body or drape one over each shoulder. Hold your arms down alongside your body while you are sitting or standing. Next, slowly draw the shoulders up, then back, and then slowly let down. You will thus bring your shoulder blades toward each other as you raise your shoulders. Repeat this movement slowly for 1 to 2 minutes twice a day (Figure 4-10).

6. *Sternomastoid stretch:* To stretch the muscles on the side of your neck behind your ear, put your right arm behind your neck and grasp your left ear. Now bend your head forward and pull it to the right with your hand and arm, thus pulling your ear away from the shoulder. You should feel a pulling sensation in the muscles radiating at the right side of your neck. Similarly, reverse and use your left arm to grasp your right ear. With your head tilted forward, draw your head to the left and feel a pulling sensation in the muscles behind the left side of your neck (Figure 4-3).

7. *Mayo head sling:* Sew the two ends of a bath towel together to make a loop. Place it on the floor beside your bed with 5 to 10 pounds of weight in the towel loop. Lie across your bed, on your stomach. Hang your head over the edge of bed. Grasp loop. Place over your head. Place hands on buttocks. Lift weighted towel loop about 3 inches with your head. Hold for 10 to 20 seconds, relax, and repeat for 2 minutes.

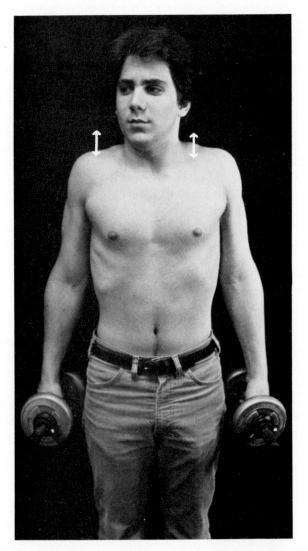

Figure 4-10.   A shoulder-shrugging exercise to strengthen the muscles
that raise the shoulders.

CHAPTER 5

The Shoulder Region

Shoulder pain is second only to back pain as a cause of time lost from work, although the shoulder is seldom a problem before age 25 or after age 65. The shoulder joint is a suspended ball and socket that is unique in many ways (Plates 5-1 and 5-2). Although muscles must rotate the shoulder through many directions, the only point of attachment is where the collarbone joins the sternum, or breastbone, in the front of the chest.

What Causes Shoulder Pain?

Many shoulder ailments come from direct injuries. One of the most common of these occurs when you fall on an outstretched arm and jam your shoulder joint. Another injury can result from throwing the shoulder beyond its tolerance. More subtle, less-direct injury can occur from repetitive arm movements such as wiping windows, polishing a car, or performing other tasks in which the arm goes to and fro like a piston. These repetitive movements can lead to frictional irritation in which the soft tissues become swollen, frayed, or pinched between adjacent bony structures. A more direct injury occurs when the shoulder is converted to a weight-bearing joint as in push-ups or pushing off a chair when your arms are lifting your body.

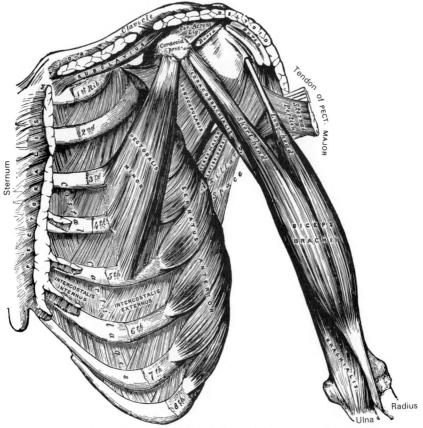

Plate 5-1.　Front view of shoulder anatomy.

RALPH S.: REPETITIVE-MOVEMENT INJURY

Ralph S., a 57-year-old businessman, provided proof that a lot of pain problems result from just plain wear and tear. He is a very competitive man, who is constantly on the move and participates in many sports, including a lot of tennis.

Such activities were temporarily out, however, for his pain was so intense that it awakened him and had invaded both shoulders. Furthermore, the pain aggravated arm movements and made almost everything difficult, from shaving in the morning to holding the evening paper. Only after three visits could he be pinned down about what had caused his problem. It had never occurred to him that the morning push-ups he did so religiously could be detrimental to his well-being. Although this exercise is supposed to strengthen the body, in an older person it can cause a repetitive-movement injury.

Canes or crutches can cause this injury too. The blood vessels to muscles that form the capsule, or cuff at the top of the shoulder, are also subject to injury. Decreased circulation leads to thin, weakened tissue. The shoulder capsule should be a very tough bag surrounding and protecting the joint and the muscles must give the capsule a lot of strength, but if they are prematurely thinned, a capsule tear can occur quite easily. If you are out of condition, sagging muscles can lead to pinched nerves and blood vessels as they pass through three tunnels located across the shoulder-joint region. These three tunnels, collectively known as the *thoracic outlet*, lie between the neck and the chest wall beneath the collarbone. Figure 5-1 represents the bony joint of the shoulder with the adjacent muscles and a bursa. A bursa provides a cushion between the muscles and the shoulder's bony part. Figure 5-2 shows the three tunnels that make up the thoracic outlet. When muscles sag and the shoulder drops downward and forward, these tunnels

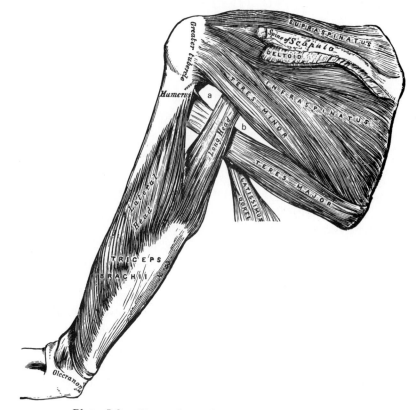

Plate 5-2.   Rear view of shoulder anatomy.

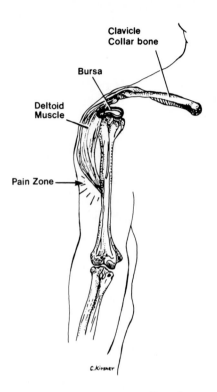

Figure 5-1.   The shoulder. The bursa lies above and toward the outside. The deltoid muscle lies above the bursa. Bursitis pain (arrow) is felt where the muscle attaches to the arm bone.

can become too small or too narrow for the nerve and blood vessels they encase. Many doctors aptly label this condition the "droopy-shoulder syndrome." The droop may be accentuated by heavy arms and heavy, unsupported breasts. (According to the December 5, 1985, issue of the *Toledo Blade,* an estimated 80 percent of American women wear incorrectly fitted brassieres!)

Shoulder pain may result from arthritis, bursitis, tendinitis, inflammation, and capsulitis, or inflammatimoid scarring of the capsule. Other causes include actual tears of the shoulder cuff (capsule) and painful muscular disorders arising from the shoulder-blade area or neck, or from a thoracic-outlet syndrome. These disorders will be described in this chapter. In most disorders of the shoulder capsule, motion in all directions is restricted or painful. Conversely, in cases of tendinitis, motion is usually not as painful, and normal motion is possible (Figure 5-3).

However, you should also be aware that shoulder pain can arise from diseases located in some distant organs. Examples are disorders of the cervical (neck) disc, gallbladder, diaphragm, lung, or adjacent shoulder bones.

The blood vessels supplying the muscles that move the shoulder are very easily damaged; and when damage does occur, the decreased blood supply results in thinned and weakened muscles. A surgical examination of the shoulder often reveals this premature aging process. It has not been determined whether such a process results from specific injury, from overuse, or from genetic factors; but if it does

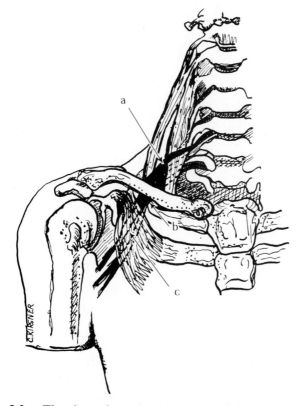

Figure 5-2. The thoracic outlet is a series of three tunnels (*a, b,* and *c*) through which nerves and blood vessels travel from the neck toward the arm and hand.

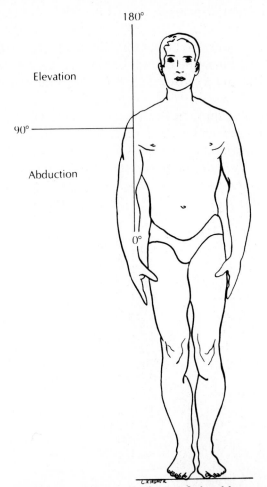

Figure 5-3.   The normal arc of shoulder movement.

occur, a shoulder injury can fail to recover completely. Similarly, if diagnosis has been delayed, a torn and untreatable shoulder capsule may result.

   The shoulder joint is a very complex area of the body. At the end of this chapter, a danger list is provided to help you detect serious problems (Table 5-1). Self-examination techniques are outlined in Table 5-2. Tables 5-3 to 5-5 will help you recognize and manage the more easily treated disorders and identify common aggravating factors that can lead to shoulder pain and disability. Table 5-6 lists exercises that may prove helpful in relieving discomfort.

Bursitis

Acute bursitis is a common, often severely painful disorder. Acute bursitis will be considered separately from chronic, or subacute, bursitis.

JOHN W.: ACUTE BURSITIS

John W., who has worked hard at a desk job for 10 years, is 33 and concerned that he is growing flabby. When the boys at the office suggested forming a baseball team recently, John eagerly volunteered to pitch. A coworker, Bill, who lives in the neighborhood, suggested they begin warming up John's arm the following Tuesday morning. The men tossed the ball around a couple of hours, testing their various skills and having a fine time. That night John was awakened by severe pain in his shoulder, pain that was bursting and intense. Fearful of moving his arm, John found that just getting out of bed was a major task. He took some aspirin and applied an ice bag to the shoulder, but by 7 A.M. John realized he couldn't go to work. He couldn't even turn on a faucet. Any arm movement caused severe and reverberating pain.

That afternoon John's internist said that this was acute bursitis that had begun with an inflammation in a tendon lying just above the bursa at the top of the shoulder joint. Often inflammation in the tendon will spill over into the bursa. Then the sac becomes swollen and inflamed. This inflammation, in turn, causes the deltoid muscle to contract and leads to pain and tenderness at the point of attachment of the deltoid muscle in the upper third of the outer arm. The pain is so acute that medical attention is almost always sought. The condition is usually self-limiting and lasts 3 to 7 days. Pain medication, nonsteroidal anti-inflammatory drugs, or a local injection by your physician can be helpful (see Chapter 15). The cause is almost always a strain brought on by attempting a new task or a new sport without adequate warm-up. In the present example John would probably have benefited from a more gradual conditioning program before trying to pitch.

In subacute, or chronic, bursitis one of several bursal sacs in the shoulder region becomes irritated and inflamed in a more gradual fashion. You may feel the discomfort in the upper third of the outer arm, in the front of the shoulder, or diffusely throughout the shoulder. Self-examination may reveal points of tenderness either at the outer tip of the shoulder over the bursa or near the outer tip of the coracoacromial, or collarbone, bursa. The pain is not as intense, but it is usually present both night and day. Shoulder motion is possible, but you suffer pain during movement—particularly in raising the elbow from down at the side of the body to out, away, and up (as in combing your hair). Because the condition cannot be easily distinguished from tendinitis and because the treatment is pretty much the same for either chronic bursitis or tendinitis, more detailed discussion of treatment follows the case of Debbie W.

Tendinitis

You will recall that tendons are cordlike structures at the ends of muscle. Tendons are protected and nourished by the tendon sheath (a moist envelope), which covers the tendon. Irritation and injury of the tendon result in fraying of the tendon fibers or in swelling of the sheath. The pain of tendinitis is usually less severe than that of bursitis—a dull aching, worse during arm movement, but relieved during rest. The *painful-arc syndrome,* as tendinitis is often called, can occur in swimmers on the side of the body on which they breathe and in tennis players who develop the "King Kong arm": a shoulder droop on one side and muscle hypertrophy (increased size) on the other. Ordinarily, tendinitis will not awaken you. The pain is felt in the shoulder, but not on the side of the arm; the ache can be in front, on top, or just behind the shoulder.

If you have tendinitis at the shoulder, you often can do a self-examination to determine which tendon or muscle is involved. A thumb-rolling test for tendinitis of the biceps muscle along the front of the shoulder is helpful (Figure 5-4). This thumb-rolling test, with comparison of the opposite side, can reveal a swelling along the involved biceps-tendon sheath. Another frequent site for tendinitis is the supraspinatus tendon just behind the shoulder (Figure 5-5). The supraspinatus originates above the crest of the scapula, or shoulder blade. If you pinch-grasp the muscle that lies between the neck and the tip of the shoulder and then let your index finger drop about half an inch behind, you will be slightly above the shoulder blade. You should now be palpating the supraspinatus muscle. Do you detect tenderness?

Another common tendinitis is the *impingement syndrome,* a very common irritation of either the biceps or supraspinatus muscle. When the arm is used as a piston with the elbow away from the body, the tendinous portion of muscle and tendon sheaths can become pinched

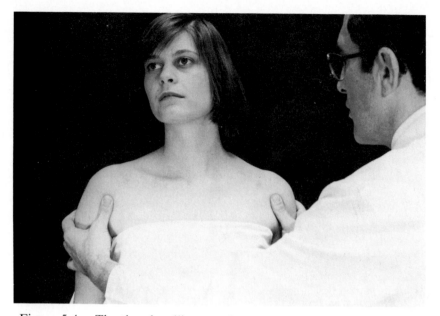

Figure 5-4.   The thumb-rolling test for tendinitis (bicipital tendinitis).

between the bones of the shoulder joint. Sometimes a spur will develop beneath the clavicle (collarbone) and acromion (part of the shoulder blade). This spur doesn't necessarily mean the impingement syndrome requires surgery. In fact, most cases of spurs get better with the exercises and joint-protection measures detailed in the tables at the end of this chapter. On the other hand, surgery may be very helpful if the acromioclavicular joint—the joint at top of shoulder—is grossly enlarged by arthritis. See Table 5-2 and Figure 5-6 for tests you can do to help diagnose an impingement syndrome.

DEBBIE W.: IS SHE A TOO-PERFECT HOMEMAKER?

Debbie W. has always done everything just right. In college she was a cheerleader and the prom queen; she also got all A's. As you might expect, Debbie's home is immaculate. So, too, is her husband. And her windows always shine brightly; in fact, the windows are kind of a fetish with Debbie. Some people might think she is too pernickety, but Debbie is willing to wash those windows every weekend, and they give her a great feeling of pride.

But if Debbie has a fault, it is probably this neatness—or this "compulsiveness," as some of her friends say. Although we don't agree with the plaque that reads "Immaculate women lead dull lives!" we do think Debbie

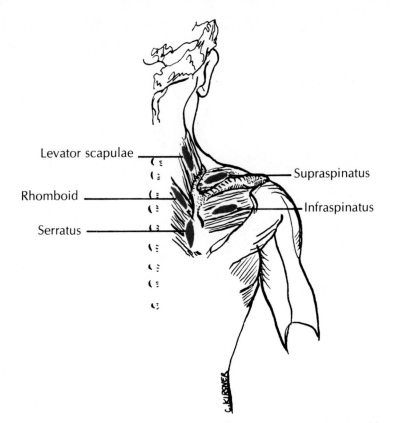

Figure 5-5. Tender points, or trigger points, in muscles near the shoulder blade.

could ease up, especially because she likes to entertain. This doubles the burden when one is too fussy.

One Tuesday when her shoulder bothered her, Debbie naturally blamed it on washing windows the weekend before. Her shoulder had bothered her a little afterward, but by the next day the pain was less noticeable. Now, her right shoulder hurt when she combed her hair or reached up into a cupboard, and there was a dull ache most of the time. However, as the week wore on, the pain wore off.

That weekend Debbie, of course, had another go at the windows, paying for it by awakening Sunday night with a dull, nagging shoulder ache. She had been sleeping with her head on her arm and, in trying to rotate the arm downward, had been awakened by the pain.

Debbie continued to have the pain, but sometimes it eased up. She found also that it was always worse on humid days, especially before it actually rained. Her mother, who has arthritis and thinks Debbie is "hyper about her housework," couldn't resist saying, "I told you so!" She suggested that Debbie ask her doctor about a shot of cortisone, thinking (as many do) that cortisone is the answer to almost everything.

Debbie did make an appointment with Dr. Granger. He, noting that this was the second time Debbie had suffered a pain like this, ordered an x-ray. She was surprised to learn that not only did she have tendinitis but also that the x-ray showed a calcium deposit. Dr. Granger, however, explained that the calcium is often the consistency of toothpaste and does not portend disaster. Sometimes it even disappears, he said, but the tendinitis will per-

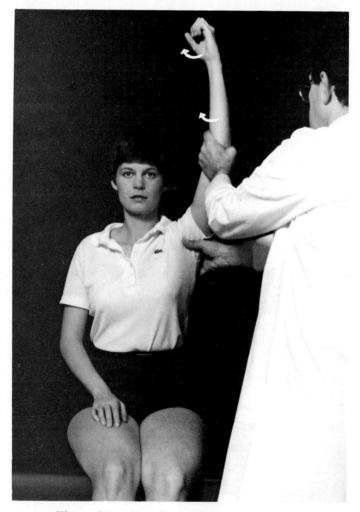

Figure 5-6.   Test for impingement syndrome.

sist. More often, though, the calcium continues to show on x-rays, but the shoulder pain subsides. Debbie also learned that calcium deposits may indicate metabolic problems in the healing process that are poorly understood. A calcium crystal, known as calcium apatite, can form in tendon attachments at the shoulder, wrist, hip, or ankle. The crystals are submicroscopic, their cause is unknown, and they are rarely found in tendons. Most tendinitis is not associated with calcification.

If such deposits do occur, there is presently no special treatment. Dr. Granger, recognizing that Debbie had habitually performed a task that, with too much repetition, commonly leads to an impingement syndrome and tendinitis, warned her that in the future she might develop acute inflammation at these locations. Dr. Granger's recommendations included a nonsteroidal anti-inflammatory agent to help reduce the swelling of the tendon sheath, local use of ice packs, a gentle stretching exercise to prevent scarring, and joint-protection measures that included general conditioning such as aerobics or any of a dozen other workout programs available in the community. He also advised Debbie to pace her household tasks and let up on the windows. He cautioned Debbie, too, to eliminate perfectionist attitudes that lead to joint overuse and suggested a proper support brassiere. Ice-friction massage of the biceps tendon is also helpful in cases like Debbie's.

Debbie followed all of the suggestions and was thankful to find so many ideas which worked. Debbie had learned that she could avoid pain if she first kept her elbow in close to her body when her work required her to raise her arm overhead. She combed her hair by keeping her elbow in until it was above her shoulder. At that point she could move the elbow out to the side and continue her arm motion. Learning this simple habit allowed her to use the arm with less pain. Doing this, you see, prevents the head of the humerus (the ball at the top of the arm bone) from pinching the tendons.

If aggravating factors are recognized and eliminated, most cases of bursitis or tendinitis will subside. Professional help is available for resistant cases. Your physician can prescribe nonsteroidal anti-inflammatory drugs or inject the bursa or tendon sheath with a long-acting cortisone preparation to hasten the healing process. Only one injection is usually necessary. An exercise to maintain shoulder-joint movement, the pendulum shoulder exercise (Figure 5-7) calls for a circular movement of the arm as it hangs out at the side. The exercise can be performed at first without any weight and then by grasping and holding 2 to 15 pounds. A circular motion about 12 inches in diameter is the usual movement. You should not use weights until movement without weights is pain-free. Additional exercises are presented in Table 5-6;

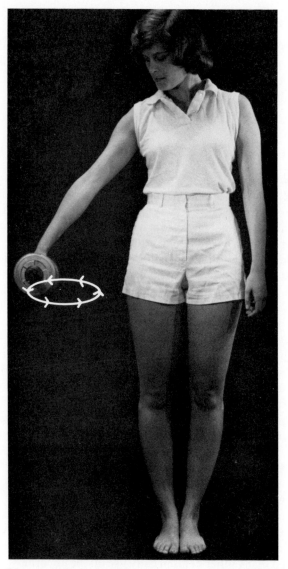

Figure 5-7.   The pendulum shoulder exercise to loosen the tissues around the shoulder joint.

particularly useful are nos. 2, 3, and 10. Application of ice to the shoulder before exercise is helpful in alleviating pain. A physical therapist can review your exercise program and can also add ultrasound, ice, or heat. Surgery for tendinitis is rarely needed unless the groove for the biceps tendon is unusually shallow and needs deepening.

Muscular Pain in the Shoulder-Blade Area

Pain that arises in the muscular tissues about the shoulder blade is common and often stubbornly persistent. Figure 5-5 illustrates the various tender points, or trigger points, in the muscles near the shoulder blade.

BILL AND ANN R.: A NEW KITCHEN BRINGS PROBLEMS

Bill and Ann, a middle-aged couple, have recently stepped up to a new home, which they enjoy. The kitchen is long and narrow with the stove and sink along one wall, cabinets and shelves opposite. Ann thinks it is ideal, mainly because the distance between the two work areas is only several feet. It had never occurred to her that something she liked so much would prove a problem. In a month Ann began to notice a nagging pain behind her right shoulder when she awakened. Because it let up as she moved about, she didn't think much about it. But when it began worsening by dinner, she was annoyed. Ann realized that her pain did not in any way limit shoulder movement, and she did not have pain during movement. Finally, she decided to meet with her doctor. Dr. Farnsworth talked with her about many of the harmful practices that result in shoulder pain, and together they decided Ann's pain must be due to some aggravating habit. Ann would watch for any movements which led to pain.

One thing she noted was that whenever she was working and needed something from the drawer behind her, she reached back instead of turning. In fact, her hand was constantly going back and forth. Also, she noticed that when she answered the phone, she kept on working, cradling the telephone between her shoulder and ear. (Do you do any of these things which cause strain on the muscles of your shoulder blade?)

Ann's new kitchen was indeed quite different from her old one in the proximity of the cabinets, and the entire arrangement was conducive to strain. Not only did she have her utensils behind her, but she also had her coffeepot and many other items in daily use on the uppermost shelves. This meant standing on tiptoe and stretching the soft tissues about the shoulder blade. She had Bill stand behind her as she sat and apply acupressure to relieve the tender points in her shoulders; with a gentle, rolling motion he massaged them into temporary relief. Then they rearranged that kitchen, moving the items she used daily to lower shelves. She made certain that she thought ahead in laying out utensils before she needed them. And she did the stretch exercise shown in Figure 5-8. Within a few days, Ann felt better.

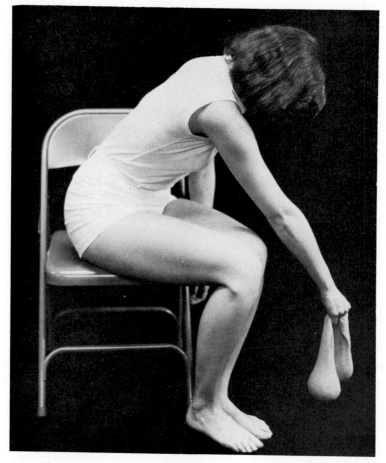

Figure 5-8. Stretch exercise for the shoulder blade.

Frozen Shoulder

A frozen shoulder, or *adhesive capsulitis,* differs from other soft-tissue rheumatic shoulder problems in that there is a loss of arm motion in all directions. This means the free movement of the involved arm is restricted even when someone else tries to move it. Thus more than pain is limiting arm movement. If dye is injected into the involved shoulder joint and x-rays are taken, creating what are called *arthrograms,* it will show the volume of the normal shoulder capsule to be severely constricted, demonstrating a shrinking of the capsule.

The muscles that rotate the arm form the capsule that covers the bony joint. This capsule normally has many folds, allowing a very loose covering for free arm movement. When the capsule becomes contracted, arm movement is lessened. As the capsule tightens, the inflammation of the bursal sacs causes progressive pain at night. Sometimes a frozen shoulder follows a spell of tendinitis, particularly biceps tendinitis. Occasionally, too, a case will follow a direct shoulder injury such as a fall or a blow. Most cases have no known traumatic cause. Sometimes a frozen shoulder is the first manifestation of diabetes, thyroid, or hyperparathyroidism (overactive parathyroid) disease. The parathyroid gland is important in calcium metabolism, and hyperparathyroidism results in a high blood-calcium level. It is a good idea to get a blood chemical battery and blood thyroid determination if you develop a frozen shoulder. Most cases of frozen shoulder begin gradually.

MARY L.'S FROZEN SHOULDER

Mary L., 56 years old, is a secretary in a large corporation, and she has just about decided that the office pool is a whirlpool. She not only types; she also files and searches records. In the evening Mary performs home-making duties and bowls as an important member of her league. She says she was just at the point of realizing that she was doing too many things, when she found her shoulder was giving her a great deal of pain. While dressing, she had difficulty fastening her brassiere. Her left arm would not go back as far as it should. And there was a nagging ache in the shoulder area when she awakened each day. Sometimes on cold, muggy days the shoulder also had a decided ache. Gradually Mary realized she was losing left-shoulder movement when she reached overhead, forward, or backward.

A little later she realized that all shoulder movement was going. Although she could not detect anything that might be the cause, she had read about the pendulum shoulder exercise. She tried this in an effort to prevent further motion loss.

Finally, Mary consulted her physician, Dr. Talbot, and her careful examination confirmed the lost motion. Fortunately, x-rays and blood tests revealed no other health problem. In fact, the x-rays were surprisingly normal. Dr. Talbot explained that the lining of the shoulder capsule had become inflamed and was tightening up the shoulder. Usually these x-rays are normal, and the best treatment is intensive passive exercises to stretch the shoulder capsule.

Dr. Talbot explained further that a frozen shoulder frequently involves both arms and that her bowling might actually prevent Mary's right shoulder from developing the condition. She advised Mary to refrain from lifting her elbow higher than her breast, because if she did, the muscles across her shoulder could actually tighten the joint more and worsen the condition. She suggested exercise, using the good arm to push and pull the bad arm through a range of movements. Mary was given wand exercises and a wall-ladder exercise (Figures 5-9 and 5-10). Dr. Talbot explained that if night pain worsened or if the shoulder movement did not show steady

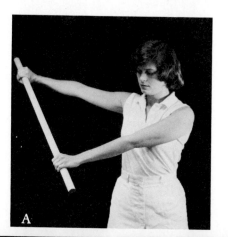

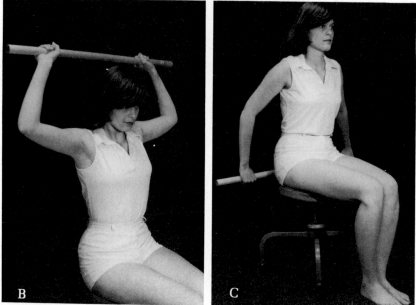

Figure 5-9.   Three wand or broomstick exercises to mobilize the shoulder.

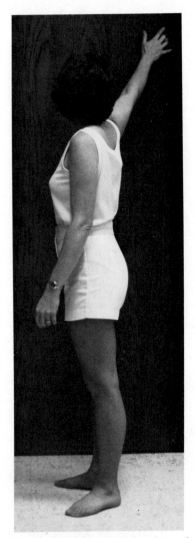

Figure 5-10.   The wall-ladder exercise for a frozen shoulder.

improvement over any 2-week period, she would inject a corticosteroid agent into the shoulder.

Not being particularly pain-sensitive, Mary preferred to try an anti-inflammatory, nonsteroidal agent that her doctor recommended. She advised her to perform the shoulder exercises several times a day and gradually increase the intensity of each exercise. The number of repetitions was not as important as the diligence with which she performed each movement. Dr. Talbot further cautioned that many patients take longer to recover if they give in to pain during the exercise. On the other hand, if the exercises should result in pain of more than 20 minutes' duration, she would be performing them too stressfully. She wanted to follow Mary's progress and emphasized that she must continue the exercise until a full range of shoulder motion was restored. She could determine this only by examination.

Mary discovered that she could cheat during the exercise by raising the arm with scapular, or shoulder blade, movement rather than with true shoulder movement. But she soon realized this was self-defeating, because there was no improvement. As she learned, true movement must occur at the shoulder joint. Mary performed the wand exercises (Figure 5-9) in front of a mirror to see that she did not use her shoulder blade to lift the entire shoulder during the exercise. It took her nearly 3 months to recover most of her shoulder movement. Although it was slow going, Mary soon realized that her discomfort was diminishing steadily. She did not mind the few minutes the exercises required each morning, afternoon, and evening. She performed them before and after work and at bedtime. Within several weeks, she was much more comfortable. (Today a frozen shoulder is rarely manipulated by the physician.)

Home Treatment

Treatment for frozen shoulder can be started at home with pain-relieving medication and mobilizing exercises. Relief is often obtained with aspirin, acetaminophen (Tylenol), or ibuprofen used on a regular-dose schedule (for example, two tablets with food or milk every 6 hours) and with ice therapy. Take six ice cubes, place in a plastic freezer bag, and apply to shoulder for 5 to 10 minutes three or more times daily. Be sure to try this just before performing the mobilizing wand exercises described below. Ice increases deep circulation and may assist the healing process. If you cannot tolerate the direct application of ice, try wrapping the ice bag in three layers of towel and applying this to the shoulder for 20 or 30 minutes. Moist heat or rub-on medications may also be helpful.

The key to pain relief, however, is to free the joint and thus release the muscle pressure. This requires pulling the shoulder joint, gradually and progressively, almost beyond your endurance. Begin with the pendulum motion for 1 minute; then go on to the wand exercises. After a moment of rest, you can try the wall-ladder exercise. Exercises 8 through 10 in Table 5-6 are similar to the wand exercises and bring similar results. Choose whichever seems less painful.

Until motion is restored, you should avoid any task requiring you to lift the arm above breast height. If movement does not improve to some degree each week, medical consultation is advised. Use the better arm to reach into cupboards and closets. Fasten your brassiere in front of you and then turn it to the proper position. Bowling and swimming may be well tolerated. Pressure on the shoulder—for instance that caused by push-ups—is harmful.

The Damage of Pain

Pain is the patient's worst enemy in recovering from a frozen shoulder. The pain means less use and movement, more muscle tightness, easier scarring, and restricted exercising. Do not give in to pain! Be gentle but persistent. If it hurts, push a little harder, but push slowly. Pain from the exercise should not last more than 20 or 30 minutes. If it does, you have overdone it and should ease up. If a physical therapist is required, always know which exercises you should be doing between your appointments. Treatment should provide gradual improvement in each 2-week period. As motion improves, the final stages of stretching (as described in Table 5-6, exercises 8, 9, and 10) are helpful. With proper care, night pain should be eliminated within the first 2 weeks. Ultimate improvement may take many months of self-help exercise, but nearly complete recovery can be accomplished in most patients. Some doctors have noted that up to 20 percent of patients with frozen shoulder have diabetes, so a blood-sugar test is a good idea. Diabetics who require insulin may have a particularly lengthy recovery from a frozen shoulder.

Do these measures work? In one study, simple home treatment consisting of salicylates or nonsteroidal anti-inflammatory drugs, rest, cold packs, and exercise improved patients in 1 week. Other researchers, in a double-blind test, tried dimethyl sulfoxide (DMSO), a solvent that is purported to have pain-killing properties when rubbed on afflicted areas. Using a 70 percent solution for the treatment group and a 5 percent solution for the control group, the researchers found no difference in the two groups after 1 to 3 weeks. About 40 percent were better in each group. But note that when exercise, joint protection, and simple pain-killing and anti-inflammatory drugs are used, twice as many improve—and more quickly, too.

Shoulder-Cuff Tear

In people under 50, a tear of the shoulder cuff generally indicates exceptional force and injury. After about age 50, the tissues that constitute the shoulder cuff may have thinned out from vascular and other aging factors. Then a shoulder-cuff tear can occur from a more trivial injury. These tears are being diagnosed more frequently because of the availability of *arthrography,* the diagnostic x-ray technique in which dye designed to show on an x-ray film is instilled into the shoulder capsule. If a tear has occurred, then the dye will leak outside the shoulder capsule. Symptoms suggesting a capsule tear include the inability to use the arm in an elevated position. Also, tasks that require raising the elbow and arm above the shoulder may exceed the shoulder's capabilities. A blow to the shoulder, a fall on an outstretched arm, as well as grasping during a fall (and thus suddenly stretching the shoulder) are common precipitating injuries.

If you suspect a shoulder-cuff tear, try the Moseley test, described in Table 5-2, item 5. If the arm gives way and drops, a significant tear has occurred. A partial tear can be suspected if the arm does stay out at the side when the helper lets go, but further arm elevation is performed with great difficulty. If the helper now applies any downward pressure as you try to raise the arm upward, the shoulder will give way. This "giving way" strongly suggests a shoulder-capsule tear. If it is diagnosed early and if the shoulder-capsule tissues are strong, surgical repair can be attempted and is often successful. The repair job is similar to the stitches on a baseball. However, the surgeon may encounter thin, weak tissue that will not recover despite surgical repair. If the capsule tissue is very thin, the sutures will pull away. There is no therapy other than gentle exercise to prevent further loss of motion. You will have to adapt your mode of living to avoid raising the arm beyond its ability. Over the years, much of the soreness will disappear in most cases.

Thoracic-Outlet Syndromes

As already mentioned, the nerves and blood vessels to the arm and hand cross through the shoulder region and travel through three tunnels. Any impingement can result in a group of symptoms strongly suggestive of a *thoracic-outlet syndrome.* These symptoms are numbness, tingling, weakness, and aching pain in the hand and arm, plus a sensation of swelling in the hand. The condition can result from a wide range of causes, including an extra rib, an overly large muscle in one of the tunnels, or scars or bands developing in a tunnel. Habits that aggravate the condition are described in Table 5-4.

WILLIAM F., WHO SUFFERED FROM SLEEPING WITH HIS ARMS OVERHEAD

William F., a 56-year-old factory worker, was always looking for ways to save money. He wasn't miserly, just careful. When his car broke down, he saw no reason to hire someone to do the repairs. A friend with a gas station let William use the garage and equipment; and each weekend William worked, arms overhead, for several hours on his car, which was raised on the hydraulic lift. Sunday and Monday night of each of these weeks William had difficulty sleeping. The muscles of his upper shoulders and at the back of his neck hurt. He had been sleeping with his arms overhead because it seemed to ease the pain, but soon he began awakening each morning with tingly hands. His condition worsened, and William began to notice that he could not tolerate handwork for more than 15 or 20 minutes. Several weeks later William was aware of a sensation of numbness, tingling, and swelling of all the tissues of both hands. Now he was finally alarmed enough to seek medical advice. His doctor, Ben Thayer, could detect no true joint swelling. Blood tests of inflammation were normal. Because the constellation of symptoms suggested a thoracic-outlet syndrome, the physician performed several examination procedures: One of them required William to raise his arms over his head for 1 minute. The numbness and tingling were accentuated. The physician then asked in what position William slept. When he heard the answer, curing William became easy.

The simple recognition of the hyperabduction syndrome, one of the three types of thoracic-outlet syndromes, required no invasive techniques and no x-rays. The relief that followed the change in William's sleeping position corroborated the diagnosis: Dr. Thayer suggested that William alter his position and, if the symptoms continued, have an x-ray for diagnostic purposes. But the symptoms diminished rapidly when William slept with his arms positioned closer to his waist.

DAVID C. AND HIS BACKPACK

David, a young man in love with camping, developed symptoms that were similar to William's. He had backpacked for a number of years with no difficulty. However, this time he had been laden for a trip of longer duration. After several days of backpacking, he developed rather profound numbness and tingling in both hands, a sensation of swelling in both, and weakness in his hand grip. He decided that his backpack must be too heavy. Lightening the load and taking frequent rest stops brought immediate relief to this backpacker.

As mentioned previously, another very common cause of thoracic-outlet syndrome is slack and flabby musculature that allows the shoulder to slope downward and forward—an occurrence in both men and women. This "drooping-shoulder syndrome" can be helped if you perform the posture-correcting neck exercise and the shoulder-shrugging exercise (see Chapter 4).

Heavy breasts and heavy arms are associated with the drooping shoulder. Vague complaints, with minimal physical-examination findings, are usually the features of a thoracic-outlet syndrome in many patients. If you are in doubt, you can use the shrugging exercise as a diagnostic test. If it relieves the arm and hand symptoms, a thoracic-outlet syndrome is as good a diagnosis as any.

Reflex Sympathetic Dystrophy and Shoulder-Hand Syndrome

A very unusual and distressing syndrome is reflex sympathetic dystrophy—in particular, one form of it, the shoulder-hand syndrome. Reflex sympathetic dystrophy should be considered if you have sensations of numbness, tingling, aching, and swelling, and, in addition, a *throbbing, burning* pain in the upper extremity. If you allow this disorder to progress, it will cause the skin to grow shiny, the hand to swell visibly, and movement to be restricted or lost. When adhesive capsulitis (frozen shoulder) also occurs, the condition is known as a shoulder-hand syndrome. See your doctor.

Shoulder-hand syndrome and reflex sympathetic dystrophy are two examples of a nerve condition that may result from trivial injury. More severe forms of these disorders can result in blockage of the blood supply with resulting discoloration of the hands (see Table 5-1 for danger signs). Nerve blocks in the neck region are both diagnostic and curative for reflex sympathetic dystrophy. Recently use of certain ganglionic blockers (blood-pressure medications), a transcutaneous electrical nerve stimulator (TENS), and exercises have been advocated. Several of our patients have avoided the need for surgical treatment in this manner. No home treatment alone will suffice.

Bony Arthritis of the Shoulder

Bony arthritis of the shoulder joint is not common, probably because the shoulder is not used as a weight-bearing joint. Bone is not often rubbing against bone as happens in joints of the lower extremities. Nevertheless, arthritis sometimes does develop and leads to a loss of movement and pain. A grating noise or sensation in the shoulder can suggest the presence of true arthritis. But noises can also occur in the shoulder region from tendon snapping, tight muscles, loose jointedness, or sagging musculature. Noises without pain probably do not require medical attention. Easy rule to remember: if it's not broken, don't fix it! See Table 5-6, exercise 1 to prevent further joint damage.

Shoulder-area pain can also result from gallbladder disease, hernias of the esophagus or diaphragm, and neck problems. Tender points, limitation of shoulder motion, and recognizable aggravating factors are not usually present when shoulder pain is referred from deeper or more distant problems. (A self-examination and other simple examination maneuvers already described are detailed in Table 5-2.) You should consult your physician if none of the above disorders is apparent.

After Recovery

When you recover from an attack of shoulder pain, you will have to pace the use of your arm. You may have to reeducate yourself for sports or hobby activities, using a conditioning activity beforehand. After the pain has subsided and a full and active range of movement is present, you can begin gentle weight lifting. Tasks that require repetitive arm motion such as raking, sweeping, wiping, polishing, or stirring should be interrupted every 10 to 15 minutes. If you are a compulsive person, start a timer before you begin any such tasks. A 5-minute break may be all that is needed. If you have acute pain, apply ice to the site; this is possibly the best quick-relief therapy. A half dozen ice cubes in a plastic bag placed directly on the site can be tolerated for as long as 10 to 20 minutes. Repeat this as often as every 3 or 4 hours. Certainly aspirin should be used if tolerated. Acetaminophen and similar products are good pain relievers, but they do not reduce inflammation in cases of tendinitis or bursitis. The anti-inflammatory prescription medications take several days to build up an effective dosage. There are some prescription drugs that work on inflammation faster, but they are more likely to cause side effects. Your physician may prescribe them after due consideration. The pendulum exercise can be performed safely in most situations. Less severe and more lingering pain may respond to counterirritant, rub-on types of medications (see Chapter 15).

When to Seek Professional Help

Certainly pain almost beyond your endurance should prompt medical consultation; and failure to respond to self-administered treatment within a reasonable period of time should also lead you to a medical consultation. How long should you wait? A dull, aching pain that is intermittent is not nearly as serious as pain that is constant, severe, and worsening each day. Visible swelling of the hand is decidedly more serious than an intermittent sensation of hand swelling without visible evidence. A sensation of swelling, such as "my rings feel tight," is not as serious as swelling that is more visible.

If your physician chooses to inject a corticosteroid agent, always refrain from any sport or repetitive-movement task for at least a week afterward; tissues are temporarily weakened by corticosteroid agents. You can actually tear a tendon completely apart when cortisone has been recently injected nearby. Although cortisone is a great help in hastening healing and bringing pain relief when used judiciously, you should be cautious about it being used locally in your tissues. The physician should not repeat the injection more than three times (although most patients will need only one injection); injections should be spaced several weeks apart. Cortisone medications taken by mouth do not often achieve a therapeutic level at the site of local inflammation, and therefore physicians rarely recommend them for these conditions.

Physical therapy can be helpful in any disorder that has persisted beyond 4 to 6 weeks. Local application of heat, ultrasound, ice packs, or massage followed by active and passive exercise may be helpful in resistant cases. Gentle manipulation of the shoulder can be performed by a physical therapist for a resistant frozen shoulder. The occupational therapist uses a joint-protection plan to aid you in preventing further damage to the joint tissues. Suspect that an aggravating habit is the cause if you have had several attacks of shoulder pain that have spontaneously improved. If you cannot identify such a habit or aggravation, an occupational therapist is often helpful. A rare frozen shoulder will require a pressure-fluid injection, called *bresement therapy,* or manipulation and loosening of the shoulder while the patient is under general anesthetic. This is usually performed by an orthopedic surgeon only after all other treatments have failed. Risk of permanent shoulder-capsule tear from manipulation under an anesthetic is of great concern to the orthopedic surgeon. The natural history of an untreated frozen shoulder often evolves through stages of "freezing," "frozen," and "thawing." Thus, time favors the patient. But spontaneous improvement is seldom complete. Early treatment is essential in order to restore good shoulder motion.

Summary

In summary, pain and muscle spasm can restrict active arm movement, but in those situations, *passive* (assisted) arm motion is normal unless arthritis, tendinitis, or adhesive capsulitis (frozen shoulder) is present. Whenever there is shoulder pain, it is a good idea to examine yourself. Begin checking for swollen glands in the neck area and above the collarbone on the involved side. Then move on to the armpit, and if any lymph glands are as hard as a green olive, bring them to your physician's attention. Look at the shoulder in a mirror and compare it with the other shoulder for abnormal swelling. Because of the overlying musculature, it is very difficult to feel swelling by direct examination. Read the danger list in Table 5-1. Consult your doctor promptly if any of these warning signs is present. If you have persistent or recurring problems, then an aggravating habit may still be present.

Table 5-1
Danger Signs in the Shoulder

Any visible swelling
Fever and chills
Constant and progressive pain
Disturbances of the stomach or bowel that are new
Pain in the armpit under the shoulder
Numbness and tingling at the shoulder
Inability to maintain the arm out at the side after passive arm elevation
Shoulder pain that is aggravated by neck movement

Shoulder pain that is not aggravated by arm motion
Color change in the hand
Visible loss of muscle tissue in the hand

Table 5-2
Self-Examination of the Shoulder

1. To perform active arm elevation, let your arm hang down; then raise it out and up to an overhead position. Watch your motion in a mirror (Figure 5-3).
2. To perform active arm rotation, start with your elbow at the side of your body; bring the hand to the chest, then away from the chest.
3. For passive arm elevation, you will need a helper. Maintain a limp arm while the helper lifts the arm from down at your side, to out at the side, and finally to up overhead.
4. For passive arm rotation, you will again need a helper. Your helper holds your limp arm straight out at the side of your body; then, with the elbow bent, he or she rotates the arm so the palm goes downward, facing the floor, and then upward, always keeping the elbow at the level of the shoulder and out to the side.
5. A helper raises your arm out at the side of your body, level with your shoulder; then, when the helper releases the arm, you try to hold it at this position. If you are unable to do so, this suggests a shoulder-cuff tear.
6. Have a helper gently roll his or her thumbs across the front of the shoulders on each side to detect swelling or pain. Keep the thumbs vertical as shown in Figure 5-4. If you feel pain or if the helper detects vertical sausage-shaped tendon-sheath swelling, this suggests tendinitis of the upper end of the biceps tendon.
7. Raise your arm forward—not outward—with the elbow out from the body; then repeat the movement with the elbow kept at the side of the body. Pain is usually worse with the first motion. Another technique is to raise the arm straight overhead, hand in a fist and palm forward. Now rotate fist and thumb toward midline. Pain may be accentuated with either of these tests if you have an impingement syndrome (Figure 5-6).
8. Grasp your hands in front of you and make a circle with your arms. Raise this circle and your hands over your head and hold it for 1 minute. If your arms and hands become numb and tingly, a thoracic-outlet syndrome may be present.

Table 5-3

Possible Causes of Shoulder Symptoms

Complaint	Possible Cause
Pain in the shoulder and upper one-third of outer arm	Bursitis; tendinitis; impingement syndrome
Pain throughout shoulder (no numbness or tingling)	Arthritis; tendinitis; rotator-cuff injury
Pain in the shoulder-blade area	Muscular injury (myofascial pain with trigger points)
Aching of shoulder and entire arm, numbness, tingling, and a sensation of swelling anywhere in the arm or hand	Thoracic-outlet syndrome

Table 5-4

Possible Causes of Persistent Shoulder Problems

Complaint	Possible Aggravation
Pain in the shoulder and upper one-third of outer arm	Sudden forcing injury that jams the shoulder; sleeping with arms overhead; sport activity with thrusting motion such as pitching overhead; repetitive arm movements such as raking, sweeping, shoveling, etc.
Pain throughout shoulder (no numbness or tingling)	Repetitive arm movement, as when washing windows or polishing an auto; weight lifting or doing push-ups
Pain in the shoulder-blade area	Carrying a heavy object such as a suitcase; reaching backward repeatedly (e.g., traveling sales agents who reach for their briefcase in back seat); cradling a telephone with the shoulder rather than holding it with the hand

Complaint	Possible Aggravation
Aching of shoulder and entire arm; numbness, tingling, and a sensation of swelling anywhere in the arm or hand	Sleeping with the arm overhead; obesity, heavy breasts, improper brassiere, or poor posture; carrying heavy objects at the side of the body; backpacking; cradling the telephone with the shoulder; repetitive hand use while sitting; prolonged sitting or standing

Table 5-5

What's Harmful, What's Helpful for the Shoulder

Harmful	Helpful
Repetitively moving the shoulder to and fro while holding the elbow out to the side pinches tendons inside the shoulder.	Frequently interrupt such tasks as washing windows, vacuuming, and working on an assembly line. Keep the elbow close to the body during to-and-fro movement. When raking or sweeping, hold the rake or broom out in front of the body. Doing so changes the angle of shoulder motion.
Sleeping with the arms overhead can pinch muscles and nerves in the shoulder region.	Sleep with the arms below the level of the chest.
Similarly, working with the arms overhead for prolonged periods can be injurious.	Take frequent breaks when working with the arms overhead.
Using the shoulder as a weight-bearing joint (e.g., when leaning on crutches or canes or pushing off from chairs) can lead to shoulder injury.	See that crutches fit 2 in (about 5 cm) below the armpits; carry weight on ribs. A forearm cane may be preferred. When arising from a chair, push off with thigh muscles, not the hands.

(continued)

Harmful	Helpful
Reaching sideways and backward into the back seat of a vehicle to bring a briefcase, grocery bag, or other object forward is a common cause of pain in the shoulder-blade region.	Face the object and draw it forward.
Repetitively reaching behind for a kitchen utensil and bringing it forward has a similar effect.	Turn the body, not just the shoulder, and grasp the utensil.
Placing the hands on top of the steering wheel for long periods can be irritating to nerves and muscles in the shoulder region.	Keep the hands below the 3- and 9-o'clock positions on the wheel. If possible, use a steering wheel that tilts.

Table 5-6
Exercises for the Shoulder Region

1. *Pendulum exercise:* Stand or sit, leaning slightly toward the painful side. Then, while grasping a 2- to 5-pound weight, swing the arm in a small circle the size of the top of a pail. Proceed slowly in a smooth, circular motion for a minute or two every few hours (Figure 5-7).
2. *Wand exercise to stretch biceps tendon:* Grasp a yardstick or broom handle with your hands wide apart. The good or better arm is always used to push the bad arm. You must keep the painful side limp and let the wand perform the motion. The wand is held across the chest and then used to force the involved arm out, away, and slightly back. Push gradually, with increasing force, to loosen scar tissue. After 1 minute, slowly draw the arm back down (Figure 5-9).
3. *Additional wand exercises:* Lift the wand upward and overhead. Keep the wand close to the head, bending the elbows to do so. Try to get the wand over and then behind the head. Hold the position a moment and then repeat 10 times. Next, put the wand behind you and, with the elbows straight, try to raise the wand backward and upward. The movement is performed slowly and steadily for 1 minute (Figure 5-9).
4. *The wall-ladder exercise:* Stand sideways to the wall, reaching out to the wall with the involved arm. Stand away from the wall so just the fingertips reach the wall; then begin to walk your fingers

up the wall, keeping your body sideways. Don't turn the shoulders or chest toward the wall. The arm must be kept directly out at the side from the trunk. Begin climbing the fingers upward and slightly backward. When you can go no higher, note the location that you have reached; stay at this extreme position for 1 minute, then slowly slide the hand back down the wall. *Do not drop* the arm abruptly, or you may tear the rotator cuff. If this cannot be performed sideways, begin it by facing the wall and reaching forward, walking the fingers straight up the wall. Each week, if you are improving, try this sideways technique (Figure 5-10).

5. *Shoulder-blade stretch:* Sit in a chair and grasp a 2- to 5-pound weight with the hand on the painful side. First reach out straight in front, then slowly cross the arm until it is over the knee on the opposite side. Slowly bend your body straight forward and draw the weighted hand beyond and to the outside of the opposite foot. You should end up bent forward, your head centered and looking down, your arm crossed to the other side, and the weighted hand about 6 inches from the floor—12 inches in front and 12 inches to the outside of the opposite foot. For example, if the right shoulder blade is painful, the right hand holds the weight and crosses beyond and to the left side of the left foot. The position is held for 20 seconds and the exercise is repeated three times in succession several times a day (Figure 5-8).

6. *Shrugging exercise:* Shoulder shrugging can begin with 2- to 5-pound weights, gradually increased to 7- to 15-pounds for each side. You can hold the weights at your side or place them over your shoulders. (Soft weights can be made with athletic socks, freezer bags, and sand.) Raise the shoulders slowly upward, backward, and then downward. Repeat for 1 or 2 minutes, several times daily (Figure 4-10).

7. *Ice-friction massage:* Fill a cone-shaped paper cup with water and pinch the top together; clip or staple the top and then freeze. Grasp the frozen ice cone with a towel at the broad end and use the tapered end in deep, stroking massage along the biceps tendon. Move slowly up and down the tendon.

8. *Shoulder-capsule stretch:* Sit on a high-backed chair, drape your bad arm over the back of the chair. Lean against the back and with your good arm, grasp the bad one above the elbow and begin a rhythmic downward pull (Figure 5-11).

9. *Arm stretch:* Stand next to a ledge or fireplace mantel and lay the arm on it, palm down. Now lower your body to stretch the

(continued)

straight arm. The body position can be forward and then sideways to the mantel or ledge (Figure 5-12).

10. *Rotation stretch:* Stand in a doorway and place the back of the hand on the door frame with your elbow bent at 90 degrees. Slowly walk forward, stretching the shoulders. Now back up and repeat with your palm flat on the door frame (Figure 5-13).

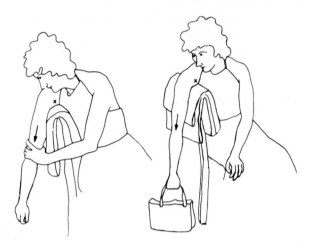

Figure 5-11.   Shoulder-capsule stretch. (*R. M. Kessler and D. Hertling, Management of Common Musculoskeletal Disorders, Harper & Row, Philadelphia, 1983.*)

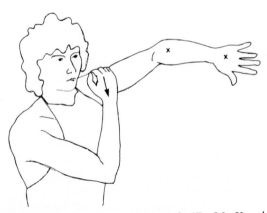

Figure 5-12.   Arm stretch with arm on a mantel. (*R. M. Kessler and D. Hertling, Management of Common Musculoskeletal Disorders, Harper & Row, Philadelphia, 1983.*)

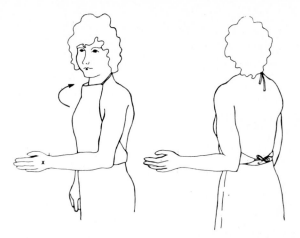

Figure 5-13.   Rotation stretch. (*R. M. Kessler and D. Hertling, Management of Common Musculoskeletal Disorders, Harper & Row, Philadelphia, 1983.*)

CHAPTER 6

The Elbow

The elbow is composed of three bones that allow bending and straightening of the joint and rotation of the hand from palm up to palm down. The elbow allows the arm to act as a piston, or a lever, and to perform tasks in many directions and with a variety of degrees of power. However, the elbow does not tolerate prolonged repetitive movement.

If you stand with your arm hanging at your side, palm facing forward, the part of the elbow closest to the body is the inner side or medial aspect, and the part aligned with the thumb is the outer aspect (Figure 6-1 and Plate 6-1). When the elbow is mentioned, most people think first of the "crazy bone." Their second thought is probably "tennis elbow." This latter term most often refers to pain and irritation about the outer aspect of the elbow. Bursitis, on the other hand, often occurs behind the elbow or on the outer side, or thumb side, near the head of the radius. Another bursa can become inflamed beneath the biceps muscle that attaches directly in front of the elbow. When arthritis occurs, the swelling will not allow the joint to fully straighten. However, in the early stages of arthritis only painful motion may occur, without swelling.

Some people have too much elbow motion. These persons with

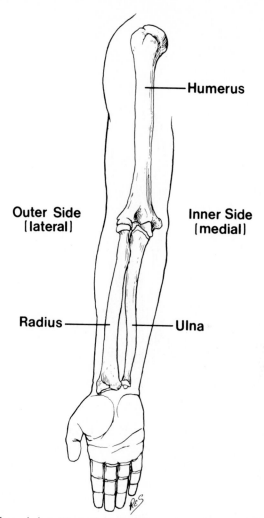

Figure 6-1. Elbow joint. Note that the elbow is composed of three bones joined together.

loose-jointedness can overextend (hyperextend) the arm, bend over and touch the floor with their palms while keeping their legs straight, and bend their wrist until their thumb touches the forearm of that side.

Don't overdo extensions like these. At the present time elbow joints are not readily replaceable, so don't wear them out! If you show respect for your elbow, it can serve you a very long time. This chapter will provide information about tennis elbow and other con-

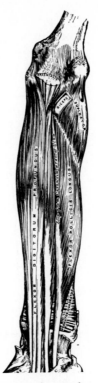

Plate 6-1.   Muscles of the anterior (palmar) aspect of the left forearm.

ditions that mimic tennis elbow. We will also give some pointers on bursitis and pinched nerves in the elbow region.

At the end of this chapter are tables outlining danger signs in the elbow (Table 6-1), self-examination techniques (Table 6-2), possible causes and aggravating habits that induce pain (Tables 6-3 to 6-5), and exercises for the elbow region (Table 6-6).

Tennis Elbow

The term "tennis elbow" is often applied to any elbow pain; but, in fact, it refers to a group of soft-tissue disturbances that lie outside the elbow joint. *Tendinitis* is the most common cause of tennis elbow. The pain of this affliction is detected on the outer side of the elbow. "Golfer's elbow" is a term applied to pain and tenderness of the inner side of the elbow.

The average case of tennis elbow has persistent symptoms for up to 8 months. Most of that time the pain is bad only after hard or repetitious use. As mentioned, tennis elbow refers to elbow disturbance with pain at the outer aspect of the elbow. Elbow movement is normal, although painful. Physicians sometimes label tennis elbow as *epicondylitis*. The pain may be acute and severe, but more often it is intermittent or chronic with aggravation during hand use such as in grasping an object, shaking hands, or turning a tool such as a screwdriver. It occurs most often in racket-sports participants, carpenters, gardeners, dentists, and politicians; and it seldom involves both arms. Most of these people are between 40 and 60. Numbness and tingling do not occur, and visible swelling should not occur. The hallmark of tennis elbow is tenderness at the outer border of the elbow.

To identify which tendon is affected, you can examine the tendons by contracting each individual muscle and then noting which is painful: place your good hand over the back of your bad hand and try to draw the back of the hand upward against your good hand. If this is painful, one or more of the wrist-extensor-muscle tendons are involved. If this is not painful, try to turn the bad hand against the good hand, first with thumb upward and then thumb downward. That too involves wrist-action muscles. If that is not painful, then draw each finger and thumb upward against the opposite hand. If none of this is painful, then tendinitis is not likely a cause, and a bursitis or a pinched nerve may be a consideration. Sometimes tennis elbow is due to a pinched nerve in the neck or carpal tunnel (Chapters 4 and 7), but most of the cases arise from one of the tendons that control wrist extension.

Tennis elbow results from injury, and it may be an accumulation of many strains or one single event. Most often it is a cumulative injury in our old friend, the "I'll-finish-this" person. It often occurs in homemakers during canning season or after the performance of an unusual task requiring hand tools such as a screwdriver, pliers, or wrench. Sometimes it happens to a worker who is on an assembly line that requires strong, repetitive movements, such as tightening bolts. Other causes may be gripping a racket too tightly because it is too small, improper playing technique such as pointing the elbow to the net for a backhand shot, hand clenching from anxiety, caffeine sensitivity, driving with an overly tight grip, reading, or telephoning.

Tennis elbow is more common in loose-jointed individuals, especially those who play tennis.

Self-Treatment

Try to determine what you have done wrong and try to exchange a bad habit for good body mechanics. Rest is important until severe pain has subsided, but studies have shown that tennis players who continue to play despite mild pain have the same rate of healing and duration of pain as those who stopped playing to "rest" the sore elbow. Aspirin and stretching exercises before play are advisable. Also, some means of maintaining muscle tone must be continued in spite of pain. Harsh activities that require gripping should be curtailed until tenderness ceases.

Acute pain can respond to ice massage followed by forearm stretching. Perform ice massage with a cone of ice: Fill a paper cup with water and clamp the top with a paper clip or staple. Then place in the freezer until frozen. Put the cone of ice in a towel and use the tip to massage deeply into the muscle tissue of the forearm. You may also start at the elbow. Be sure to include the points of maximum tenderness. Massage 2 or 3 minutes, then follow the ice treatment with forearm stretching, as described in Table 6-6, exercise 2 and Figure 6-2. As you perform this twice daily, notice the level at which the pulling sensation occurs. Use the good arm to note what your normal level is. Make sure you keep the back of your hand, not just the fingers, against the door so that the wrist is fully flexed.

Follow this movement with the mobilizing exercise, as demonstrated in Table 6-6, exercise 1 and Figure 6-3. The exercises should be kept up twice daily until no tenderness exists.

A helper can try cross-friction massage, using a deep kneading of the underlying tendons (Figure 6-4). A helper can locate the most tender area, then rub across the arm with increasing pressure. Begin gently at first, then use progressive pressure with a slow back-and-forth motion for 2 or 3 minutes. If symptoms are unchanged, an occupational therapist can be consulted to review work, home, and hobby activities. Rub-ons and DMSO have not proved helpful in double-blind studies. However, use of aspirin before an activity may be helpful in preventing more inflammation and irritation. Nonsteroidal anti-inflammatory drugs such as ibuprofen may be helpful in resistant cases.

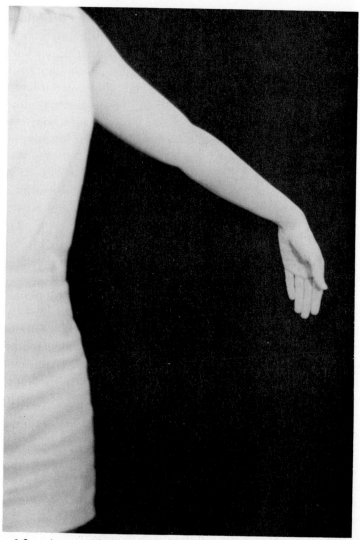

Figure 6-2.   A stretching exercise for the forearm muscles. With the back of the hand against a door, hold the arm straight and raise it slowly. The forearm muscles are stretched until you feel a "pulling" sensation.

Professional Treatment

If 2 weeks of treatment does not provide relief, then other measures and consultation should be considered. X-ray of the elbow is rarely of help; but if you cannot fully straighten the elbow, you should seek medical consultation. The physician's examination may indicate

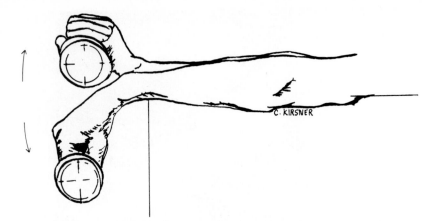
C. KIRSNER

Figure 6-3.   A mobilizing and strengthening exercise for forearm muscles.

findings that require an x-ray examination. If any of the danger signs for the elbow region is present, medical consultation should be obtained right away. Ultrasound treatments are beneficial, and one or two local corticosteroid and procaine injections may result in rapid healing of an otherwise intractable case. A physical therapist is sometimes specially skilled in performing friction massage. Tennis-elbow bands come in numerous styles; one is as good as another (Figure 6-5). Tight-fitting sleeves of elastic may be injurious if you have bursitis or a pinched nerve. Tennis-elbow splints will probably remind you to use less force in your work and play.

Surgery for tennis elbow is rare. Occasionally x-ray can show a spur near the attachment tendon, or a careful examination may reveal a nerve trapped by scar tissue. This can give rise to symptoms similar to those of tennis elbow. A specialist would be needed to perform the examination, but the problem is rare.

Pain at the inner side of the elbow, which indicates golfer's elbow, can result from overuse too. Treatment is similar, but stretching is performed with the back of the hand to the door (Figure 6-6 and Table 6-6, exercise 3), followed by the strengthening exercise (Table 6-6, exercise 1).

How effective is conservative therapy? A Canadian clinic reports that 95 percent of the patients benefited from therapy within 8 weeks; 50 percent had complete relief; others improved markedly. In a large series treated at Georgetown University School of Medicine, only 7 percent (88 of 1213 cases) failed conservative treatment and required surgery. Our experience is similar.

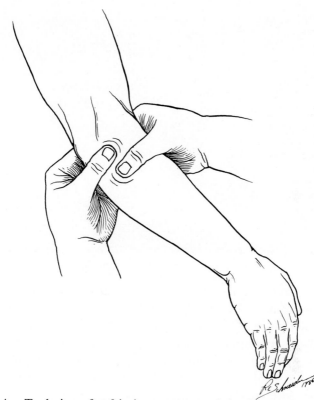

Figure 6-4.   Technique for friction massage of the forearm tendons and muscles.

Bursitis

Bursitis is an inflammation of one of the small sacs that protect muscle from the underlying bone prominence. Figure 6-7 demonstrates a typical case of olecranon bursitis.

The most common cause of bursitis is direct traumatic pressure such as leaning on the elbow while seated or using the elbow to push off when arising from bed. Other cases may result from occupational trauma (for example, in carpet layers or electricians). Occasionally bursitis results from sports activities such as throwing darts. Also, falling on an elbow could cause both pain and an accumulation of fluid in the elbow. One of us once slipped and fell on the ice with most of his weight landing on his elbow. It was painful for a couple of months and cleared up only after the fluid was aspirated and two shots of cortisone had been injected. Redness and swelling would

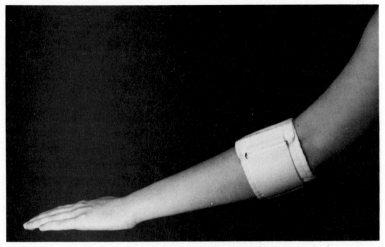

Figure 6-5.   A tennis-elbow band.

also signify the need for medical consultation to rule out infection, gout, rheumatoid arthritis, and other forms of inflammatory disease. Swelling without much tenderness or internal pressure may gradually subside without any treatment. If swelling persists or if the bursa is tense, diffusely painful, or associated with any other symptoms listed in Table 6-1, you should immediately seek consultation. Only a skilled physician should aspirate the fluid contents of a bursitis, and when this is performed, the fluid should be submitted for tests to rule out a low-grade infection. Certainly the elbow should be protected from pressure. This can be done by using padding in bed, avoiding improper resting positions, or altering work habits.

Pain in the front of the elbow may result from tendinitis or bursitis near the attachment at the lower end of the biceps muscle. If you hold your arm straight out, you can note tenderness right in the middle of the elbow crease. This can be treated with ice massage for 2 to 3 minutes and a stretching exercise (Table 6-6, exercise 5). This biceps stretching will hasten healing. It can be repeated 10 times, twice daily (Figure 6-8).

Arthritis

Bony enlargement can lead to painful movement with the inability to fully straighten the arm. Two worthwhile exercises are the triceps muscle strengthening (Figure 6-9 and Table 6-6, exercise 4) and the

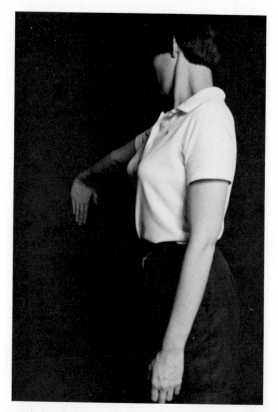

Figure 6-6.   Stretching exercise for golfer's elbow.

hammer rotation performed as described in Table 6-2, item 6, but used as an exercise. Rotate the hammer slowly for 1 minute twice daily.

Nerve Entrapments

Nerve entrapments in the elbow region are very rare but must be considered in any chronic, persistent elbow pain. These nerve disorders are often associated with numbness and tingling. As shown in Figure 6-10, the supinator muscle in the forearm overlies the radial nerve, and the pronator muscle, attached to the ulna and radius in the forearm, overlies the median nerve. Either structure can trap the nerve as it passes through the muscles. These nerve entrapments can be detected by the pain produced from pressing deeply in front of the elbow at the inner or outer aspect, about 1 inch to either side

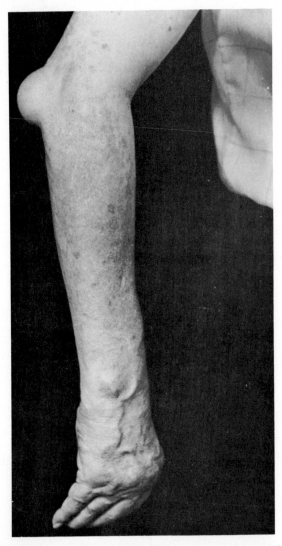

Figure 6-7.   Bursitis of the elbow (olecranon bursitis).

of the midline. Sometimes such a nerve entrapment will result in popping sensations about the elbow, as well as numbness, tingling, and weakness. A good test is the aggravation of pain when the long finger is pressed upward against resistance with the opposite hand. Surgical consultation is necessary in such cases. Numbness and tingling may be detected anywhere in the forearm, in the case of radial-

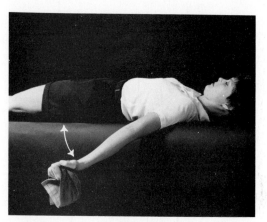

Figure 6-8.   Biceps muscle stretch.

nerve entrapment, or into the thumb, index, and long fingers, in the case of median-nerve entrapment.

When to Seek Professional Help

The pain of tennis elbow is a dull aching that gradually subsides, at least to some degree, during rest. It is certainly aggravated when you perform movements with hand gripping. If tenderness and a sensation of tightness are not detected or if pain is out of proportion to what has been described, then medical consultation is indicated. The physician will examine the neck, shoulder, elbow, and wrist

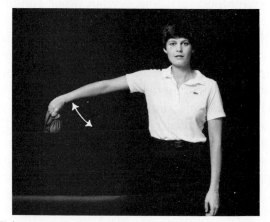

Figure 6-9.   Triceps muscle strengthening to restore power to the elbow.

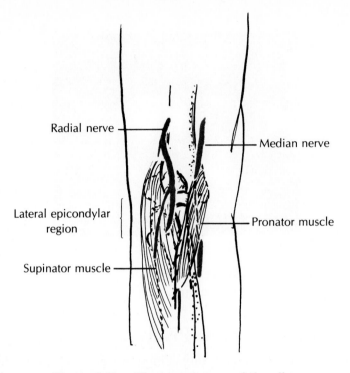

Figure 6-10.   Nerve pathways of the elbow.

regions to detect signs of impairment resulting from these structures. An x-ray will be made, if there is pain on passive motion,
swelling, or restricted active motion. The doctor might also test for
gout, excessive blood fats, and certain other conditions that can
result in chronic, persistent elbow pain and/or swelling. We have
mentioned the importance of studying fluid from an inflamed or unusually uncomfortable bursitis. The physician may recommend the
use of anti-inflammatory agents or muscle relaxants or suggest consultation with a physical therapist. If your physician detects a bursitis or tendinitis, an injection with a corticosteroid agent may be
useful. He or she might also recommend Fluorimethane, a pressurized spray coolant, followed by a stretch routine.

Consultation with an occupational or physical therapist might
also be helpful. The physical therapist begins with a careful muscle
assessment and then starts treatment using physical-therapy modalities such as ultrasound followed by a stretching program. Other
treatment might include ice or friction massage; as many as 12 treat-

ments are sometimes necessary. The occupational therapist can review joint-protection measures.

Bursitis at other sites about the elbow is much less common and can be diagnosed only by a skilled physician. However, whether the cause is a bursitis or tendinitis (which is a condition involving elbow pain when turning the hand from palm up to palm down), the condition can be treated almost the same as tennis elbow. But, in addition, an exercise performed with a hammer can be helpful: grasp it close to the end of the handle and rotate the wrist from palm up to palm down, back and forth, allowing the weight of the hammer to rotate the arm with it. Spend 1 minute at this exercise, twice daily.

Sometimes a tennis elbow is complicated by other conditions. For example, this patient had a coexisting problem.

JACK A.: DOUBLE ELBOW TROUBLE

Jack A. is 39 and a traveling sales agent. Though he enjoys his work, he believes it contributes to flab. Staying thin is a constant struggle for Jack. Because he has to spend so much of his day in the car, he has taken up jogging. He is gone most of the week, but he tries to jog each morning wherever he is. Weekends he spends on chores around the house, and on a recent Saturday he assembled a set of lawn furniture that required the extensive use of a screwdriver. The following Tuesday Jack became aware of intense discomfort in his right elbow when grasping his sample case. Jack consulted Dr. Frazer, who diagnosed his problem as tennis elbow. He recommended rest and exercises. When 10 days had passed and still he felt no improvement, he returned to his doctor. Jack told Dr. Frazer that each morning upon arising he had numbness and tingling in his arms and a sensation of swelling in his hands. This subsided within several hours, but would recur whenever he had driven a long distance. Now he had additional symptoms which were not part of tennis elbow.

From the doctor Jack learned that a sensation of swelling and numbness that lasts less than a day may indicate a thoracic-outlet syndrome. He also began to realize that his conditioning program took care of only his lower limbs, not the sagging of his shoulders, which was aggravated by prolonged sitting and driving.

So Jack came to realize that his tennis elbow was aggravated by a thoracic-outlet syndrome that was more subtle. Therefore, he began conditioning the upper limbs with shoulder-shrugging exercises, and he held his shoulders in a more elevated position while driving. He has continued the tennis-elbow program and is rapidly improving. Jack also jogs with hand weights part of the time. Thus, he is now conditioning both upper and lower extremities. Persistent symptoms such as Jack's may be due to continued, aggravating habits.

Summary

The elbow is a three-part joint flanked behind by a bursa and in front and on the sides by muscles, tendons, ligaments, and nerves. An amazing array of movements is possible, but your elbow does not tolerate long or repetitive motion. Tight hand clenching in the performance of a sport or work activity may give rise to tennis elbow, golfer's elbow, bursitis, or tendinitis. Treatment includes rest and the cessation of aggravating activities. It also should entail stretching, conditioning, and strengthening exercises. In addition, using a tennis-elbow splint, massaging with ice, and taking nonsteroidal anti-inflammatory agents for pain relief will be of value. Aspirin can be taken before you engage in a stressful activity. Most of these conditions begin gradually, get worse gradually, and only improve gradually. But they seldom cause constant pain.

Table 6-1
Danger Signs in the Elbow

Swelling and redness
Fever and chills
Swollen glands under the armpit
Loss of muscle tissue
Pain that is gradual, progressive, and spreading throughout the arm
Numbness, tingling, and persistent loss of sensation anywhere in the arm or hand

Table 6-2
Self-Examination of the Elbow

1. With your arms straight, note whether the elbow fully straightens. If not, arthritis may be limiting movement.

2. With your elbow bent, rotate the clenched fist from palm up to palm down. When pain occurs with this movement, the likely cause also is arthritis of the elbow.

3. Note in a mirror the appearance of both elbows, looking for swelling or loss of muscle tissue. Now place one hand over the back of the hand on the involved side. Try to raise the lower hand upward against the other hand. Next, raise fingers upward against the other overlying hand. Note if pain occurs. You might identify a specific injured tendon in this manner. Tennis elbow often results from tendinitis, and can be a likely diagnosis.

4. Test forearm muscles that attach to the outer side of the elbow by performing the stretching movement pictured in Figure 6-2. Begin with the backs of the hands against a door, arms straight. Place the arms at body length, with the backs of the hands approximately waist high. Now slide each arm upward slowly until a pulling sensation is noted in the forearm region near the elbow. Is the painful side perceived as tight compared with the nonpainful side? If so, this suggests tennis elbow caused by tendinitis.

5. If the inner aspect of the elbow is painful, perform the same procedure as in item 4, above, but with palms to the wall and fingers pointed down (Figure 6-6). Slide palms up and note any pulling sensation in the muscles of the involved arm, which would suggest golfer's elbow.

6. With the elbow bent, gently hold a hammer straight out, thumb on top. Now slowly rotate the hammer with the thumb moving downward; then reverse. Note if there is pain at the outer aspect of the elbow. While doing this, touch the outer aspect of the elbow and gently poke deeply while turning the elbow. Is there a grating feeling or a rubbery sensation? These suggest inflammation.

7. If you notice numbness and tingling, use the opposite long finger and tap over the middle of the wrist on the involved side. Does a tingling sensation jump up to the elbow and/or down into the hand, signifying a carpal-tunnel syndrome?

Table 6-3
Possible Causes of Elbow Symptoms

Complaint	Possible Cause
Pain in outer elbow with use	Tennis elbow
Pain in inner elbow with use	Golfer's elbow

(continued)

Complaint	Possible Cause
Pain and numbness of elbow, forearm, and hand	Pinched nerve in neck; thoracic-outlet syndrome; carpal-tunnel syndrome; or other nerve entrapments
Swelling behind elbow	Bursitis
Pain in front of elbow (middle)	Tendinitis
Cannot fully straighten elbow	Arthritis

Table 6-4
Possible Causes of Persistent Elbow Problems

Complaint	Possible Aggravation
Pain at the outer elbow; no visible swelling	Twisting and forced motion such as hand shaking, use of tools (screwdriver, pipe wrench), improper gripping, unconscious hand clenching while driving, sleeping, or telephoning
Swelling and pain at the tip of the elbow	Injury and possible infection; injury; repeated rubbing; or pressure; gout; rheumatoid arthritis; high fat content of blood; infection
Aching and pain at the elbow with numbness and tingling	Pinched nerve in the neck; carpal-tunnel syndrome; nerve pinched under the collarbone from droopy shoulder; falling asleep with the arm over back of chair; use of crutches too high in the armpit
Pain at the inner aspect of the elbow	Prolonged golfing; grasping of a tool; hand clenching; droopy-shoulder syndrome with nerve pinched under the collarbone; wristy backhand and/or lobs in volleyball, tennis, or squash

Table 6-5
What's Harmful, What's Helpful for the Elbow

Harmful	Helpful
Using the elbow to push the body up when arising from bed or to prop it up when sitting can result in pressure injury to nerves at the elbow.	Use the abdominal muscles to help roll the body out of bed; when sitting, keep the elbows in space.
Repeatedly using tools that must be twisted and forced (e.g., screwdriver, pipe wrench) may injure tendons near the elbow. Improperly gripping golf clubs, rackets, or other pieces of sport equipment may be injurious to the elbow.	Grip tools less tightly; use foam-plastic pipe insulation (sold at hardware stores) on tool handles; take frequent short breaks. Learn the proper techniques for gripping various pieces of sport equipment.
Unconsciously clenching the hands while sleeping or driving may produce elbow pain.	Wear stretch gloves (seams to the outside) to bed. Use a padded steering wheel. Learn to use relaxation techniques.

Table 6-6
Exercises for the Elbow Region

1. *Mobilizing exercise for tennis elbow:* Place your arm on the kitchen table. Grasp a 1- to 3-pound weight and allow your hand to hang over the edge of the table, first palm down and then palm up. In each position let weight pull your hand down below the table; then raise it back up. Repeat 50 times palm down, then palm up for 1 to 2 minutes twice daily (Figure 6-3).
2. *Forearm stretching exercise for tennis elbow:* Stand facing a wall; extend the involved arm toward a door. Put the back of your hand on the door, fingers toward the floor. Start with the wrist at about belt level, then slide the wrist and hand slowly upward until you feel a pulling sensation near the elbow. Hold this position for 1 minute and repeat twice daily (Figure 6-2).

(continued)

3. *Stretching exercise for golfer's elbow:* Perform as in no. 2, but place palm on the door, pointing fingers to the floor. Slide upward until you feel a pulling sensation near the elbow. Hold this position for 1 minute and repeat twice daily (Figure 6-6).

4. *Triceps strengthening exercise:* Grasp a 1- to 5-pound weight. Hold your elbow bent out at 90 degrees, shoulder height. Now raise your arm to extend the elbow to 180 degrees, in line with your shoulder (to strengthen triceps). Repeat, slowly, 3 to 10 times twice daily (Figure 6-9).

5. *Biceps stretch:* Lying on a bed on your back, with the elbow at the edge of the bed, grasp a 5-pound weight and raise this, keeping the elbow against the edge of the bed. Thus, the shoulder and arm lie on the bed, elbow at the edge of the bed, hand upward—holding the weight. Now let the weight draw the arm straight out. This will pull on the side of attachment of the biceps tendon. Repeat slowly, 3 to 5 times twice daily (Figure 6-8).

CHAPTER 7

The Wrist and Hand

Many people develop enough arthritis with bony knobs on their fingers to cause impairment and to necessitate medical consultation. Others with arthritis will have an impairment of their hand resulting from disturbances of the soft tissues—including the nerves, tendons, ligaments, and muscles. When these are added to a knobby arthritis, it is common for a *mistaken* diagnosis of arthritis to be given as the sole cause of the disturbance, but the arthritis may be only a minor contributor to the problem. This chapter will help you sort out the very common soft-tissue ailments of the hand and wrist.

Some bumps about the wrist may be herniated cysts called *ganglions*. Other lumps and bumps can be *fibromas,* which are benign tumors composed principally of fibrous connective tissue; arthritic cysts; and only rarely, tumors. Sometimes a patient will complain of pain and swelling of the veins on the back of the hand. This actually may result from an underlying tendinitis. The "locking" of a tendon may result in a *trigger finger*. Often when awakening in the morning, a patient may find either the thumb or one of the fingers locked in a bent position. The digit can be pulled into a straight position and, with a few additional movements, the locked joint seems to improve. As you will learn, the locking frequently seems to be in the finger joint. However, you will also learn where to look for the cause of the troubled joint in the tendon. Tendons act as pulleys. These thick stringy ends of muscle are the cords that travel across the front and back of the hand. They have a tube-like covering, a sheath, that lubricates the tendon (Plate 7-1).

Often a pinched nerve in the neck, thoracic-outlet area, elbow, or wrist can cause great distress in the hand. For example, a carpal-

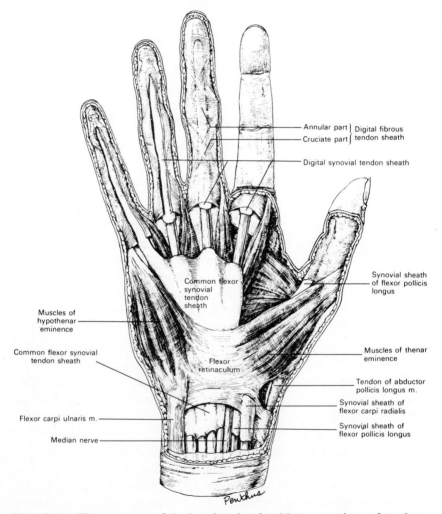

Plate 7-1.   The anatomy of the hand and wrist. Note coverings of tendons that cross the palm. See how confined the wrist is beneath the flexor retinaculum, a strong bandlike structure.

tunnel syndrome or a thoracic-outlet syndrome can cause numbness, tingling or weakness, painful use, and altered coloration.

Symptoms of significant arthritis include morning stiffness of 30 or more minutes' duration in the small joints of the hand, joint tenderness, visible swelling of more than 1 day's duration, or constitutional symptoms such as generalized fatigue, weight loss, and joint symptoms that move from place to place. Table 7-1 at the end of this chapter lists features that indicate the need for urgent medical attention. These danger signs should not be ignored. This chapter will deal with those conditions that afflict the hand and wrist and result from injury to or mild structural impairment of tendons, ligaments, loose joints, and ganglions. Table 7-2 outlines self-examination techniques. Tables 7-3 to 7-5 list the symptoms and causes of many of these hand afflictions and the habits that may ease or aggravate pain. Table 7-6 provides helpful exercises.

Self-Examination

Please study Table 7-2. Inspection of the hand involves simple testing of the muscles and ligaments by bending each finger or thumb onto itself, as in Figure 7-1. The hinges or ligaments can be tested by attempting to rock the joint from side to side, as demonstrated in Figure 7-2. Inspection for muscle wasting, particularly as a feature of the carpal-tunnel syndrome, should be performed when numbness and tingling or other hand discomfort is present at night. The round ball of the hand between the wrist and thumb should be inspected by looking at the hand palm upward. Raise the hand until

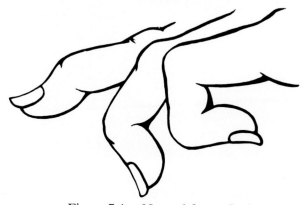

Figure 7-1.   Normal finger flexion.

the ball of the hand is at eye level. From the palmar crease to the thumb, there should be a gradual rounded slope. If it is flattened or indented, muscle wasting has occurred. Similarly, turn the hand over and look at the space between the thumb and index finger. If the muscle tissue adjacent to the web of skin is indented, muscle

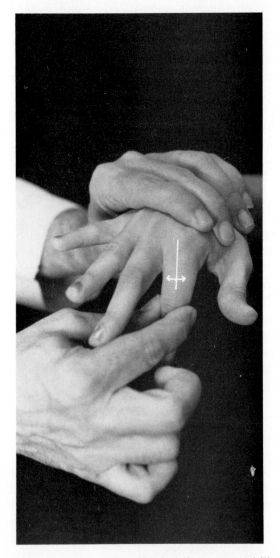

Figure 7-2. Metacarpophalangeal collateral ligament stability test. The finger is flexed to 90 degrees at the MCP joint in order to tighten the collateral ligament. Normally, lateral finger motion is minimal in this position.

wasting may have occurred. Similarly "valleys" between each of the finger tendons are a sign of muscle atrophy. If a digit cannot be flexed upon itself, either arthritis or tendinitis is likely. Knobbiness of a significant visible degree may impair this movement. Another cause for loss of finger flexibility is swelling into the palmar aspect of the finger. If the pad located between the first knuckle and the palm is felt on the palm side of the digit and compared to all the other digits, you may be able to detect a thickening or fullness to that region of the involved finger. This would signify tendinitis. Marked redness in the palm nearest the thumb suggests a systemic illness such as rheumatoid arthritis or liver disease. Dusky blueness in the hand that only occurs while the hand is dangling may not be serious, but it does require medical attention. Episodes of color change with discomfort upon exposure to cold is known as Raynaud's phenomenon and consists of blue, white, and red color changes. Also characteristic of the phenomenon is a return to normal coloration within minutes after warming. This sequence is brought on by cold *or emotion* in persons with Raynaud's disease.

Wrist Disorders

The two bones of the forearm are the radius and the ulna, the outer bone and inner bone, respectively, when the palm faces out. These are joined by a long ligament. Sometimes this is disrupted, allowing a looseness at the end of the ulna. This results in *piano-key wrist,* as demonstrated in Figure 7-3. When this knobby protuberance is pressed, it acts like a piano key, popping back up. If it is painful and of recent origin, you can use an elastic wrist band to protect the wrist. Strengthening exercises for the wrist and hand are helpful (Table 7-6, exercise 6).

Similarly, *loose-jointedness* of the wrist can be a problem. Hypermobility of the wrist allows you to bend the wrist and bring the thumb against the forearm (Figure 7-4). Loose-jointedness, as demonstrated, can also result in wrist discomfort. Strengthening exercises as presented in Table 7-6, exercise 3, will be helpful.

Calcific tendinitis of the wrist may result from a generalized metabolic derangement known as calcium apatite deposition disease. This results in a toothpaste-like deposit of calcium in tendinous regions of the shoulder, wrist, hip, or ankle. Attacks of redness, swelling, pain, and impairment are temporary. Ice massage may help to

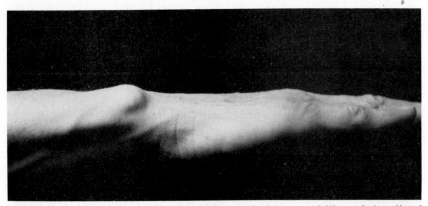

Figure 7-3.   Piano-key wrist. Posttraumatic hypermobility of the distal ulna. Examination with downward pressure results in "piano-key" movement of the distal ulna.

alleviate the pain and swelling. Fashion a cone of ice from a paper cup as described in Chapter 6. With a towel, grasp the ice cone and place the narrow end of the ice along the tendon. Rub deeply and slowly, chilling and stroking the tendon. This can be done for up to 20 minutes several times a day. Also, treatment with oral anti-inflammatory agents is usually helpful.

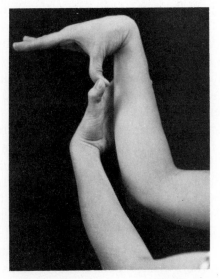

Figure 7-4.   Loose-jointedness, or hypermobility test of the wrist.

Strains, sprains, and other ligament injuries are often the result of a sports injury or a blow to the wrist. Any of these conditions should be treated immediately with ice or an elastic bandage, or splinted by simply wrapping the area with a magazine to prevent further injury. If movement is painless after 20 or 30 minutes of ice, then serious injury is unlikely.

Afflictions of the Thumb

Pain at the base of the thumb, where the wrist joins the hand on the thumb side, is often the result of *arthritis*. If "pinch-grasping" (grasping with the thumb and index finger) is painful, particularly at the base of the thumb, you can bet this is a symptom of arthritis and that the joint is under pressure. A simple exercise to loosen this joint is provided in Table 7-6, exercise 5 (Figure 7-5). This should be performed twice a day. Pinch-grasping or repetitive hand use, as in knitting or crocheting and other handwork, must be paced. See Ta-

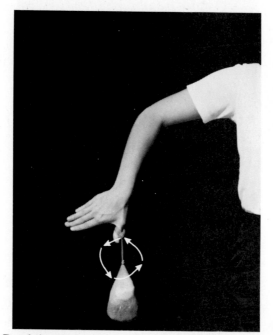

Figure 7-5.   Pendulum thumb stretch. A 1- or 2-pound weight placed in a stocking and tied with a loop knot allows a pendulum or circular motion. This stretches the thumb joint and adjacent tendons.

ble 7-4 for aggravating factors that cause recurrent wrist and hand symptoms.

If using the thumb causes pain, it may be the result of *washerwoman's tendinitis*, also called *de Quervain's tendinitis*. In Figure 7-6 a technique for reproducing discomfort, and thus enabling the diagnosis, is demonstrated. Tendinitis is an injury which results in swelling of the wrapper surrounding the tendon. This can actually be seen in the two tendons that pull the thumb outward from the palm. When the thumb is pulled away to form an L, these tendons stand out.

They are noted where the thumb joins the wrist. To check them, feel for any swelling of these tendons and compare them with the tendons of the uninvolved hand. Sometimes there will be a squeaky feeling as the thumb is bent and straightened during the time you are feeling the tendon, or you may feel a thickening of the tendon when you compare it with the opposite side (Figure 7-7).

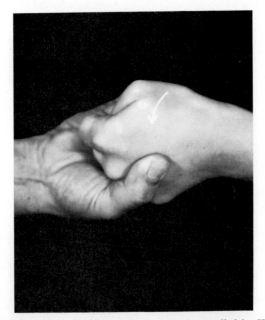

Figure 7-6.　Finkelstein test for washerwoman's tendinitis. With the thumb drawn into the palm and the fingers folded over the thumb, the other hand is used to draw this hand away bending the wrist away from the thumb. This will stretch the involved tendon and cause pain if tendinitis is present.

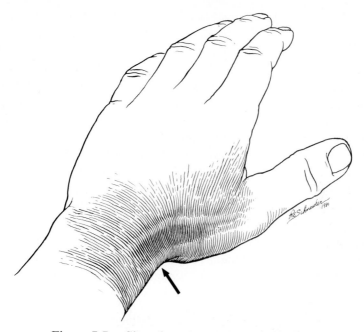

Figure 7-7. Site of washerwoman's tendinitis.

When tendinitis is present, the thumb should be put to rest by wrapping the wrist and thumb with an elastic bandage to hold the thumb outward, forming an L. A 2-inch elastic bandage can be used, leaving the last segment of the thumb unwrapped. Thus a gentle pinch-grasp with the tip of the thumb and index finger is still possible. This bandage should be applied each day after bathing and after the completion of exercise. Exercise 1 in Table 7-6 should be performed twice daily. A pendulum-type of exercise, as shown in Figure 7-5, will stretch the tendon and help free any adhesions. Ice massage, with deep stroking of the tendon sheath for 1 to 5 minutes several times a day, may hasten healing. Attention to joint-protection measures is important in preventing recurrence. If this treatment does not provide relief, then an experienced physician can inject a corticosteroid agent parallel to the tendon. Such an injection will result in relief if it is followed by exercises. Sometimes the tendon sheath has to be surgically incised. If the condition occurs in both hands, it may result from rheumatoid arthritis.

Some bowlers develop hard, painful calluses of the soft tissues at the base of the thumb, in the web of skin. Pain, stiffness, and a hard lumpy skin may result, a condition called *bowler's thumb*. When this occurs, the bowling ball holes may have to be beveled in order to reduce the friction.

Snapping thumb is an irritating trigger-thumb condition, which results in either a thumb stuck in a bent position or brief locking of the thumb in the morning, after the patient has rested. When the-thumb snaps free, the sensation is perceived in the thumb joint nearest to the nail. However, the real trouble lies in a tendon at the junction of the thumb and the base of the palm. The cause is the formation of a split-pea-sized swelling on the tendon or a closing of the tube that covers the tendon. Sometimes this can be freed with ice massage applied to the tissue deep in the palm at the base of the thumb. The thumb should then be pulled away from the hand to stretch the tendon. Do this treatment twice daily and, if it is not successful, consult a physician experienced in injecting the tendon sheath. Please see *trigger finger*, which follows, for further details.

Finger Problems

Trigger finger is similar to snapping thumb, but it usually affects the third or fourth finger, with locking of the digit in flexion. This usually occurs when one arises in the morning and is the result of repetitive finger movement. Figure 7-8 shows the location where the tendon locks up. Trigger finger is of increasing concern because of its economic impact on health costs in industry. The culprit is usually the type of repetitive tasks we have mentioned; the number of movements that the tendon performs per unit of time and the degree of clenching during use are important. Sometimes tasks are performed at home that aggravate tasks performed at work.

If your job requires repetitive hand movements, then you shouldn't choose hobbies or participate in sports that require similar repetitive finger movements. Here is one simple method of providing rest for the tendon: Obtain a 2-inch roll of gauze that sticks to itself (Kling gauze is one brand). Make five turns around the finger joint nearest the palm. Reapply this each day, removing it only when bathing. Meanwhile, each day draw the finger backward slowly and then hold it extended for 10 seconds. Repeat often each day. Also, you can ice massage with a corner of an ice cube, rubbing deeply up and down on the tendon. This self-care recovery program may take up to 6 weeks. Try to use

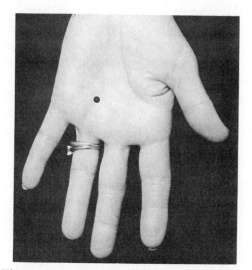

Figure 7-8.   Site of trigger finger disorder.

conservative treatment. It works in three out of four cases. If your job does consist of repetitious hand and finger motions, you might prevent tendinitis with exercise 6 in Table 7-6.

Recently, diabetes has been found to cause thickening of the tendons in the hand, called *cheiroarthropathy*. Trigger finger may also result from diabetes. However, trigger finger rarely results from rheumatoid arthritis, ochronosis (a blue or brownish blue pigmentation of cartilage and connective tissue), degenerative arthritis, or injury from a finger pulled too far backward.

Unconscious *hand clenching* (making a fist) may occur in anger and other emotionally charged states. Wrist pain, finger pain, trigger finger, carpal-tunnel symptoms, and hand discoloration may result. Dark beverages including tea, coffee, colas, and chocolate may push the nervous system and result in unconscious jaw clenching or hand clenching. Hand clenchers tend to be jaw clenchers. Hand clenchers may go so far as to develop the *clenched-hand syndrome* with resulting hand fatigue, carpal-tunnel syndrome, and/or tendinitis. Such persons have hand symptoms that are worse after they arise from sleep. Often, they have suffered from jaw clenching in the past. They describe themselves as "heavy-handed" persons. One way to break that habit of nocturnal hand clenching is to wear nylon stretch gloves, such as spandex or Isotoner, with the seams turned to the outside when sleeping. A less-common syndrome, the *clenched-fists syndrome,* occurs in extremely emotionally charged individuals who suffer a minor injury. Their clenched fists cannot be extended unless they are given a general anesthetic. Laceration of the skin of the palm, with increased perspiration, may lead to infection.

Writer's cramp may result in persons who are otherwise heavy-handed, or it may result from a neurologic disease, but this is very rare. Sufferers at times cannot grasp a pen or pencil in a normal fashion. Rather, they grasp it in a jerky fashion, they have difficulty picking up the pen, and they may grip it with a closed fist instead of in the ordinary manner. Behavior modification and biofeedback have helped in some cases. Most people need only to use a thicker pen or pencil or to obtain a plastic triangle penholder from a stationery store. These holders slip over the pen and keep the fingers in the proper position and cost about 25 cents each.

Most children and many adults today do not hold a pen correctly, often gripping it in a fist with the thumb wound around the index finger. In addition to the possible pain, these children will be at a tremendous disadvantage when they are required to take notes in class. A friend who tutors says five of six students hold a pen or pencil in a tortuous fashion. Most children who do hold the pen wrong absolutely hate to write. Unless this changes by the time they reach college, they will not be able to keep up with professors who lecture.

Holding the neck and back straight and the shoulders up when writing so that the nerves to the arm muscles are free in the thoracic-outlet area will help prevent writer's cramp.

Hypermobility, or loose-jointedness, affects 5 percent of our population. As previously mentioned, these individuals can overly flex or extend the hand and wrist. Similarly, they can draw the little finger backward and lay it parallel to the forearm. The *hypermobility syndrome* refers to symptoms that occur in loose-jointed people, whose muscularity is weak or flabby. Hippocrates noted the inherited predisposition of loose-jointedness. He described the Scythians as so loose-jointed that they were unable to draw a bowstring or hurl a javelin! If hypermobile people fail to maintain good muscle tone and then perform hard hand use, they may develop symptoms of painful hands associated with morning stiffness and a sensation of swelling in the finger joints. However, the symptoms improve within

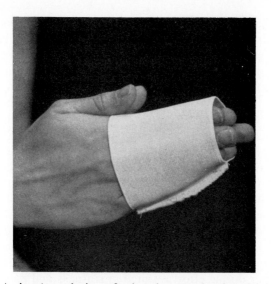

Figure 7-9.   A simple technique for hand strengthening. Finger-extension exercises are performed using a band made from foundation elastic. The band is sewn to fit snugly. The patient inserts eight fingers into the band and allows the band to cover the distal end of the fingers; he or she repetitively extends the fingers against the elastic band while keeping the palms together.

hours and will respond to strengthening of the hand as demonstrated in Figure 7-9. See also Table 7-6, exercise 3.

CAROLINE P.: WAS IT REALLY ARTHRITIS?

Caroline is a 27-year-old secretary-typist. She loves to dance, both modern dance and ballet. But, not long ago, after 3 months of pain while dancing, she had become demoralized. She had all of the symptoms of rheumatoid arthritis, including stiffness, pain, and swelling of her finger joints and knees. Her case did fit the diagnosis of arthritis until we looked more carefully at her problem. Was the swelling actually visible? Not for sure. Each morning Caroline's fingers felt swollen and her rings were tight. Did it last for several days or longer? Not really. The fingers did get stiff and feel swollen each day, but it lasted only for about 4 hours.

   True inflammation of joints doesn't come and go in less than a day. The 4-hour duration is an important clue, for the hypermobility syndrome can mimic arthritis, cause symptoms for several hours each day, but then can disappear and not recur until the next day. When the cycle of joint swelling is less than a day, gout; rheumatic fever; flare-ups of osteoarthritis, rheumatoid arthritis, lupus; and the many other disorders can be ruled out.

Caroline's problem began to fall into place. She had had a baby 8 months earlier, given up all of her conditioning and dance activities, and become sedentary. Just before the hand symptoms began, the family moved from an apartment to a house, and Caroline had done all the packing. This was in addition to caring for the new baby. Just after settling into her new home, Caroline was asked to return to work.

In addition, Caroline is loose-jointed. She was not aware that she had this joint feature, nor was she "double-jointed." But her finger joints could be cocked from side to side, she could draw her thumb into apposition with her forearm, and her little finger could be bent backward and parallel to her arm. As she became more sedentary, her muscle tone diminished. Then when she had to perform more strenuous tasks, her muscles did not provide the needed support for her finger joints. That added joint activity was too much for the joints. Presumably, increased friction from the bones slipping upon each other during effort resulted in stiffness and pain.

Tests for arthritis were normal. Exercises to condition the hands resulted in progressive improvement. Had Caroline been told, "You have arthritis, and you need to get more rest," the advice would have had dreadful effects. People with joint laxity and the hypermobility syndrome must keep up a good conditioning program for life.

Disorders of the Palm Area

A number of disorders will give rise to a tightening of the palm of the hand, particularly in the tissue of the outer portion of the hand closest to the little finger. In younger (and some older) persons it can be a sign of diabetes and, as mentioned earlier, is known as cheiroarthropathy. In older persons Dupuytren's contracture may occur, or it may result from an inherited predisposition combined with exposure to vibrating tools or repetitive hand clenching as seen in race-car drivers or in persons who ride horses (Figure 7-10). The condition can cause severe scar tissue to be laid down under the palm, which can result in completely bent fourth and fifth fingers that cannot be lifted out of the palm. One should attempt to prevent this. Palm stretching may be beneficial: lay the fingers on the edge of the table and draw the palm upward while pushing the digit pads into the table. This stretches the soft tissue that lines the palm. Perform this maneuver twice daily, indefinitely. Advanced cases will require surgery to remove scar tissue. Unfortunately the problem may recur.

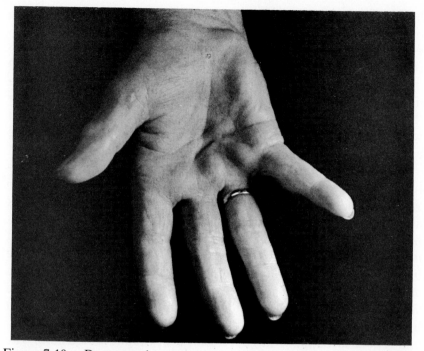

Figure 7-10.   Dupuytren's contracture (nodular scars on the palm). This condition results in a shortening of the tissue lining the palm. The fourth and fifth fingers are pulled into a bent position, often touching the palm.

Carpal-Tunnel Syndrome

The nerves, blood vessels, tendons, and muscles to the hand travel through a tunnel whose outer walls are bone and the inner walls, ligament. This unyielding tunnel may be too small if the bones enlarge from arthritis, if the muscles enlarge because of excessive use, if the space is invaded by fluid as in pregnancy, or if it is filled up with other substances in such diseases as rheumatoid arthritis, conditions of the blood, or low thyroid. The most common cause is a mechanical constriction of the nerve by a tightened band. In young individuals, this sometimes results from repetitive finger movement or hand clenching. In middle age, rheumatoid arthritis and degeneration of the ligament are common causes. In the older people, the condition can arise from pushing off from chairs or using a cane. Although this phenomenon is poorly understood, we know that the resulting irritation of the nerve is most common in the early morning hours. The patient is awakened with an intense numbness, burning, tingling or aching sensation usually into the thumb and index fingers, but sometimes involving the whole hand. The patient often shakes the hand and wrist for relief. A tap test (Figure 7-11) or the Phalen maneuver (Figure 7-12) can help diagnosis. Sometimes the numbness and tingling go upward into the arm and shoulder, and even into the neck. Once set off, carpal-tunnel syndrome may recur each night with distressing regularity. If you have a carpal-tunnel syndrome and are a compulsive person you have a difficult problem.

Persons who suffer tendinitis, washerwoman's thumb, or carpal-tunnel syndrome often are compulsive people, who will finish a job whatever the consequences and who enjoy performing handwork such as knitting. Such people must practice less compulsive behavior, balance work and rest, and plan ahead. Application of heat or ice or rub-on substances is not helpful. In an effort to loosen the ligament, this exercise may be helpful: With the hand and fingers straight, press the ends of your fingers against the opposite forearm with a maximal force while slowly raising the wrist and bending it upward as shown in Figure 7-13. Hold this position 5 seconds, relax, and repeat three times in succession every hour, as feasible. The

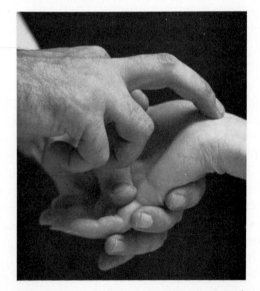

Figure 7-11. A tapping test over the carpal tunnel to detect pinching of the nerve. Numbness and tingling that spreads out to the digits or up the arm as the nerve is tapped confirms a constriction in the carpal tunnel.

tensed bowstringing of the flexor tendons during the exercise can stretch the ligament and can result in benefit within 6 weeks. Also see Table 7-6, exercise 7. Many physicians prescribe a wrist splint that rests the palm, and used at night, it may provide relief. The use of pyridoxine (vitamin B_6) has been recommended as a treatment for some cases of carpal-tunnel syndrome. However, excessive use of this vitamin can cause a *serious* neuritis of the whole body. Any treatment of carpal-tunnel syndrome that does not involve surgery must be tried before there is loss of the muscle in the ball of the hand. Anyone who suffers from carpal-tunnel syndrome should frequently observe the muscle ridge between the crease of the palm in the center and the base of the thumb and note any flattening of this normally rounded muscle tissue. Any evidence of muscle loss indicates a need for surgery. Fortunately, most cases don't progress to muscle loss. Consider the use of joint-protection measures, as listed in Table 7-5.

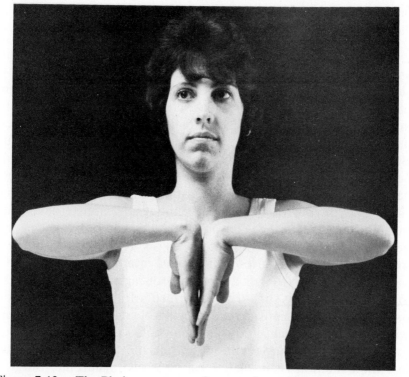

Figure 7-12.   The Phalen maneuver for carpal-tunnel syndrome. Holding this position for 1 minute will result in increased numbness and tingling when a carpal-tunnel syndrome is present.

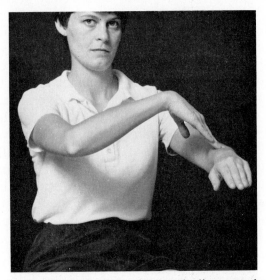

Figure 7-13.   A stretching exercise to loosen the ligament that compresses the carpal tunnel.

Failure to obtain relief within a relatively short period of time should lead to consultation with an experienced physician. The physician will conduct an examination to be certain there are no signs of a systemic inflammation such as rheumatoid arthritis. He or she may conduct blood tests for inflammation, or order tests for defects in metabolism. X-rays of the hands and wrists are seldom helpful. Because electrodiagnostic testing is so expensive, this test should be used only in difficult cases or if surgery is contemplated. It does help to differentiate neuritis from carpal-tunnel syndrome. The physician may begin treatment with splinting and nonsteroidal anti-inflammatory agents. The conservative treatment program can prevent the need for surgery in as many as two of three cases. If these measures fail, then a series of injections into the carpal canal of a local anesthetic mixed with a corticosteroid agent may provide lasting relief. Again, this should be performed before any loss of muscle tissue is evident. If there are two attempts at conservative treatment without benefit, surgical consultation should generally be considered. The surgeon may require electrodiagnostic testing to be certain the condition is, in fact, a carpal-tunnel syndrome. Surgical removal of the ligament crossing the nerve often requires good visible examination that is not possible by microsurgery techniques. About 10 percent of surgically treated patients have recurrences.

This occurs even more frequently if there was not good conservative management in the first place. Persons who continue the aggravating hand tasks are often the ones who have surgical failures. If the surgeon has failed to identify the hand clencher or the over user, he or she is making a serious mistake in operating first and asking questions later. Consultation with an occupational therapist for splinting and joint-protection review may be helpful in resistant cases.

Raynaud's Phenomenon

As previously mentioned, this neurovascular disturbance results in paleness and duskiness to the digits and even to the palm of the hand, lasting 5 to 10 minutes after exposure to cold or after an emotional upset (Figure 7-14). The discolored areas may be red and white, red and blue, or white and blue, alone. *Raynaud's disease* is the term used when no other underlying condition is discovered. *Raynaud's phenomenon* implies that another entity is causing the disturbance. Connective-tissue diseases, hypothyroidism, frostbite, exposure to vibrating tools, use of certain drugs, or compression of the vessels within the thoracic outlet are common causes. Certainly a physician should be consulted to detect any underlying cause.

A number of simple treatments are helpful. Avoiding cold to any part of the body is at the top of the list. Drugs that block the autonomic nervous system, biofeedback, and (rarely) surgical clipping of the nerves can bring relief. Treatment measures include dressing warmly. However, exposing even the face to cold may still cause the condition to occur in the hands. Doing shoulder-elevation exercises as described in Chapters 4 and 5 may be useful. Through biofeedback, an individual can quickly learn to raise his skin temperature 8 to 10° Fahrenheit and maintain it at that level. This will block the spasm that occurs within the blood vessels. Medical management with drugs that block the nervous system—calcium-channel blockers, reserpine, guanethidine, and phenoxybenzamine—may also prove helpful.

Ganglions

Nodules of many kinds occur about the hand and wrist. A *ganglion* is a cystic swelling that can be transilluminated. To do this you take a small penlight and place it up against the skin of the nodule. The

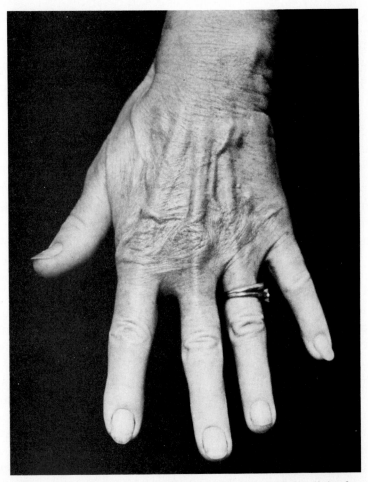

Figure 7-14.   Raynaud's disease. Despite blanching of the digits from the metacarpophalangeal joints to the fingertips for many years, this patient's hands failed to show evidence of atrophy or other features of connective-tissue disease.

entire nodule will light up. This is because of the jellylike substance in the center of the nodule. A ganglion is a cystic swelling that often results from a herniation of a tendon or joint (Figure 7-15). It usually occurs before age 50 and often will gradually and slowly disappear. It can be treated surgically, but recurrences are common. *Smashing a ganglion with a book is an old remedy that is destined to result in a recurrence.* Often the best treatment is to let it alone unless it is causing significant symptoms.

When to Seek Professional Help

Certainly if any of the features considered dangerous (Table 7-1) occur, it is urgent that you consult with a physician promptly. If your condition fails to respond to self-administered treatment methods within a reasonable period of time, you should also seek medical consultation. Most cases of tendinitis, trigger finger, carpal-tunnel syndrome, and ganglia do not require surgical treatment. If surgery is performed without first establishing an aggravating factor or factors, then recurrences are likely. Also people with a carpal-tunnel syndrome may return with a tendinitis or trigger finger, or vice versa.

Physical therapy, including ultrasound on involved tendons, is sometimes of value and may help you proceed along a self-help program that has previously failed. The occupational therapist may assist in discovering the cause for recurrences that has remained unrecognized. An occupational therapist may also apply splints for recurrent thumb disorders. Such splints may be fashioned of heat-moldable plastic that is lightweight, easily padded, and easily removed. Be sure to use such a splint—don't put it in a drawer. Some occupational therapists have experience in teaching relaxation techniques. This may be of value to the hand, jaw, or fist clencher.

Above all, if you have any persistent symptom involving the hand, you should see a competent physician to rule out systemic

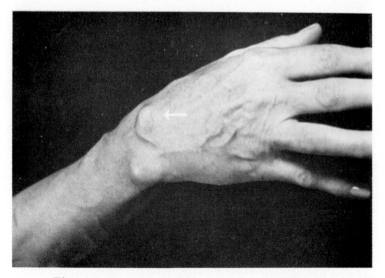

Figure 7-15. Ganglion on the back of the wrist.

disease that sometimes involves a hand complaint. Other regional pain syndromes resulting in hand symptoms may also be considered, such as nerve-root impingement in the neck, thoracic-outlet syndrome, or nerve entrapment at the elbow.

Carpal-tunnel syndrome can be a very expensive problem to industry. If you have suffered this disorder, please pay close attention to Table 7-5. Read it and reread it and try to identify any aggravating factor that could contribute to recurrences.

Table 7-1
Danger Signs in the Hand and Wrist

Fever and chills
Lymph-gland swelling
Dusky blueness of the fingertips
Crampy sensation after or during use
Swelling or warmth and redness about the hand
Numbness and weakness, with sudden onset
Loss of muscle tissue on palm or back of hand
Pits at the tips of fingers when Raynaud's phenomenon is present

Table 7-2
Self-Examination of the Hand and Wrist

1. Place both hands flat on a table in front of you. Notice the color, muscularity, and knuckle size. Look at the color beneath the nails.
2. Now turn the hands over and inspect the palms for color and muscularity. In particular, look at the slightly rounded muscle that serves the thumb, located in the palm between the thumb and wrist. If the slight roundedness has flattened, it could signify a pinching of the nerve above the hand. Arthritis at the base of the thumb can cause similar loss of muscle.
3. Flex the thumb, then sweep it over to the base of the little finger and back, noting full motion. Bend the four fingers onto themselves, but not into the palm. If motion is restricted, arthritis or tendinitis may be present. If a bent finger or thumb gets stuck and won't straighten, then a trigger finger is likely.

4. Tap over the nerve at the wrist on the palm side and right in the middle. Tap just as you would a piano key, but with a little more quickness. Pain and tingling into the fingers or up the arm signify a constriction in the carpal tunnel (Figure 7-11).
5. Put both arms in front of you at shoulder height and press the position for 1 minute. Tingling indicates a carpal-tunnel syndrome (Figure 7-12).
6. Can you draw the thumb into apposition to the forearm? If so, this signifies hypermobility, or loose-jointedness, of the wrist (Figure 7-4).
7. Fold your thumb into the palm, close the fingers over the thumb. With your other hand covering the thumb, push the hand outward toward the side of the little finger to stretch the thumb side of the wrist. Pain signifies a tendinitis (Figure 7-6).

Table 7-3
Possible Causes of Hand and Wrist Symptoms

Complaint	Possible Cause
Wrist	
Mild swelling, painful use	Tendinitis
Cyst, almond-sized swelling	Ganglion
Swelling, morning stiffness	Arthritis
Back of hand	
Swelling and redness	Deep infection
Cool, numb, throbbing, burning	Reflex dystrophy
Veins stand out	Tendinitis
Palm of hand	
Redness, mottled	Systemic illness
Numbness, swelling	Carpal-tunnel syndrome, thoracic-outlet syndrome, or reflex sympathetic dystrophy
Hollow muscle near thumb	Carpal-tunnel syndrome (late)
Nodules and cords	Dupuytren's contracture or cheiroarthropathy
Fingers	
Bumps at distal (farthest) joint	Osteoarthritis
Bumps/swelling at middle joints	Osteo- or rheumatoid arthritis
Swelling at one side of middle joint	Callus from overuse
Single finger swollen	Psoriatic arthritis or tuberculosis

(continued)

Complaint	Possible Cause
Fingers turn blue, white, and red	Raynaud's phenomenon or disease
Trigger finger or locking	Tendinitis with trigger finger
Tight rings, tender joints, lasts about 4 hours	Hypermobility syndrome
Thumb	
Painful motion of entire digit	Washerwoman's tendinitis
Snapping, triggering	Trigger thumb
Painful calluses	Bowler's thumb

Table 7-4

Possible Causes of Persistent Hand and Wrist Problems

Complaint	Possible Aggravation
Osteoarthritis in finger joints	
End joint	Usually inherited; repetitious action
Middle joints	Probably inherited; repetitious action
Thumb	Repetitious use: knitting, canning, tools, etc.
Inability to make a fist	Tendons inflamed, usually no joint swelling, but often the beginning of rheumatoid arthritis
Trigger thumb, painful thumb use	Tendinitis following repetitious use
Trigger finger	Tendinitis following repetitious use
Callus on side of finger	Tendinitis following repetitious use
Carpal-tunnel syndrome	Tendinitis following repetitious use; pushing with outstretched palm from chair; heavy reliance on a cane; hand clenching when driving, sleeping, phoning, or reading; inflammatory or infiltrating diseases
Ganglion	Not well known—possibly strain or birth defect

Table 7-5

What's Harmful, What's Helpful for the Hand and Wrist

Harmful	Helpful
Repetitively moving the fingers excessively, in typing, peeling vegetables, knitting, needlepointing, playing cards, and some assembly-line work, is the most common cause of carpal-tunnel syndrome, tendinitis, trigger finger, and trigger thumb.	Restrict repetitive tasks to 20-minute periods separated by a short break. Keep the hands flat and open rather than making tight fists. Pad the handles on utensils and tools and the steering wheel with pipe insulation. Use stronger, larger joints for assistance. Use the palms and forearms to carry heavy objects. Push, slide, or roll objects instead of lifting them. Use both hands as much as possible when lifting heavy objects.
Writing, stapling, or using scissors for long periods can cause hand injuries.	Use pencil holders and pad the stapler. Take frequent breaks.
Pushing off from chairs, clenching the hands, writing for prolonged periods, or doing work that requires repetitious wrist or hand motion can result in carpal-tunnel syndrome.	Keep the hands off chairs when rising; be aware of hand clenching and wear gloves to bed if necessary; interrupt lengthy writing sessions. Consult an occupational therapist about work-induced problems.

Table 7-6

Hand and Wrist Exercises

1. *Thumb stretching:* Grasp the affected thumb with the other hand wrapped around that thumb and pull the thumb straight away from the forearm.
2. *Finger-flexor tendon stretch:* Grasp the involved finger and gently pull it backward until a pulling sensation is noted in the palm.

(continued)

3. *Finger-strengthening exercise:* Obtain a piece of elastic at least 2 or 3 inches wide. Foundation elastic can be found in "notions" at department or fabric stores. Sew a band large enough for the four fingers to be inserted. Sew at an angle to keep the band tight at the little-finger side. The fingertips should be within the top of the band. Then keep the palms together and pull the fingers apart against the band. The band should be snug so that the fingers cannot be drawn farther apart than 1 inch. Repeat for 1 minute twice daily, holding only a second or so for each motion (Figure 7-9).

4. *Palm-flexor stretching:* Place the fingers on a table, palm down. While pressing the finger pads into the table, slowly draw the palms up, thus stretching the ball of the hand. Do this slowly and to maximum tolerance. Hold 10 seconds; repeat five times.

5. *Thumb stretch:* Place a 1- or 2-pound object in the toe of a woman's stocking; tie a loop knot above the heel of the stocking. Slip this over the interphalangeal (middle) joint. Then, with the forearm held vertically and the thumb pointed downward, direct the back of the hand forward, with the thumb, tendon, and forearm all aligned with the weight tugging downward on the tendon. Slowly twirl the thumb for 1 minute clockwise and then 1 minute counterclockwise. Do this twice daily (Figure 7-5).

6. *Wrist strengthening:* Grasp a 7- to 10-pound weight; rest your arm upon a table with the wrist hanging over the edge, palm down; raise the weight as high as possible without lifting the arm from the table (Chapter 6, Figure 6-3). Perform for 7 to 15 repetitions with increases in the weight and the repetitions each week. Exercise each hand with 7 pounds until you are able to do 15 repetitions; then increase weight to 8 pounds and 7 repetitions, etc. A second exercise is performed similarly, but with the palm up and raised as high as possible and the forearm maintained on the table.

7. *Carpal-tunnel stretch:* With the fingers straight, press them against your other forearm with maximum force, while slowly flexing the involved wrist and holding that position about 5 seconds. Be careful to keep the wrist tented at a 45-degree angle. Return to starting position, relax, and repeat three times in succession every hour throughout the day, as feasible (Figure 7-13).

CHAPTER 8

The Chest and Upper Back

Chest pain is a frightening experience. When it occurs, you should immediately consider any other symptoms you may be having. The pain may not even be a heart pain but rather may arise from disturbances within the chest cavity; in the chest wall; from the spine, neck, abdomen; or from psychological stress. We can help you recognize and manage chest pains that arise in the muscles, ligaments, and bones that compose the chest wall and the spine.

Tables outlining danger signs in the chest and upper back (Table 8-1), self-examination techniques (Table 8-2), possible causes of discomfort and aggravating factors (Tables 8-3 and 8-4), commonsense solutions (Table 8-5), and helpful exercises designed to alleviate pain (Table 8-6) are listed at the end of this chapter.

One of our colleagues, Dr. Lala Mohan, an emergency room physician who works with one of us, recently kept track of 50 consecutive patients who came to the emergency room with chest pain. Only seven of them had a serious disease. The others had mostly chest-wall pain; a few had stomach ulcers or hiatus hernia (swallowing tube) problems.

Many heart specialists think the most important physical examination for chest pain is that of the physician pressing his fingers on chest-wall structures to check for a simple chest-wall pain disorder. The examination can save the patient expensive, needless diagnostic testing.

When chest pain does occur, you can quickly assess whatever else is happening. Is the pain in the center, the back, or at the side of the chest? What is going on outside of the chest? Do you notice numbness, tingling, or congestion in the hands? Is the pain aggravated when you move your neck forward and backward or from side to side? Have you been having indigestion? If you have, determine whether the chest pain travels into the neck and is accompanied by a choking sensation, or whether the pain spreads into inner aspects of the arm, particularly on the left side. These pains would indicate heart disease.

Have you been coughing? Does it hurt to take a deep breath? If it does, then consider whether the pain is relieved by holding your breath. If so, this would be consistent with pleurisy, an inflammation of the lining of the lung. If the pain is aggravated by twisting the upper trunk to the right or left or bending to the right or left, a spinal or rib condition is probable. Should you have reason to think that your pain is arising from the heart, lungs, stomach, or neck, seek prompt medical attention.

Our concern, however, is to help you recognize the most common form of chest pain: pain that arises within the musculoskeletal structures of the chest wall. Figure 8-1 presents the more common trigger points that, upon palpation, will reproduce or accentuate a chest-wall pain syndrome. But even if these trigger points are present, a serious medical condition still has to be considered.

Most people with chest pain immediately think heart trouble, yet, as we have pointed out, statistics show this is not likely. Heart pain, or angina, sometimes is perceived as merely indigestion. True heart pain usually is a squeezing, choking, or heavy sensation felt in the middle of the chest and often in the neck and throat and down the inner part of the arms. It arises from effort, a large meal, or exposure to cold wind and may be accompanied by sweating or a sensation of imminent death. Usually it lasts only a few minutes. However, the chest pain in rheumatic conditions described in this chapter usually continues or gets worse during rest; lasts for hours, days, or weeks; and has none of the features that usually would suggest a more serious disease.

Chest pain resulting from stress has a long and interesting his-

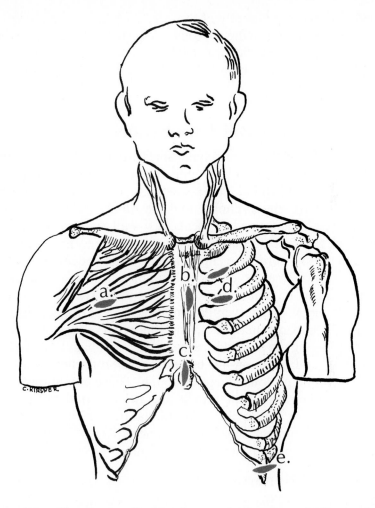

Figure 8-1.   The chest wall with trigger-point locations. (*a*) Pectoral muscle; (*b*) sternum (breastbone); (*c*) xiphoid (tip of sternum); (*d*) costosternal (rib-sternum) joint; (*e*) rib tip.

tory. In the past, during times of military service, soldiers would collapse with chest pain and suffer profound fatigue. This "effort syndrome" was later recognized in civilians following World War I and became known as "neurocirculatory asthenia." Today, persons having complaints of chest discomfort, fatigue, shortness of breath, palpitations, rapid heart beat, anxiety, and anxiousness of a severe degree probably suffer from psychological chest pain. The pain, palpitations, shortness of breath, and rapid heart beat are very real, but they may arise independently of the heart. There is conflicting evidence for an alteration in the nervous system in such patients. Some patients require mild medication that blocks the nerves to the heart. Relaxation techniques are probably of value for those who dislike using medication.

Chest-Wall Pain Syndromes

Included in the chest-wall pain syndromes are the *costosternal syndrome* (pertaining to where a rib joins the breastbone, or sternum), *sternalis syndrome, xiphoidalgia* (pertaining to the lower one-third of the breastbone, the xyphoid), and the *rib-tip syndrome*. These disorders are characterized by local chest-wall tenderness with accompanying aching pain ranging from a dull ache to throbbing and intense. In these disorders, pain is present when you are at rest and during chest movement such as twisting or reaching; it lasts up to several hours or days and may be slightly aggravated by a deep breath. Anxiety and hyperventilation (rapid, uncontrollable breathing) may accompany the attack, and the hyperventilation can be stopped by having the patient breathe into a paper bag. Episodes are usually brief and self-limiting, but on occasion a chest-wall pain syndrome can be prolonged and disabling. These conditions could coexist with other chest pain from angina, thoracic-outlet syndrome, a hiatus hernia, or peptic ulcer. Additional trigger points could lie in the upper abdominal muscles, the other chest-wall muscles, or even in some of the muscles along the spine.

Costosternal Syndrome

Here pain occurs in the front and slightly to the side of the breastbone. It may spread out widely in the front of the chest and can be aggravated by a deep breath. Pain usually is intermittent, lasts several days, and recurs over many months or years. Often the patient feels a bandlike tightness in the chest wall. Tenderness occurs at a costochondral junction (Figure 8-1*d*). In the presence of this chest pain, you can use the self-examination techniques detailed in Table 8-2. It is a good idea to perform each of the nine points of the examination. When you perform item 6, note any tenderness both at the pectoralis major (Figure 8-1*a*) and at the costochondral junction (Figure 8-1*d*). This would suggest costosternal syndrome. Sometimes physicians call this condition "costochondritis." However, true costochondritis is a feature of inflammatory arthritis, and the tenderness and pain occur along *both* sides of the sternum. The hallmark of myofascial (muscular rheumatism-type) chest-wall pain and each of the individual syndromes is the presence of aching chest-wall pain *and tenderness* limited to one side of the chest wall. Treatment of these syndromes will be discussed later.

Sternalis Syndrome

In this disorder chest pain occurs throughout the anterior chest wall, and a trigger point in the middle of the breastbone (Figure 8-1*b*) reproduces pain in both sides of the chest. The pain is a less-intense aching and more constant than the costosternal syndrome.

Xiphoidalgia

In this condition you can definitely feel localized pain and tenderness at the lower end of the breastbone (Figure 8-1*c*). The trigger point at the tip of the breastbone, at a projection known as the *xiphoid*, is a point where many muscle fibers attach. This pain is often aggravated by eating a heavy meal, lifting, stooping, bending, or twisting.

Rib-Tip Syndrome

This condition differs from the others because the pain is often severe and lancinating (shooting or tearing). Clicking may be heard and this is known as the clicking-rib syndrome; the condition probably results from an injury at the end cartilage of one of the floating ribs, the tip of which may be loose. The diagnostic maneuver, the "hooking maneuver," is demonstrated in Figure 8-2. A helper is required. Breathing quietly, you must lie on your back with knees bent so that the abdominal muscles are relaxed. Curling the fingers under the rib edge, the helper gently pulls upward. A click or snapping sensation will sometimes occur in the rib tip.

Management

Once you have identified a trigger point in the chest wall, that alone can provide reassurance that the condition is not serious. The corner stretch exercise (Table 8-6, exercise 1 and Figure 8-3) is helpful. Simply performing this exercise often relieves the tight muscle that in turn is putting pressure on the joints of the chest wall. The exercise can also be helpful in cases of intercostal neuralgia (see Table

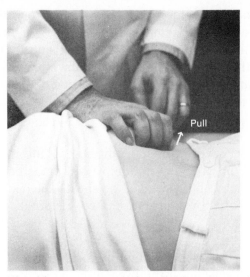

Figure 8-2.   The "hooking maneuver" for clicking-rib syndrome (rib-tip syndrome).

8-3). Aggravating factors to look for include repeatedly lifting heavy objects and transferring them across the front of the body instead of turning with the feet to place the object. Another aggravating factor is smoker's cough. Certainly anyone with repeated bouts of chest-wall pain should avoid smoking. Another aggravating condition is working without regard to posture. Typing, bookkeeping, and similar tasks undertaken for particularly long periods are also detrimental. When performing motions that repeatedly bring the arms across the chest (such as stacking logs or taking groceries from the bag and stocking them in the cupboard), you should position your body so there is little movement in which the arms cross the chest. Otherwise such action fatigues the pectoral muscles.

When chest-wall pain occurs in association with a thoracic-outlet syndrome, consider your sleeping position (Table 8-5).

For more persistent or stubborn cases, Janet Travell, M.D., of Washington, D.C., recommends use of Fluorimethane spray. This pressurized coolant is sprayed across the involved chest wall to help relieve the pain. It is a prescription item and can be demonstrated by a knowledgeable physical therapist. The technique requires a helper. You should stretch the muscles by grasping your hands behind you, thrusting your shoulders backward until you feel the involved muscle in front of the chest beginning to stretch. Then the

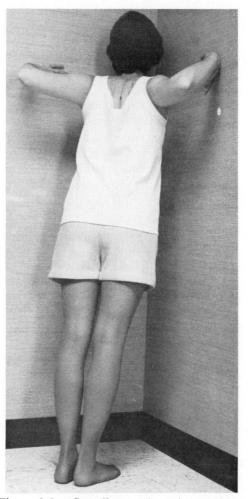

Figure 8-3. Standing push-up in a corner.

helper marks the involved trigger point, as depicted in Figure 8-1, and begins to slowly spray from the trigger point outward to the pain area in a zigzag, up-down fashion across the painful area. Two slow sprays lasting about 30 seconds each should be applied. Then proceed to the corner stretch.

WILEY J.: TOO MANY JOBS?

Wiley J. worked in a plumbing-supply store and was having a hard time making ends meet. To help Wiley conquer his finances, friend Bill, who ran an auto-repair service, gave Wiley a part-time job in his garage. After several months, Wiley noted an aching pain in the left side of his chest, a crampy aching that seemed to occur at the end of the day. It was also uncomfortable when he tried to sleep. After several days, Wiley consulted his physician because he wanted to be sure it wasn't heart disease. Because Wiley smoked, the physician ordered a chest x-ray and an electrocardiogram, both of which revealed normal findings.

Because Wiley had no history of stomach disturbance and because he knew Wiley was working hard at two jobs, his physician decided the problem was the result of anxiety. He recommended a muscle relaxant. Despite this medication, the pain continued. As winter wore on and the pain grew more severe, Wiley mentioned the problem to Bill, who often visited Wiley's home. Bill knew that Wiley was using a fireplace for which Wiley would buy a cord of wood and then stack it outside his home. Every few days Wiley carried some of the firewood into the garage, always transferring the logs from right to left across his chest. Bill wondered if this task might be creating the chest pain.

Wiley, thinking this was logical, went back to his doctor. A brief examination identified a costosternal syndrome with chest-muscle tenderness and spasm. Teaching Wiley to use better body mechanics when transferring the wood and also to stretch the chest wall solved the problem. This was not a case of anxiety, but simply improper body mechanics with the resulting muscle strain of the chest wall.

We have seen many similar cases further complicated by the presence of a pinched nerve in the neck, shoulder, or wrist areas, in which the irritated nerve causes reflex spasm all the way up the arm into the neck and the chest!

If after several weeks the condition has not responded completely, then medical consultation is in order. If the doctor confirms a chest-wall pain syndrome, the pain-spasm-pain cycle can be eradicated with an injection of a local anesthetic mixed with a small amount of a corticosteroid medication, and with an exercise program. If sleep is greatly disturbed, we often use amitriptyline or similar drugs (see Chapter 15).

Arthritis of the Chest Wall

Two conditions are important. *Costochondritis,* as we mentioned previously, is a term used loosely. For us, this condition represents a generalized inflammation that happens to involve the chest-wall joints. A very important finding on physical examinations is tenderness in each side of the breastbone at the rib joints, equal on both sides. *Restriction* of chest expansion is another finding. A simple measurement of the chest cage can be performed by a helper with a tape measure, as described in Table 8-2, item 7. If restricted chest motion is noted, your doctor may perform a test of inflammation and, sometimes, a bone scan to help diagnose such conditions as ankylosing spondylitis, Reiter's syndrome, and (occasionally) rheumatoid arthritis.

Another condition, *Tietze's syndrome,* presents as a visible enlargement of one of the costosternal or rib joints at the side of the breastbone, usually at its upper end. The swelling is at the point of tenderness, feels firm to bony-hard, and is slightly elongated or (less often) round. This feature of swelling does not occur in any other chest-wall syndrome. Medical consultation is necessary to rule out a tumor, infection, or a healing rib fracture.

Upper-Spine Disorders

The age of the person developing discomfort in the upper spine is important for diagnostic considerations. For example, teenagers may have "poor posture" and upper-back discomfort. But their real problem is a developmental disorder of the vertebrae that causes wedging at the front end. This, in turn, results in a forward rounding of the upper back that slopes forward. It is often an inherited manifestation. This forward curvature, known as a *kyphosis,* can be improved somewhat through the use of exercises. In adults, a similar rounded back can occur (Figure 8-4). The examination technique as described in Table 8-2, items 1 and 2, can be helpful in diagnosis. The exercise that is helpful is exercise 2 in Table 8-6. As the exercise is performed over several weeks, the muscles that help maintain an upright posture are strengthened. But then they must be used; one old-fashioned method is to walk around as if balancing a book on your head.

In the middle years (30 to 60), postural strain is the most common cause of upper backache. Sometimes bursitis in the center of the back can occur. This condition is seen in persons who habitually rise from a chair with their chest overly straight or who work with arms up and overhead so that the upper spine is arched backward. Two

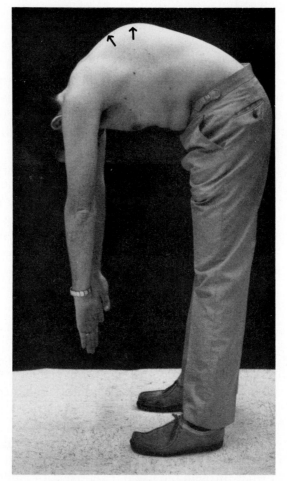

Figure 8-4.   Adult round back.

adjacent vertebral spines start touching and rubbing, thus creating a bursitis between them. The pain is a dull, diffuse ache in the midline of the spine. During forward bending, a helper can poke along each of the vertebral spines and detect exquisite tenderness at the site of the bursitis. Giving up the improper arching will usually allow healing; if not, a small dose of cortisone can be injected into the bursa. It is important that the danger signs in Table 8-1 be reconsidered in cases of upper-back pain. Tuberculosis can occur at this location, as can spinal tumors. In these instances, pain at night and other symptoms often occur.

Older people may suffer from *osteoporosis*, or thinning of the vertebrae (Figure 8-5). This is becoming the most common spinal problem of elderly women, and lately much has been written about it. Osteoporosis may begin as early as 2 years after menopause, and it tends to occur in women of northern European ancestry. It can result from many factors: inheritance, inadequate calcium intake throughout life, age at menopause, amount of walking the person

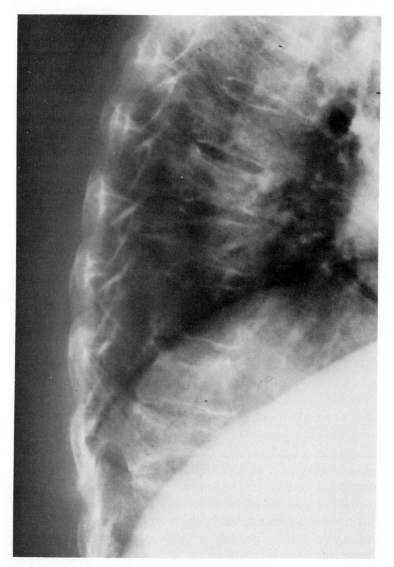

Figure 8-5.   X-ray showing osteoporosis with fractures of the vertebra.

has done during life, inability to absorb vitamin D, and other factors yet to be understood. The use of estrogen and progesterone after menopause has been recommended. If you are concerned about osteoporosis and are approaching the age of menopause, consult your physician. Nearly everyone agrees that women should begin calcium supplementation to the diet after age 35. From 1000 to 1500 milligrams of calcium is recommended. Those who have milk allergies or milk aversion should begin calcium supplementation earlier. There are many calcium supplements on the market including calcium lactate, calcium citrate, calcium carbonate, calcium gluconate, and oyster-shell calcium. If the body does not need the calcium, it will block the absorption. If you have had kidney stones, check with your doctor. Current research is trying to determine which of these products will be best absorbed by the body. Your physician or pharmacist can advise you regarding the cost, potency, and number of tablets per day needed to supply your daily requirement for calcium.

Other treatments proposed for osteoporosis include vitamin D, fluoride, and exercise. Presently a number of researchers are evaluating the use of vitamin D in very large doses (50,000 to 100,000 units or more per week). Cod-liver oil is a dangerous source of vitamin D because the amount of vitamins A and D it contains may vary widely and may even include toxic amounts. Many experts recommend fluoride but its use should be limited to a six-month treatment. Calcium may not add to the strength of bone unless a significant amount of exercise is performed by the patient. The exercise is thought to stimulate the bone in picking up the calcium. Currently most researchers recommend 45 minutes of brisk walking at least 3 days a week.

Table 8-6, exercise 2, can help avoid the humpback that occurs in some women with osteoporosis (Figure 8-6).

Psychogenic Chest Pain

As mentioned earlier, chest pain may result during times of severe anxiety. Such pain is bizarre in that it is far out of proportion to the medical conditions that cause it. Furthermore, you often feel threatened by the pain to the point of being disabled. Sometimes the pain is an unconscious need, as when you have stress so great it cannot be faced. Instead, your mind creates chest pain to divert attention and

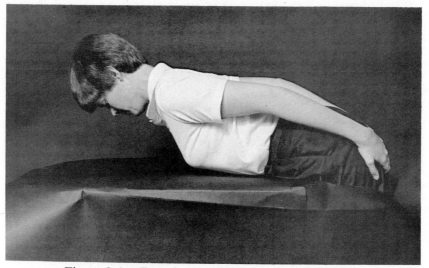

Figure 8-6.   Exercise to straighten the upper back.

allow you to avoid the real stress. In fact, your mind may block out the true stress so that you deny its existence. If that is the case, psychotherapy will be needed. However, in most cases you can handle the stressful problem and the reaction to stress in a more appropriate manner. In order to get a handle on your problem, the first goal is to sort out the factors. These may include the chest-wall pain, the anxiety that it creates, your real stress (we like to call it "the brick wall"—stop knocking your head against it!), and potential solutions to the problem. Sometimes just knowing how somebody else would deal with such a problem can be a big help. One family-counseling session can often provide this information. Dealing with the anxiety can best be handled through relaxation techniques. Simply practicing yoga-style breathing may suffice. Meditation techniques are also helpful. Biofeedback relaxation is yet another technique that has proved helpful in patients with intractable psychogenic chest-wall pain.

Pain syndromes have been associated with mitral valve prolapse (a very common condition of elongated mitral valves). It remains uncertain whether this pain arises in the nervous system or is an unrelated psychologic chest pain disorder. We have found that these patients benefit from exercise and relaxation techniques. Many also benefit from taking beta blockers. However, some beta blockers have been noted to induce shoulder stiffness and pain. You should check with your doctor.

When to Seek Professional Help

Consult a physician at once if any of the danger signs listed in Table 8-1 are present. Also, chest pain that has persisted or that awakens you in the night should cause you to consult a doctor. A physician may order a chest x-ray and electrocardiogram, a blood test for inflammation, or possibly a bone scan depending on the findings from a comprehensive office examination. If the physician detects a trigger point, he or she may try a nonsteroidal anti-inflammatory agent, aspirin, physical therapy, or an injection with a local anesthetic and a corticosteroid mixture into the trigger point in the involved chest muscles. If chest-wall pain persists, then you may find the advice of a physical therapist and an occupational therapist valuable because they may identify a continuing improper habit or body use. If an intercostal neuralgia is diagnosed, you may require a nerve block.

Table 8-1

Danger Signs in the Chest and Upper Back

Fever and chills
Swollen lymph glands
Pain that spreads to the neck, or the left arm, or both arms
Numbness and weakness in an arm
Pain that radiates to the middle of the upper (thoracic) spine
Upper abdominal pain that spreads to the shoulder-blade area
Upper-back pain that awakens you
Coughing up blood
Pain with each breath; no pain when breath is held (pleurisy)
Pain that spreads to the armpit

Table 8-2

Self-Examination of the Chest and Upper Back

1. Look at yourself in profile: turn sideways to a full-length mirror and hold a small mirror to the side so you can see your side view. Is there a hump at the top of the chest? Now bend over and watch the spine. Does the spine form a hump? This indicates a malformed vertebra (Figure 8-4).
2. Use the two mirrors and inspect your backbone while standing

with your back to the full-length mirror. Does the spine curve from side to side? With a helper behind you, bend forward and try to touch your toes. Does the helper see a spinal curvature?

3. Measure your height and record it. If you are beyond the age of menopause, have you lost height? This may indicate osteoporosis.

4. Does the chest seem in balance? Are the breasts at the same level when standing upright? Curvature of the spine (scoliosis) may cause asymmetry of shoulders or breasts.

5. Rotate the neck. Does it aggravate chest pain? Sometimes a pinched nerve in the neck will cause chest pain.

6. Can you push firmly on the sides of the breastbone and accentuate the pain? If you press right on the breastbone about every inch from top to bottom, does any spot accentuate pain? At the lower rib cage are the "floating ribs." Are these tips tender? Repeat the procedure for the left side. Trigger points may be discovered and you might avoid the time-consuming and expensive studies and tests.

7. Have a helper encircle your chest cage with a tape measure at the nipple line. A measurement is taken after you exhale, emptying the chest of all air. Then a new measurement is taken after you take a deep breath and fill the chest completely. A normal female should have at least a 2-inch chest expansion and a normal male, a 3-inch expansion. If this finding is reduced by 50 percent, an inflammatory arthritis must be considered.

8. Lie on the floor on your back with knees bent and feet flat. Now gently, but firmly, press a fist into the middle of the stomach, just below the breastbone. Does this aggravate the chest pain? If painful, you are likely to have a hiatus hernia or stomach ulcer.

9. Do the corner push-up exercise (Table 8-6, exercise 1). Does this demonstrate tightness in the chest muscles on the side that hurts? This may indicate myofascial (costosternal) syndrome.

Table 8-3
Possible Causes of Chest and Upper-Back Pain

Complaint	Possible Cause
Aching chest pain; arm weakness; numbness	Pinched nerve in neck
Aching chest pain; both arms numb, with or without swelling sensation in hands	Thoracic-outlet syndrome

(continued)

Complaint	Possible Cause
Vicelike (squeezing) midchest pain of less than 10 minutes' duration; heavy feeling in arms	Heart trouble
One-sided midchest pain; lasts for hours or days; tender to touch	Costosternal syndrome
Chronic midchest pain; tender along both sides of sternum	Costochondritis
Midchest pain; tender middle of sternum	Sternalis syndrome
Midchest pain at lower end of sternum; tender at lower tip of breastbone	Xiphoidalgia
Chronic midchest pain; no tenderness; indigestion	Possible stomach ulcer
Sharp, brief left-sided ache over heart; occurs any time	Intercostal neuralgia
Sharp, momentary chest pain in lower left side	Colon spasm
Ache on either side of chest; aggravated by movement	Spine or muscle irritation
Sharp pain with clicking noise on either side of chest	Rib-tip syndrome
Sharp, throbbing pain anywhere in chest; terrible when anxious or panicky	Psychological pain
Dull pain in upper back between shoulder blades; aggravated by fatigue	Adult round back
Constant pain in upper back; spreads around both sides of chest to front	Osteoporosis

Table 8-4
Factors That Aggravate or Cause Persistent Chest and Upper-Back Pain

Complaint	Aggravating Factor
Midchest pain	Obesity and hiatus hernia; peptic ulcer; gallbladder trouble; working with head drooped forward; arthritis of rib and sternal joints; cardiac or vascular disease; chronic cough from smoking
Right-sided chest pain	Pleurisy; rib fracture; neuralgia; referred pain from neck area; muscular chest-wall pain; sternocostal syndrome; chronic cough from smoking; shingles
Left-sided chest pain	Pleurisy; rib fracture; referred pain from colon, spleen, neck, esophagus; muscular chest-wall pain; sternocostal syndrome; chronic cough from smoking; mitral-valve prolapse; psychological chest pain; shingles; heart disease
Upper-back pain	Interspinous bursitis (midline); gallbladder disease; kidney stone; osteoporosis; other thoracic-spine conditions; chronic cough from smoking

Table 8-5
What's Harmful, What's Helpful for the Chest and Upper-Back

Harmful	Helpful
Carrying heavy objects (e.g., logs or grocery bags) across the chest can strain muscles in the chest-wall and cause sudden, severe chest pain.	Turn and face the object and then lift it, using your body, not just your arms, to carry it.

(continued)

Harmful	Helpful
Smoking-induced coughing aggravates chest-wall pain.	Stop smoking!
Sleeping with your arms overhead can pinch nerves, which in turn can cause chest-wall muscles to tighten up.	Sleep with the arms below the level of the chest.
Arching the spine backward during exercise or while working with the arms overhead (e.g., painting a ceiling) can lead to bursitis of the spine.	Cautiously try extension exercises; discontinue if painful. Do not arch backward while working with the arms overhead.

Table 8-6
Exercises for the Thoracic-Cage Region

1. *Stretching the chest:* Do a corner push-up by standing 2 feet from the corner of a room. Place each hand at shoulder height and 2 feet from the corner. Now press your chest into the corner until the chest muscles and ribs are stretched. Keep the chin tucked in like a soldier. As you push into the corner, you will feel the muscles of your back near the shoulder blades bunch up. More importantly, you should feel a tight chest muscle being stretched. If you don't feel it, move your hands farther away from the corner of each wall. Then push your chest toward the corner again. Maintain this stretch for 20 seconds each, for six repetitions, and perform it at least twice daily (Figure 8-3).

2. *Straightening the upper back:* Lean across a kitchen table, counter, or ironing board with the abdomen, chest, and nose against the surface. Place your hands on your buttocks. Keep your chin neutral. Draw your sholders back. Raise your head and chest together as a unit about 2 to 4 inches, while keeping your abdomen against the table. Hold 10 to 20 seconds; repeat three to five times twice daily (Figure 8-6).

CHAPTER 9

The Low Back, Pelvis, and Hips

The back is one of the most vulnerable parts in the human body, and an aching back is a common complaint. Ever since human beings assumed an upright posture, back pain has been a fact of life. Until recently any consideration of this pain centered around a structural concept such as a ruptured disc, a wearing out of the disc pads or vertebrae and the facet joints, pinching of nerves, bony overgrowth within the nerve canal of the spine, or other bony disorders. As the sciences of epidemiology, ergonomics, industrial psychology, rheumatology, neurosurgery, and orthopedics investigate and interact, we learn that previously held concepts and classification methods fail to address the majority of patients with back pain.

Tables outlining danger signs in the low back and pelvis (Table 9-1), self-examination techniques (Table 9-2), possible causes for discomfort and aggravating factors (Tables 9-3 and 9-4), common-sense solutions (Table 9-5), and helpful exercises designed to alleviate pain (Table 9-6) are listed at the end of this chapter. The muscles of the back, pelvis, and hips are shown in Plates 9-1 to 9-3. If you have a back problem, we would suggest you read through this chapter to get an overview of the pain problems. Back pain may result from several coexisting problems. If you don't have any of the

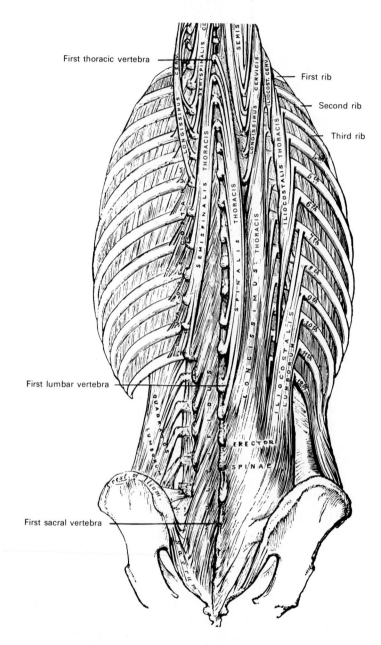

Plate 9-1.   Deep muscles of the low back.

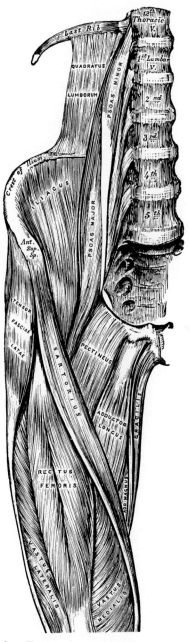

Plate 9-2. Front view of hip and thigh muscles.

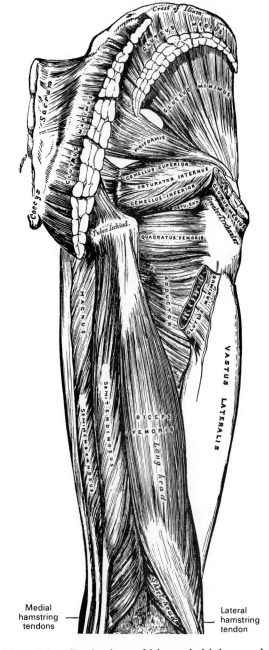

Medial
hamstring
tendons

Lateral
hamstring
tendon

Plate 9-3.   Back view of hip and thigh muscles.

danger signs, try the measures described later in this chapter. They may save you from unnecessary surgery.

Why Do Backs Hurt?

As we have mentioned, industry is interested in back pain because it is a leading cause of time away from work. A recent year saw 580,000 workers treated in emergency rooms for industrial injuries, and low-back pain was a symptom in most of them. In 1980, one-fifth of all workplace injuries and illnesses resulted from back disorders. In England, back pain was second only to bronchitis as a cause of work-time loss. In Sweden, 1 percent of all work days are lost on account of back pain each year. Overall, 80 percent of adults in western countries will eventually suffer from back pain.

Most of you are probably familiar with the cartoon of the man stretched out on the couch, while the wife says to a friend, "His back goes out more than we do." One woman we know reported that everytime something needed repair around the house, her husband had to rest his back. The truth is that women seek medical attention for backache more often than men; but they may tolerate the pain better, and surgical procedures are less often performed on them. The severity of back symptoms leads to disproportionate medical care, unrelated to the severity of the condition. For example, those who complain the most or loudest may get more extensive treatment than would be necessary.

The following factors associated with back pain may help you recognize situations that can set you up for an attack of pain.

Social and Environmental Factors

Ergonomics, also called *human engineering,* is the study of the complex relationships between people and their occupational, domestic, and leisure activities. Such studies reveal a significant correlation of low-back pain in persons between age 35 and 55; the duration of pain increases with age. Back pain is more likely to be present where there are drug and alcohol abuse, divorce, family problems, and lack of education. A ruptured disc may be more common before age 40 and is seen more frequently in relation to operating motor vehicles, whether for work or pleasure. The lack of support in the vehicle seats, mechanical factors associated with accelerating or decelerating the vehicle, and extension of the driver's leg in the direction of the floor pedals (rather than being flat on the floor) are contributing factors. Use of cruise control may be beneficial. Other risk factors outside the workplace include chronic cough and bronchitis; insufficient physical exercise; and sport activities such as baseball, golf, or bowling. Back pain seems to worsen in the spring and fall seasons.

Occupational Factors

Nearly 2 percent of the nation's work force suffer a compensable back injury each year, with significant cost to the nation's economy. Hazards at the workplace are often not the primary cause of low-back pain, but rather the workplace is the setting in which underlying disease becomes manifest. The relation of back pain to driving has been mentioned. In addition, back pain may occur in the workplace in relation to slipping or falling accidents; manual handling and lifting tasks; improper work postures while sitting; strenuous dynamic work loads such as lifting, pulling, pushing, carrying; prolonged sitting; bent-over posture; excessive bending or twisting; and frequent lifting. Exposure to vibrations (as when riding a train, bus, or subway) is associated with back pain. Stress and lack of job satisfaction were found as important to the occurrence of a back injury as were lifting or handling loads.

In a group of workers who attributed back pain to a particular activity at work, there was no significant relation between the accident record and the onset of pain. Rather, a direct correlation of back pain to the distance driven per year by these workers was noted when they were compared with their coworkers who were without back pain. A Swedish study of workers with back pain revealed only three factors that had a direct association to the pain: overtime, monotonous work, and a high degree of lifting. In another study occupations associated with an earlier onset of low-back pain included such jobs as bank clerk, heavy-industry worker, farmer, and nurse. A high incidence of low-back pain also correlated with prolonged sitting or standing the entire work day. Alternating sitting with standing was associated with the least incidence of low-back pain. Recurring back disability correlated with persistent pain in the leg, duration of the original disability of longer than a 5-week period, more than two previous symptom attacks, or an injury caused by a fall.

Psychological Factors

Anyone with persistent pain is often suspected of malingering or having major psychosocial problems. Yet, malingering is rare. More often, depression, neuroses, or hypochondriasis is detected in these patients. Work in service industries may result in more stress-related illnesses where back pain is a consideration.

Although patients with low-back pain constitute 17 percent of all disabled persons, only 2 percent of them request handicapped services; 48 percent take no medications at all. Only 20 percent see a specialist; 6 percent seek the assistance of faith healers. Thus, these patients do not overuse the health-care system.

In another study, anxiety and other psychiatric problems improved as the patient improved. Perhaps the person is psychologically impaired by the disease, and she or he then seeks medical care. A controlled study of women with backache who attended a family-practice clinic did not reveal greater anxiety or depression symptoms or other psychologic problems when compared with other patients. In comparison to persons without back pain, an aloof attitude was more frequent in back-pain patients.

Preemployment Status

Industrial physicians have not found much value in x-ray changes, back-examination findings, or worker medical histories in determining work capability. Studies now are under way that will enable matching of the worker's strength and personality with the work tasks. Three times more back injuries occurred when the worker's strength did not match the job performance or when the individual had far more capability than the job required.

Anthropomorphic Factors

Studies correlating backache with obesity, height, weight, body build, muscularity, and leg or spine structure have produced conflicting data. Most studies, on the other hand, agree that tallness, large frame, poor posture, and decreased abdominal and trunk strength all contribute to back pain. Back-muscle strength does not correlate with future back pain.

The Medical Researcher Looks at the Back

Scientists worldwide have affirmed the importance of good muscle tone, particularly in the muscles of the abdomen (stomach). Using tiny encapsulated measuring devices that can be swallowed, or pressure-measuring transducers that can be injected into discs or attached to muscles, healthy volunteers and back-pain patients have been studied. The studies have promoted the concept of the trunk as a cylinder and the importance of muscles in protecting the spine. If the pressure of this chamber is increased by compression from abdominal musculature, the cylinder can withstand greater stress. Other studies have demonstrated that sitting still and standing still are far more strain for the spine than is lifting. Weight lifters do not exceed 67 percent of ultimate strength of their spinal tissues. However, if the disc pads have fissures, a rupture might occur. Thus, heavy work is well tolerated if trunk muscles are strong and used correctly. A bad back may occur if the disc is fissured or if muscles are weak or not used.

Spinal mobility includes forward bending, backward bending, sideward bending, and rotation (Figure 9-1). Movement is restricted by various ligaments and other skeletal structures. The "stiffness" of aging is often the result of bone enlargement and spur formation, disc degeneration, and ligamentous changes. Yet the very elderly with no osteoporosis tolerate inactivity or sitting much better than those in midlife. We infer from this that much of midlife back pain results from muscle and ligament structures.

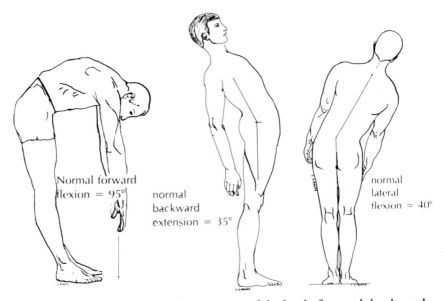

Figure 9-1.   Normal range of movement of the back: forward, backward, and sideways.

Following a back injury, reactive muscle spasm occurs in stages. Spasm is no more common than strain or fatigue but is more persistent, having an average duration of 3 weeks. Such spasm is involuntary. In some patients prolonged tightening of the powerful back muscles leads to disability. Muscles in spasm will ultimately come under voluntary control, but increased tone may persist for years if the provocative source is not removed. In prolonged spasm, elastic muscle fibers are thought to be replaced by inelastic fibrous strands. In addition, the skin, subcutaneous tissue, fascia (fibrous tissue between muscles), and muscle sheaths also are thought to deteriorate. But there are no microscopic features that support this hypothesis.

Mechanical Back-Pain Syndromes

Patients with low-back pain can be categorized into those with (1) intermittent acute low-back pain that seems to be of structural origin (mechanical low-back pain); (2) sciatica; (3) myofascial back pain; and (4) psychogenic back pain that fluctuates with internal psychic stress and is out of proportion to physical features.

We do not know whether chronic, persistent pain progresses from an acute back disorder or whether precipitating injurious events play a role in the progression to chronicity. As we have mentioned, radiographic abnormalities of the low back do not always correlate with future back pain or disability. Thus, the presence of low-back pain and a structural abnormality may have no relation to one another.

Mechanical Low-Back Pain

Back pain resulting from mechanical causes ("catches" in the back) should be suspected when pain is related to posture, minor trauma, or excessive use. This pain is episodic; aggravated by lifting, reaching, pushing, or coughing; relieved by rest; and lasts only from about 4 to 7 days. But it recurs. Often patients with mechanical back pain will describe "catches"—attacks that immobilize the patient in a slightly bent-forward position. The back may be "out of alignment" because of severe muscle spasm or locking-up of a facet joint. A listing, or tilt, of the spine occurs. The shoulders are out of line with the pelvis because the spine is pulled over toward one side. Sometimes sciatica occurs, but leg weakness does not develop. Such terms as "lumbosacral strain," "posterior joint syndrome," or "facet syndrome" are used interchangeably for mechanical back pain.

The *spinal joint* consists of the *vertebra* with bony projections on each side that connect with a vertebra above or below (creating a *facet joint*, also known as a *posterior joint*), and a *disc* between the vertebrae (Figure 9-2). The nerves to the legs come out close to the facet joints on either side. The disc pad is composed of a meshwork of fibers and cartilage. In the center of the disc is the *nucleus pulposus,* a gelatinous ball providing a cushion during spinal-rotation movement. This pad may develop a crevice or fissure that allows the contents of the nucleus pulposus to squeeze against the spinal cord. The resulting ruptured disc will lead to impairment of nerve action and weakness. Most ruptured discs are painful and give rise to sciatica. Sometimes weakness in a leg occurs without pain.

Abnormal skeletal defects are commonly associated with mechanical back pain. These include:

Degenerative-disc disease

Arthritis of the facet joints

Hypermobility syndrome

Lumbosacral-joint congenital anomalies

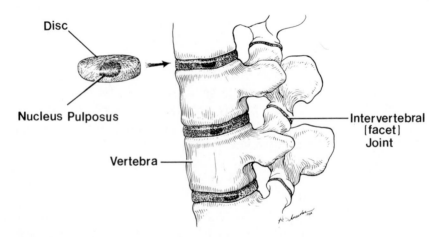

Figure 9-2.   Three-part complex of a spinal segment: vertebra, disc, facet joint.

Scoliosis, spinal curvature, does not usually predispose one to acute low-back pain. Also, many people without pain have these same skeletal defects.

Degenerative-disc disease is a very common x-ray finding in persons beyond 35 years of age. The disc does not show itself on the x-ray; rather, it is noted as a space separating each vertebra. When a disc has degenerated, the space is narrowed. Often the posterior (facet) joints have to carry more of the load. Then the facet joints show overgrowth of bone, called *osteoarthritis.* Many normal people have a narrowed disc at the lumbosacral junction that may be congenital in origin. Most can perform all activities without pain.

Facet-joint degenerative arthritis will develop in nearly all of us if we live long enough. The arthritis causes an increased stiffness when bending over. The spine is more flat during bending; and if the joint tissue swells, then the nearby nerve may be impinged and sciatica can occur. The features are similar to those of a ruptured disc except that weakness is not usual. Arching backward is painful. Some think that the "catches" of the spine result from pinching of the joint membrane. This results in muscle spasm, listing, and locking-up of the spine.

Hypermobility is a widespread loose-jointedness that was described more fully in Chapter 7. One characteristic is the ability to lay the palms onto the floor while keeping the knees straight. These people with this ability may pick articles up from the floor by bending the back and not the knees. Upon arising, they use the low-back muscles as a lever. This can result in muscle-fiber injury.

Lumbosacral-junction congenital anomalies include at least seven different defects such as spina bifida occulta, spondylolisthesis (displacement of a vertebra upon the one below), and an extra joint between the transverse process of the fifth lumbar vertebra and the pelvis. These birth defects may or may not be the source of the mechanical back pain. Surgery is rarely needed.

CLAYTON D.'S POOR BACK

When first seen by Dr. S., Clayton was 23 and working in a tire warehouse. Tall, slim, and athletic, Clayton was losing time from work because of attacks of "catching" in his back that were occurring with increasing frequency. The pain was so severe he was afraid to breathe. Two hospitalizations failed to demonstrate a need for surgery. Clayton's attacks would last from 4 to 14 days and seemed to get worse each time. Clayton was also losing muscle strength because he feared doing anything but his job. Dr. S. examined Clayton and found that his problem was the hypermobility syndrome and an extra joint connecting the left transverse process of the fifth lumbar vertebra to the pelvis. Dr. S. had considerable concern for his future.

Clayton's father had been a patient for many years with ankylosing spondylitis. Clayton, of course, was thoroughly checked for that, but tests were normal. He began to follow a very detailed exercise program, and after 2 years of care and a change in jobs to that of clerk in an auto-parts store, he was a little better.

Clayton wore a lumbosacral support at least while working. Now the attacks were less frequent and less severe. Clayton even married and had a son. He is not well, but after 5 years, he continues employment, has fewer lost work days, and can provide for his family.

Sciatica

Sciatica refers to back pain associated with numbness and tingling down one leg, usually below the knee, often into the foot on that side. Any action that increases abdominal pressure or thoracic pressure such as lifting, pushing, bending forward, coughing, sneezing, or straining to have a bowel movement may aggravate sciatica. The causes include:

Ruptured disc

Facet-joint degenerative arthritis

Spinal stenosis

Entrapment neuropathy (nerve compression)

Ankylosing spondylitis

Injury to the sciatic nerve

Ruptured disc (herniated nucleus pulposus) is the most common condition that can require surgery, but only about 10 to 20 percent will have to undergo an operation. Most can improve through careful attention to therapy and joint protection. A ruptured disc may occur slowly with, at first, just bulging of the disc against the nerve. Trivial activity such as coughing may result in a final rupture. The term "slipped disc" is incorrect. The disc doesn't ever slip. Patients with a ruptured disc have back pain, buttock pain, and pain and numbness into one hip or leg. The leg can feel heavy or weak. The examination will usually reveal flattening of the lumbar spine upon forward bending, pain upon backward arching of the back, weakness when standing on toes or heels, aggravation from prolonged sitting or driving, a positive straight-leg-raising test while seated, a positive tapping (percussion) test when tapped above the site of rupture (Figure 9-3), a positive reversed-straight-leg-raising test while lying on the stomach, and tightened hamstring muscles. Symptoms are improved by bed rest and aggravated by coughing, sneezing, or when having a bowel movement.

Runners occasionally develop a ruptured disc. In one report, runners who developed the back problem tended to be between 30 and 50 years old and had changed running styles. In 3 of 10 such runners, there was a previous history of disc disease. Only 2 to 10 required laminectomy (surgical removal of a bone or lamina of the vertebra). Eight returned to active running, one became a marathon bicyclist, and only one was unable to return to active sport activities.

Spinal stenosis is an ingrowth of spurs from the vertebrae into the spinal canal. These impinge on the blood supply to the spinal cord and pinch the nerves within the canal. Spinal stenosis is seen mostly in older persons. Symptoms begin with a gradual stiffness. Next the patient has trouble walking. After he or she has walked a few blocks, the buttocks begin to develop a crampy ache, and the legs then may begin to tingle. The legs feel increasingly heavy. Bending forward sometimes brings relief, as for example, when bending over a table or resting with knees on the lower step of a stairway with the hands on a higher step. The lower back shows little rounding during forward bending. Percussion usually causes local pain with radiation into the buttocks (Table 9-2, item 14).

In *entrapment neuropathy* the sciatic nerve becomes trapped in scar tissue, where it enters the lower limb deep in the buttock or sometimes in the back of the thigh. Pressure from horseback riding or unicycling has been reported to cause nerve damage and sciatica.

Ankylosing spondylitis is characterized by stiffness—rather than pain—upon arising after rest. (Stiffness may signify a generalized inflammation or illness and should be considered separately from pain.) In addition to stiffness, clinical findings suggestive of ankylosing spondylitis include insidious onset, symptoms of more than 3 months' duration, age less than 40 years, and pain improvement with motion.

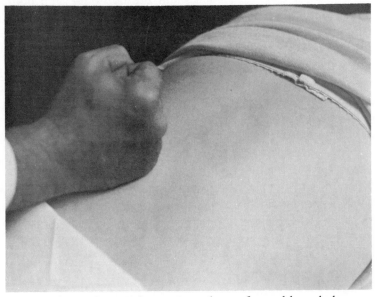

Figure 9-3.   Percussion test can be performed by a helper.

Changes on x-rays may take many years to develop. A bone scan or blood tests are helpful in diagnosis. One test that you can do is measure the circumference of your chest at the level of the breasts, with breath out, then again after a deep breath. Ordinarily your chest should expand 2 to 4 inches. In ankylosing spondylitis, it may be less than 1½ inches. Please refer to Table 9-1 for danger signals of serious illness. Ankylosing spondylitis is an important type of arthritis of the spine because it attacks younger men and women, can affect the eyes and heart, and can lead to permanent crippling of the spine if you do not treat it early. If your physician confirms the arthritis diagnosis, he will prescribe nonsteroidal anti-inflammatory drugs (several may have to be tried), physical therapy, and—most important—good posture and resting positions.

As was previously stated, sciatica is a symptom. When the sciatica symptom complex is not aggravated by coughing, sneezing, or defecating and the examination reveals normal neurologic findings with no limb weakness, the diagnosis of *pseudosciatica* is appropriate. It suggests that the cause lies outside the spinal canal, often bursitis or myofascial pain.

Pseudosciatica in most patients causes buttock pain rather than back pain, pain worse after sitting and at night, and improvement with walking. Strength examination is normal. Causes include tro-chanteric bursitis (pertaining to part of the long thigh bone) behind the hip bone (Figure 9-4) or spasm of the piriformis muscle, which lies deep in the buttock. Palpation reveals tenderness and firmness. The *piriformis syndrome* is also a common presentation in loose-jointed individuals who can easily bend over and lay their palms on the floor while keeping their legs straight. Perhaps they strain the muscle by performing such tasks or by excessive spinal rotation. Then, as they return to the upright position, the piriformis and glu-teal muscles are strained. Myofascial back pain (see below) is an-other common cause of pseudosciatica.

Regardless of how you happen to get it, sciatic pain is very stress-ful. And you really haven't felt pain until you have sciatica at the same time your sacroiliac chooses to give you fits!

Myofascial Back Pain

Myofascial back pain is probably the most common type of back-ache and, fortunately, the most preventable. Minor, repeated injury to back muscles and ligaments establishes a trigger point within one

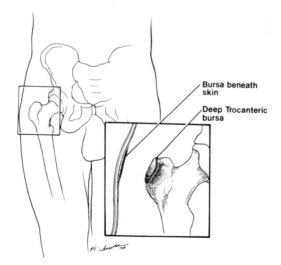

Bursa beneath skin

Deep Trocanteric bursa

Figure 9-4.   Bursitis around the hip bone. Helper first locates the outer hip bone at the side of your hip, then, pressing firmly, seeks a very painful spot. The bursitis will feel as painful as a boil. Bursitis may occur just beneath the skin overlying the outer hip bone, or deeply, about 2 inches behind the outer hip bone.

or more low-back muscles. When the tender trigger point is pressed, pain spreads into the target zone, which may lie in the back, side, buttock, leg, or foot. Figure 9-5 may help you locate trigger points. Many people with myofascial back pain have fibrofatty nodules that lie above the sacroiliac joints near the dimples of Venus (Figure 9-6). These are not likely to be the cause of pain. Rather, trigger points lying beneath the fibrofatty nodule are a more likely cause of backache. Pain is usually a deep ache in the low back or one or both

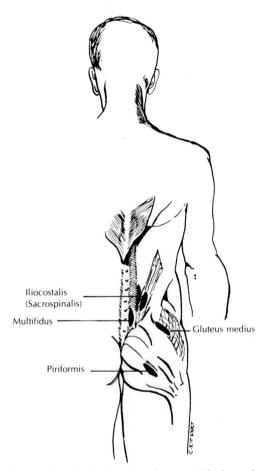

Figure 9-5.   Trigger points in the low-back area. A helper should use moderate thumb pressure and compare with similar pressure on muscles in the middle of your thigh. Trigger points are painful; pain radiates away from them.

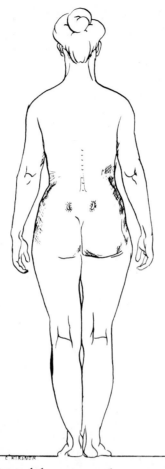

Figure 9-6.   Fibrofatty nodules commonly occur near the sacroiliac joints and on the dimples of Venus.

buttocks. Typically, the pain is worse after sitting or lying down and improved by movement. Lifting or pushing may be an aggravation, but work usually doesn't aggravate myofascial back pain. Other aggravating factors include having a short leg, standing on an uneven surface, or sitting unevenly as a result of one side of the pelvis being smaller. Many physicians believe that muscle spasm results from injury to the spinal ligaments or discs.

The iliopsoas muscle, which lines the back within the abdomen, may be the source of pain that is distributed along the lumbar spine close to the midline and into the front of the thigh. The taut muscle is discovered when performing the thigh stretch, or Ober test demonstrated in Figure 9-7 (Table 9-2, item 17).

As noted above, trigger points within the buttock muscles are very common and often cause pseudosciatica. They may result from bending with knees straight and then using the back as a lever to straighten up. Joint laxity may accompany the condition. Some have called it the *iliac crest syndrome* when the upper rim of the pelvis, in back, is the point of maximum tenderness. Another buttock muscle, the gluteus minimus, may refer pain into the side of the hip and down the side of the leg.

SHIRLEY G.: HARD WORK NEVER HURTS?

Shirley, 38 and single, had worked as a grocery clerk for many years. Her work required occasionally handling cartons and stocking shelves. Mostly, she worked as a cashier, which required prolonged standing. Her back problems began years earlier after an auto accident in which she received multiple contusions. She hated to get up in the morning because her back was always sore and stiff. However, walking seemed to help and so did moist heat or lying in a tub bath. After a few years in the grocery store, she noted progressive worsening. The back pain now interfered with her sleep. Her physician had stated that x-rays revealed minor arthritis findings, but they didn't explain her pain and suffering. He sent her to a physical therapist.

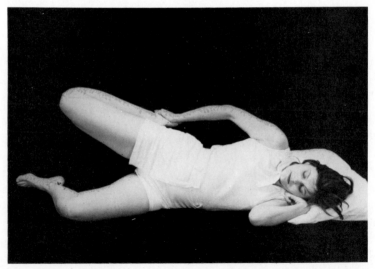

Figure 9-7.   Thigh stretch (Ober test) for tight thigh muscles.

The therapist told her that her back was very "tight." She did not practice any calisthenics; and when she finished her work in the evening, she either watched television or read for a few hours, then collapsed into bed. The worse her back became, the less rested she felt in the morning. A vicious cycle of pain-spasm-pain had developed. She quit her job and sought our (R.S.'s) assistance.

After following comprehensive back education and an exercise plan, Shirley was directed to the Bureau of Vocational Rehabilitation, which sent her to study motel management. This job would allow her to change body positions frequently, without severe back strain. Shirley completed the program, got a job in a motel in Florida, and has been "in control" for the past 12 years.

Psychogenic Back Pain

Sometimes people get an aching back when their actual problem is an aching mind. They often can feel their back tighten up like a vise. Although true psychogenic back pain is uncommon, a number of types of psychogenic backache can be detailed.

"Low-back losers" have a history of previous hard labor and poor education. They will deny depression, but they have all its features. In addition they usually have very abnormal psychologic-test results. These patients perceive themselves as very ill. Often homebound, their illnesses are used to manipulate others, and their illness behavior is as hard to break as alcoholism.

The "racehorse syndrome," reported by Dr. Ian McNab of Canada, describes people who are tense, hard-working, and hyperreactive to others. Such patients also may hyperextend their spine with exaggerated upright posture.

McNab also describes the "razor's-edge syndrome" for persons on the razor's edge of emotional stability who present outlandish appearances and complaints.

Dietrich Blumer and Mary Heilbronn while in Detroit described the "pain-prone disorder," which occurs mostly in women of all socioeconomic classes and ages. The features include:

Somatic complaints: continuous pain of obscure origin, hypochondriasis, preoccupation with and desire for surgery

Solid citizen syndrome: denial of conflicts, idealization of self and family, compulsive work or relentless activity

Depression (after pain): fatigue; lack of initiative; inability to enjoy social life, leisure, or sex; insomnia, depressed mood, despair

History: family history of alcoholism and depression, past abuse by spouse, a relative may have chronic pain or be disabled

These patients may present with perplexing backache. Most psychogenic-backache patients have pain out of proportion to the doctor's findings. Also, when they are well, they are very well. Two questions can suggest serious depression or a guarded outlook:

1. Have you lost weight?
2. Have you lost interest in sex?

Chapter 12 on chronic generalized pain syndromes can be read for information in dealing with psychogenic pain syndromes. Often, a personal physician can assist the patient through the stressful time.

Self-Diagnosis

You can ask five basic questions about low-back pain in order to entertain the various modalities of diagnosis and treatment:

Where is the pain? Many clinicians recommend the use of a pain drawing, such as Figure 9-8. Is the pain perceived as deep or superficial?

When does it hurt? Continuously or intermittently? Unchangingly or does it wax and wane? At night does it awaken you from sleep? Is it worse upon arising? When walking, bending, reaching overhead, or sitting? Has it happened in the past? When was the first episode? How long has this episode lasted?

How did it start, and *why* is it aggravated? Was there a definite injury? Does it begin or is it worse after certain movements or after coughing, sneezing, or bowel movement? After driving a certain distance? After a particular sport activity?

What gives relief? How long does it take before the pain settles down? What movement aggravates pain while you are working on the job, hobby, or housekeeping chore?

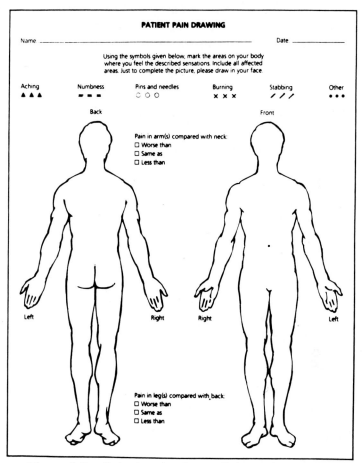

Figure 9-8.   Pain drawing for outlining pain pattern.

   The pain drawing provides a permanent record of the location, quality, type, depth, and intensity of pain. It can also suggest psychologic disturbance. Not all back pain arises within the back. Serious vascular, bowel, kidney, and other organ diseases can refer pain to the back. Apply your answers to Table 9-4. In most cases you will narrow your possible diagnosis.

Self-Examination

Your self-examination should yield such objective findings as back or pelvic asymmetry, unequal leg length, spasm, scoliosis, loss of range of motion, loss of muscle mass, weakness, or abnormal re-flexes. Follow Table 9-2. You should also note spinal movements as in Figure 9-1 and hip movement as in Figure 9-9. Remember that the value of the back examination lies in its use as a screening method for disease identification, not its severity or prognosis.

Trigger points may be identified during percussion (Table 9-2, item 14) or by deep pressure. If percussion is not revealing, then have a helper begin pressing deeply into your back with thumb pressure while you are bent across a table or ironing board. Each area, as presented in Figure 9-5, should be examined. The trigger point may be tender, but more importantly, the thumb pressure will cause

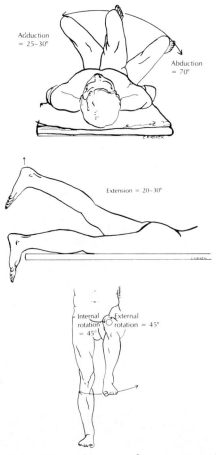

Figure 9-9.   Normal range of movement of the hip.

pain in the area that has been hurting. Be sure that the areas above and within the buttocks are examined.

Limb strength and circumference (size of thigh and calf) above and below knee should be determined and compared. Try the Patrick test (Figure 9-10) to be sure hip arthritis is not a problem (Table 9-2, items 9 through 12). Self-examination may help you detect a mild structural abnormality that can be corrected, such as a short leg or mild curvature. If you note weakness, then see your physician and you can save a lot of time and misery. When pain occurs in the front or side of the hip and not in the back, then the thigh stretch (Ober test) and another stretch test demonstrated in Figure 9-11 (Table 9-2, items 17 and 18) for a tight fascia lata (a membrane that separates the front thigh muscles from the back thigh muscles) may detect tightness in myofascial elements of the leg.

Are You Disabled?

Examinations for purposes of disability determination do not have to be difficult if the examination includes appropriate consideration for objective information. The Code of Federal Regulations defines *disability* as the inability to engage in any substantial gainful activity by reason of any medically determinable physical or mental impair-

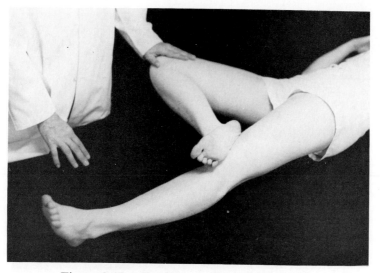

Figure 9-10.   Patrick test for arthritis of hip.

ment or impairments that can be expected to result in death or that have lasted, or can be expected to last, for a continuous period of at least 12 months. *Impairment* is defined as damage that results from anatomic, physiologic, or psychologic abnormalities that are demonstrable by medically acceptable clinical and laboratory diagnostic techniques. Statements of the applicant, including the applicant's own description of the impairment (symptoms), are alone insufficient to establish the presence of a physical or mental impairment. In the determination of disability, primary consideration is given to the severity of the individual's impairment, age, education, and work experience. Norton Hadler, M.D., of Chapel Hill, North Carolina, states that medical considerations alone (including the physiologic and psychologic manifestations of aging) can justify a finding that the individual is under a disability if her or his impairment is one that meets the duration requirement and is listed. Disability payment is made for the amount of "disease," whereas "illness" may be independent, according to Dr. Hadler. He accepts low-back pain as a disease, but the *illness impact* on behavior may result from such other factors as lifestyle, quest for medical attention, and other attributes. Illness is often how we perceive our disease.

According to Hadler, physicians should not have a role in judg-

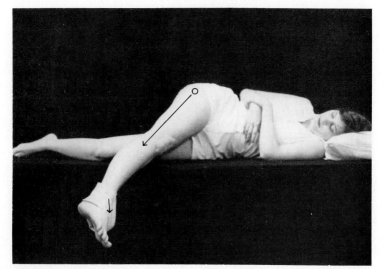

Figure 9-11.   Stretch test or treatment for tight fascial band in thigh.

ing whether a particular injury arose out of or during work; neither can they determine causality with any degree of precision. Unfortunately, physicians are given the task of stating the causality in industrial cases. As has been pointed out, more than an injury is often involved when disability occurs. *Impairment* can be considered as an anatomic or functional loss, and *disability* as the loss of capacity to work in gainful employment. Physicians have to assist in determining:

1. Compensability, a subjective assessment
2. Termination of the healing period (when no further medical recovery is feasible), also subjective
3. Degree of permanent impairment

The American Medical Association (AMA) guidelines for rating disability (permanent impairment) use only objective determinants. Most orthopedists use this guide but also add other attributes that are subjective. Problems lie in the fact that injury allegedly may result from "normal" work in which the repetitive task or activity results in degenerative-disc disease and is complicated by job stress. Often injury is not really definable and separate from other underlying or predisposing causes.

Self-Management of Back Pain

Treatment depends on your immediate condition, for example, whether you are in acute spasm, or "locked up"! If you have an acute attack in which you can't straighten up, we find the fastest relief is to get down to the floor, or onto a bed, on your back with your legs up on a chair. This position reduces the pressure within the back to the lowest levels attainable. Acetaminophen (an analgesic), aspirin, ibuprofen, or prescription analgesics can help. As you feel the spasm let up, begin a rocking motion with your knees drawn to your chest as in Table 9-6, exercises 4 and 5. This is like self-manipulation! Try this for several minutes. Acute back strain should *not* be treated with bed rest for longer than 2 days because so much muscle weakness results from any longer bed rest. Get walking and moving as quickly as possible and avoid sitting positions. A little pain is no reason to avoid going back to work. In fact, persistent but tolerable back pain does *not* mean future trouble! Most cases of acute back pain will have recovered completely within 2 weeks.

If you have recurrent or persistent back pain, then our message to you is "brains, not brawn!" Think before you act. Get your belly button down to whatever you are going to lift and keep it close to the item as you lift it back up. So what if your knees creak? Bend *them*, not your back. Get on with helping yourself and being independent. Less than 2 percent of backache patients are problem patients.

GERALDINE S.: PERSISTENCY AND A POSITIVE ATTITUDE KEEP HER MOBILE

Geraldine S. is 58 years old and has had back and hip problems for a number of years. She has been a patient of Dr. S. for nearly 2 years. Ten years ago, when her problems started, she had pain in both her back and fingers. She found both conditions very annoying; her two great loves are tennis and her beautiful, extensive yard with its lovely flowers.

In the previous 10 years Geraldine had visited a series of doctors. Blood tests had determined that she did have arthritis. At times she felt almost normal, but she says that she never really felt that anyone had a handle on her case. Finally, when her nails began peeling and became soft from her medications, she was discouraged.

In addition to this annoyance, she had severe pains in her left hip. Even though she felt terrible, Gerry insisted on keeping active. Finally, though, this was impossible. The doctor hospitalized her, and rest and an injection of a steroidal drug put her back in operation.

Again she was hospitalized for back pain. Rest and some prescription drugs helped.

For a reason which she has never disclosed, Geraldine decided to find a new doctor and came to Dr. S. After examining her, Dr. S. took her off all oral medication except buffered aspirin. A steroidal injection ended her recurring hip pain. It was now recommended that she take calcium and do some exercises regularly.

A short time later Gerry couldn't get out of bed. Again she was hospitalized, and this time she was suffering from a ruptured disc. Little wonder that the pain was so intense. This time surgery was the key that let her out, and she went home much relieved in mind and body.

Geraldine began attending one of the well-known exercise clubs religiously three times a week when her pain would permit. (She still had arthritis in her back.)

Dr. S. had told her that it was OK to do anything she could do without too much discomfort.

And she did try many things. One of the things that helped a lot was hanging from a bar. So, too, did water exercises, which she learned with the help of a book from her branch library.

All in all, Gerry felt much better. About the only thing she had to be careful about was sitting for more than half an hour at a time. Sometimes, too, riding in a car was painful.

The following spring, Gerry suffered a severe attack of pain when scar tissue rubbed against a nerve. She was willing to try an experimental drug, and fortunately it worked well.

As time goes on, she continues to have problems but never seems to be daunted by them. Recently she suffered an attack of arthritis with severe hip pain. A nonsteroidal drug brought her quick relief.

Geraldine believes that she must keep moving. In fact, she says the keys to her feeling well are a good rheumatologist and moving as much as possible. Whatever her problems, Gerry has had an exemplary attitude, and she never stops trying. Consequently, she gets the maximum benefit from treatment and stays at her optimum for endurance.

Geraldine walks a great deal. Another thing she has tried is placing a piece of elastic around her fingers and then working her hand.

This helps because when you exert force on the bones, it strengthens the muscles that hold the bones in place and keeps the tendons moving. Tendons run to the ends of fingers. If the tendons shorten, the fingers will shorten and become stiff.

Modified sit-ups are another thing by which Gerry swears. If you have Gerry's problems, you may benefit from bending over a table and stretching your back. This helps your sacroiliac. While in this position, pick up your chest and shoulders; stretch your arms back to your fanny (Figure 8-6).

As you have probably guessed, Geraldine also has quite a bit of osteoarthritis. She also has rheumatoid arthritis. And sometimes it seems to Gerry if one isn't hurting, the other is. But she plays tennis—more easily, she believes, if she takes two aspirins first.

Gerry says she tries very hard to keep her body in tune and to have a positive attitude. "You can give in or you can fight. And I'm not a quitter. If we aren't careful, I think we can very easily turn into grouches" says Gerry.

What can you do to help yourself, you ask. Surprisingly, you can not only treat yourself in most cases but also, we hope, find much that can prevent future attacks of back pain. Two important treatment measures are joint protection and exercise. Joint protection should be thought of as preventative (see Table 9-5). Exercise is needed to break a pain-spasm-pain cycle, as well as to condition and strengthen the trunk "cylinder."

Joint Protection

When a specific cause for pain can be found, treatment is straight-forward; but this is uncommon. Most instances of back pain are of myofascial origin, and these in turn often are the result of improper habits while working, resting, or playing. Therefore, special atten-tion should be given to Table 9-4. This details many aggravating activities that are often substituted for more ideal body mechanics. Good posture helps. Strong abdominal muscles that are used also help. Punch yourself in the stomach every morning; then keep the abdomen "sucked in" all day long. This is one way to emphasize the conscious use of the abdominal wall to strengthen the entire trunk cylinder.

Look at your activities at home, both at play and at work:

1. Do you have any fears such as that of returning to your job?
2. Are you dissatisfied with your job or life situation?
3. Do you have aggravating factors that involve unnecessary lifting, climbing, stooping, bending, prolonged sitting, or strains from a new hobby?
4. Do you wear high-heeled shoes?
5. What is your posture like when you sit or lie down?
6. Do you use an improper sitting angle? Is the body's trunk/thigh correctly situated at an angle of 105 degrees (i.e., tilted slightly backward)?
7. Does your work chair have a support across the lumbar region?
8. Is the chair height comfortable as you work or read?
9. Do you need a lower chair for your desk?
10. Is your eye-to-work distance as long as the distance from your elbow to your extended long finger?
11. Do your feet rest squarely on the floor when you are seated?
12. Do you lie on a sofa with your head cocked forward on the arm of the sofa? (HARMFUL!)

13. Do you work or live on a concrete floor? If so, do you wear shoes with shock-absorbing soles?

14. Do you sleep on your side or back? Most people do best on their side with arms lower than breast level.

"Back schools" have become popular recently. These programs teach groups of patients the management as well as the prevention of symptoms. Analysis of specific job tasks must be provided. Patients have a fair degree of satisfaction with this approach, but they must be able to comprehend the information. In one study, employees' performance doubled after back-school education.

Exercises

Choosing the right exercise for the person with a bad back is important. The following seem to be generally helpful:

For mechanical back-pain disorders, see Table 9-6, exercises 1 through 4 and 7 through 11. For preventing attacks try exercises 9, 10, and 11 twice daily. The addition of lateral rotation of the trunk to the abdominal strengthening (exercise 2) is helpful. When tested electrically, this exercise shows strong activation of the oblique muscles in the abdominal wall. Ten-second holds with 10 repetitions performed twice daily are recommended.

For sciatica-related trouble in the acute stage, see Table 9-6, exercises 1, 3, and 4; then, as the condition eases, add exercises 2, 5, 7, and 10.

For myofascial back pain, see Table 9-6, exercises 1 through 7, and 9.

Inversion exercise in which the patient is suspended upside down, using a commercial frame, has proved dangerous because inversion doubles intraocular pressure, pressure within the eyeball. Headache may also be a troublesome complication.

Psychogenic back pain can be helped with an aerobic-conditioning program, because significant muscle tone may have been lost. Also, exercise stimulates endorphin production and release, which may relieve pain.

Exercises may be painful at first. As a rule of thumb, the pain is acceptable if it lasts less than an hour after exercising and does not lead to increased discomfort or stiffness the following morning.

Extension exercises have been advocated for patients with the limited lumbar movement associated with muscle spasm. See Table 9-6, exercises 10 and 11. R. A. McKenzie, a New Zealand physical therapist, reported that 80 percent of patients could abort an attack and felt generally improved if they used these five times daily. Another technique we use is described in exercise 11. This is particularly useful in patients with an adult round back or thoracic kyphosis, which is a backward angular deformity of the spine in the thoracic area.

Researchers at New York Hospital have developed group exercises for the YMCA, and they report results in 12,000 enrollees who completed a 6-week program: pain and trunk strength improved in 80 percent of patients irrespective of whether surgery had been performed in the past. Success was directly proportional to maintenance of strength. In another program, a group exercise included flexion exercises, pool therapy, and back-school education for patients receiving compensation (half of whom had had previous back surgery). This resulted in 72 percent becoming employed during the next 6 months. Half the patients had symptoms of longer than 3 months' duration before entry. A small study compared flexion versus extension exercise in young persons with backache; the results favored extension exercises.

When to Seek Professional Help

Diagnostic Techniques

Professional help will depend on acuteness, mode of onset, duration, and cause of the back pain. Table 9-4 may help you consider some of the causes for persistent back pain. If you can present answers to the questions we posed earlier and perhaps complete the pain drawing, your physician may be able to more rapidly provide a diagnosis and begin treatment. Let's see what the doctor can do and what value there is in it.

X-rays can be costly and also expose you to the x-ray beam. The sun and earth also shower us with x-rays. Routine roentgenographic back examination should be considered for persons with a history of major trauma: those with a physical-examination abnormality, those who are older, or those whose medication (such as steroids) or treatment could result in skeletal disorders. In one study, x-ray findings of a narrow disc space, degenerative arthritis, and spur formation bore no relation to type of work, absence from work, sex, race, or sport activity. The findings correlated only with age.

In *scintigraphy* a harmless dose of a radioactive element that is picked up by bone is injected into your arm. Three hours later a type of Geiger counter is used to put an image of your skeleton onto x-ray film. This usually shows the circulation and bone turnover, both of which are affected by infection, inflammation, and tumors. It may be of value if the doctor suspects a sports injury to the smaller back bones in which a stress fracture might have occurred, inflammatory arthritis of the spine, osteoporosis with fracture, osteomalacia (failure of formation of bone due to lack of calcium), osteomyelitis (bone infection), disc-space infections, cancers, or Paget's disease (probably viral in etiology, although it can lead to cancer).

In *computed tomography,* known commonly as a *CAT scan,* the x-ray pictures are rearranged by a computer. This can provide a three-dimensional view of the spine. It has been helpful in diagnosing many diseases of the spine including herniated disc, facet degeneration, and spinal stenosis (constriction or narrowing). Sometimes a *myelogram* (injection of iodine-type dye into the spinal canal) is combined with a CAT scan or performed separately. Myelograms are usually performed only if conservative treatment has been tried and has failed. Myelograms on rare occasions have some complications, including infections and allergic reactions to the dye used in the procedure.

Magnetic resonance imaging is the new kid on the block. Magnetic waves are used to rearrange the body's molecules, and the waves can then be measured and reconstructed by a computer into a beautiful three-dimensional view. It can be particularly helpful in the diagnosis of disc degeneration, disc-space infection, and soft-tissue lesions.

Thermography simply measures heat given off by the body with the very sophisticated measurement of infrared detectors. Cold or warmth may signify injury and sometimes spasm. Studies at this point are encouraging, but the technique is not yet reliable. Thermography has had great technical enhancement in recent years but remains a tool of uncertain value. Certainly it does not stand alone in the diagnosis of back-pain etiology.

Arthrography of facet joints with steroid injection under fluoroscopic imaging has some proponents. The joint capsule nearly always bursts following the procedure! Others state that arthrography findings do not differentiate a pain-producing joint from a normal one. We do not now advocate this technique for diagnosis or for treatment. In our opinion it remains an investigational technique.

Electrodiagnostic studies, commonly known as EMGs, are examinations that measure the rate of nerve transmission, the health of the nerve, and the nerve center in the spinal cord. The reliability of electrodiagnostic testing is correlated with the clinical expertise of the electromyographer.

Treatments

None of our tests is perfect or infallible. What, you then ask, can the doctor do? What treatment can be ordered?

The first thing a doctor might do is *prescribe rest*. Remember that sitting still and standing still are hard work. Rest can be at home lying on a proper bed arranged as in Figure 9-12. Bed rest with the lumbar spine flattened by elevating the legs seems most helpful. As mentioned above, in acute stages, when a "catch" has occurred, we sometimes suggest that the patient get down on the floor and put the legs up on a chair. A few hours of this may allow the spasm to subside. Prolonged bed rest may be harmful to the elderly, resulting in osteoporosis and thrombophlebitis (inflammation of a vein associated with a blood clot).

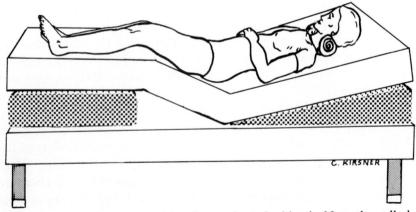

Figure 9-12.   Proper bed position for resting a bad back. Note the rolled towel under the neck.

Pelvic traction is often helpful, but perhaps the benefit is more restful than physiologic. The body should be in the same position as in Figure 9-12, and the amount of weight should gradually be increased to between 15 and 30 pounds. Pelvic traction is applied using a canvas pelvic belt. The desired weight is fastened to a floor-stand at the foot of the bed and a simple pulley system is set up to create traction. (This apparatus can be rented from a surgical supply store.) How long and how many days should be based on your improvement. When bed traction aggravates sciatica, we have found this to signify a ruptured disc of significant size or other spinal conditions that severely compress the spinal nerve structures.

The *lumbosacral corset* with a heat-molded plastic insert has been in wide use recently. In one 8-week study, the corset relieved symptoms to a greater degree when the insert was included than when the binder alone was provided. We use the support in older patients with osteoporosis, those with lumbosacral junction anomalies, or in young patients with loose joints until they develop good abdominal tone with exercise.

Pain relief begins with the physician reassuring you that she or he has found no structural damage that would cause lifelong pain. Conversely, the examination should convey to you the fact that you can improve. Changes in daily living habits, posture improvement, weight control, and other physical improvements will be helpful. Pain relief is only an adjunct to the exercise and behavioral changes that must occur.

Oral medication has a limited role in the treatment of back pain. However, some people may certainly get a lot of relief with a medication that another person finds to be of no benefit. The drugs often used include relaxants, which work on the spinal nerve pools; antidepressants, which have a direct effect on the brain centers that sense pain; and the nonsteroidal anti-inflammatory drugs, which act both to stop inflammation and to kill pain. None of these is addicting. Chapter 15 reviews these medications.

Ice massage on trigger points can be beneficial but requires the assistance of another person. Similarly, pressurized coolant spray (Fluorimethane) can be used. Fluorimethane sprayed in a slow sweep from the trigger point to the pain area, with not more than two sweeps per treatment, while the patient performs a muscle-stretching exercise, may break the pain-spasm-pain cycle.

Shots of procaine or cortisones, or both, may provide temporary and sometimes permanent relief. An experienced physician can locate a trigger point with the needle tip and eradicate it with this treatment. In one study of 22 patients with recurrent myofascial pain treated for an average of over 10 years per patient, 79 percent had good results when the sacroiliac region was involved, 76 percent when other areas of the back were involved, and 59 percent when myofascial pain was complicated by a degenerative-disc problem. Overall, the 22 patients received 115 trigger-point injections over a 10-year period with a 77 percent good or fair result. No side effects other than transient local pain were noted. Some experts like the longer-acting local anesthetics for treatment of trigger points, and these practitioners report good results.

Caudal blocks, epidural blocks (meaning, blocks injected into the spinal membranes), epidural steroids, radiofrequency denervation (cutting off the nerve supply), and posterior rhizotomy (surgical division of a nerve) have been advocated but are investigational in the opinion of many authors and clinicians. Complications following epidural steroid therapy, although rare, may include bacterial meningitis, anesthetic toxicity, and steroid toxicity. Improper needle placement may also occur.

Patients should attempt *physical therapy* as soon as they obtain relief from severe pain. The therapist may begin with gentle stretching exercises and relaxation techniques. Once pain is controlled, the exercise can begin. The physical therapist should be permitted to individualize the home-exercise program. Many patients are also started in water-aerobic classes, group exercise, and a back school or individual back-protection instruction by an occupational therapist.

Do You Really Need Surgery?

When surgery for a ruptured disc is necessary, delay can result in prolonged injury to a nerve. And even when surgery is carried out, continued and persistent pain and weakness may result. Surgery should generally be considered on the basis of signs of nerve injury, in addition to pain. There should be objective abnormalities either with reflex nerve signs, signs of weakness or wasting of muscle in one leg, a distinct abnormality on electromyography, or typical diagnostic findings on myelogram. Often a radiologist has provided a second opinion in noting a significant abnormality on myelography.

On occasion a surgeon may sense that despite the lack of an abnormality, surgery is necessary. We have seen cases in which even
though all radiographic and electrodiagnostic tests were normal, the
patient did have a tumor, an abscess, or a severely ruptured disc.

Chemonucleolysis (dissolution of the nucleus pulposus) with injected chymopapain has been approved for selected patients with
established ruptured discs. These patients are being selected very
carefully. Complications of the procedure may include recurrence
of the ruptured disc, allergic reactions, internal bleeding, or sudden
death.

Pain Syndromes of the Pelvis

Osteitis pubis, an inflammation on each side of the pubic bone, may
result from the spread of inflammation following prostate, bladder,
or hernia surgery (Figure 9-13). Also, it often follows pregnancy.
The condition causes pain that travels widely across the lower abdomen and down into the inner aspect of both thighs. The condition
may result in a duck-waddle walk. There is local tenderness over the
mons pubis in the center of the body. X-ray changes may be a late
development. Sometimes the condition occurs in association with
inflammatory arthritis. Often the condition is self-limited, and symp-

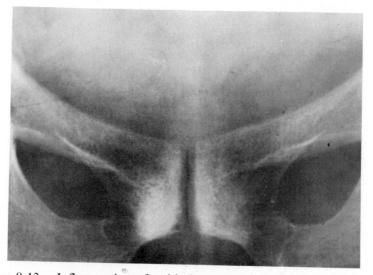

Figure 9-13.   Inflammation of pubic bone may result from injury or infection during childbirth, sports, prostate problems, etc.

tomatic benefit may be obtained from use of nonsteroidal anti-inflammatory drugs. On occasion, local injection of a corticosteroid and anesthetic medication is given. A sacral belt to stabilize the pelvis may be of benefit. Traumatic osteitis pubis, the *gracilis syndrome,* is a fatigue fracture near the pubic symphysis. The pain radiates deep into the pelvis and into the inner aspect of the thigh. Athletic activities associated with traumatic osteitis pubis include fencing, basketball, track, hockey, soccer, and bowling.

Coccygodynia is the name for a painful tailbone. The coccyx comprises three bony segments, the last of which may become fractured, dislocated, or deformed. Coccygodynia may result from referred pain arising in the bowel, rectum, or the genital-urinary tissues. The result is regional muscle spasm in the rectal muscles that lie near the coccyx. Sometimes a lumbar-disc rupture may result in coccygodynia. When the condition is thought to be of local origin, local treatment measures that are helpful include avoiding contact with a hard surface. Use of a thick, soft foam-rubber cushion about 3 inches thick with a hole 3 inches in diameter cut out of the center may provide comfort. A water-filled cushion has also been helpful.

Going down a slide and landing on the buttocks resulted in coccygodynia for one patient. Another had the condition after a friend had, in fun, applied a poorly aimed foot to that area. Riding in a car was painful for years, and the patient said she usually rode backward, sitting on her knees.

"Weaver's bottom," "tailor's bottom," or "lighterman's bottom" are vernacular terms for *ischial bursitis* and represent pain in a bursa overlying the ischial prominence. The ischium is the very bottom of the pelvis forming the two lower poles that we sit on. The ischial prominences lie deep in the lower buttocks. When the tissue becomes irritated, the sciatic nerve may also become inflamed. The patient often has exquisite pain when sitting or lying. An improper sitting position is a common cause. Also, performing exercises on the floor may aggravate the ischium. Tenderness can be noted by deep palpation. Sometimes the condition may arise from prostatitis, or from ankylosing spondylitis. A cutout cushion may be helpful. The cushion should have two holes cut for the ischial prominences. Each hole should be about 3 inches in diameter and about 3 inches apart. Ischial bursitis is very intractable, perhaps lasting many months. Exercises that are helpful include stretching, as described in Table 9-6, items 5 and 6.

Pain Syndromes of the Hip

Patients often interpret low-back or presacral pain or ischial-gluteal (pertaining to the bone upon which the body sits) discomfort as "hip pain." True hip pain usually presents in the front at the groin or in the inner aspect of the thigh and even down the knee. Hip pain can also cause back pain. True hip disease will have the associated complaint of limitation of movement, for example, loss of the ability to rotate the leg in order to put on a slipper or stocking in the morning. This in essence is the Patrick test, which is described in Table 9-2, item 10. Arthritis of the hip most often causes a painful limp during walking. The pain is relieved by lying down. However, we have seen some people with severe arthritis on x-rays of the hip who had good hip movement and no pain! The x-ray may have been taken as part of a bowel x-ray or kidney x-ray. Thus, x-ray changes do not always correlate with the findings. Surrounding the hip bone are two bursa sacs, the superficial and deep trochanteric bursas.

The *snapping-hip syndrome,* in which the hip emits a painless but annoying noise, often results from a taut fascial band slipping over the hip bone. Stretching this band for a few moments twice daily may be helpful (Table 9-6, item 13).

Fasciitis is an inflammation of the thigh fascia, a tough gristlelike tissue at the side of the thigh that separates the front muscles from the back muscles. Runners often develop an overuse syndrome, but we have also seen many older people with inflammation of this tissue. The patient may describe vague discomfort upon rising in the morning and after prolonged walking. The discomfort is a dull ache over the lateral hip and thigh region, and it radiates down the lateral thigh through the lateral knee region. Stretching that tissue, as in Table 9-6, item 14, will temporarily exacerbate the discomfort, but it can be used as treatment.

Bursitis, an inflammation of the bursa, often results from the spread of inflammation from an injured tendon of one of the gluteus muscles. Bursitis characteristically causes pain at night more severe than in the daytime and may cause sciaticlike symptoms. Often the patient cannot lie on the involved hip. Point tenderness over the bursa may require probing deeply behind the hip bone with a finger. The tenderness usually lies approximately 1 inch behind and 1 inch upward from the prominent hip bone. The bursa is actually located about 3 inches deep in the skin. Aggravating factors include obesity, a compression injury from a fat wallet, or bending over with straight knees and then having to use the gluteus muscle as a lever to straighten the body. Although local measures such as ice or rub-ons may be helpful, most cases require either an oral nonsteroidal anti-inflammatory drug or a local corticosteroid injection.

We can't talk about the hip without mentioning a most dreaded orthopedic disturbance, the *hip fracture*. Patients do not always recognize hip fractures at the time they occur. Sometimes an elderly individual will forget having had a traumatic incident. Hip fractures will cause painful walking. Moving the hip to perform the Patrick test (Table 9-2, item 10) will also exacerbate the pain. Sometimes x-rays fail to demonstrate a fracture. If management of any supposed soft-tissue disorder fails to provide benefit and an x-ray of the pelvis fails to demonstrate an abnormality, the doctor may proceed to a bone scan. We have seen pelvic and hip fractures that did not even show up on a bone scan but became obvious a month or so later. Constant pain in the hip or groin should raise suspicion of such a fracture. Of course, many other conditions may cause groin pain, including an abscess, hernia, hematoma (a tumor or swelling containing blood), lymphoma (a tumor of the lymphatic tissues), or a vascular disturbance.

Neuralgia is acute pain along the course of a nerve. In the hip, neuralgia caused by entrapment of a nerve and causing pins and needles over the lateral thigh is known as *meralgia paresthetica* (Figure 9-14). The entrapment occurs over the brim of the pelvis and may become impinged by a belt, a seat belt in a car, a holster, or some other object worn on a belt. Leaning over a workbench or table that pinches this area can also cause the problem. A heavy roll of fat can pinch the nerve, or sometimes a pelvic tilt that results from a short leg may be the cause. Prolonged sitting with crossed legs has been known to create this condition. Most cases will respond to local corticosteroid injection at multiple sites where the nerve emerges through the ligaments and spreads into the tissues.

Some patients have a tight hip capsule with *arthritis*. Although the Patrick test (Table 9-2, item 10) is painful for them, the limb can be taken through a normal range of movements. In such patients we have found an exercise that stretches the hip capsule to be helpful. The pendulum exercise is described in Table 9-6, item 13.

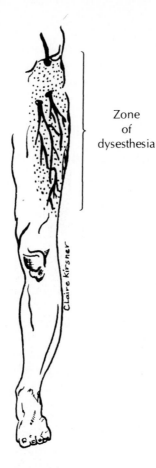

Zone
of
dysesthesia

Figure 9-14. Site of nerve pinch causing neuralgia.

Table 9-1

Danger Signs in the Low Back, Pelvis, and Hips

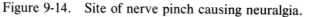

Fever, chills, weight loss
Bladder or bowel pain or dysfunction
Back pain that awakens you from sleep
Weakness or stiffness of a leg or foot
Persistent numbness at the side of the leg
Persistent numbness anywhere in the foot

(continued)

Wasting of thigh muscles
Inability to place your heel on the opposite knee
Prominent veins on the abdominal wall
Crampy ache in the buttocks if you walk any distance

Table 9-2

Self-Examination of the Low Back, Pelvis, and Hips

1. To check your alignment, stand in front of a full-length mirror. Are your shoulders and hips level? If not, you may have scoliosis or deep spasm (listing).
2. To measure lordosis, or the forward curvature of your spine, back up to a wall and, with your hands, make an approximate measurement of the space behind you at your waist. Your waist should be just an inch from the wall. If not, you may have to strengthen your abdominal muscles and learn to keep your abdomen tucked in for support.
3. To test spinal nerve SI, stand up on your toes 10 times. If you note weakness, the SI nerve may be in trouble.
4. To test spinal nerve L5, balance on your heels for 10 seconds. If you note weakness, this nerve may be pinched within the spine.
5. The modified Schober test measures the mobility of your lumbar spine. Stand erect and have a helper mark your skin in the midline of your back at the level of the lumbosacral junction, which is in line with the dimples of Venus (Figure 9-6). She or he then places another mark 4 inches above the first and a third mark 2 inches below the first. Now, bend forward as if to touch your toes. The helper measures the distance between the upper and lower marks. A normal distance is greater than 8 inches. This test is an objective way to determine whether the backbones are moving apart normally. In addition to ankylosing spondylitis, less common arthritis disorders and severe myofascial pain disorders may limit spinal movement.
6. Bend forward and try to touch your palms to the floor while keeping your knees straight. The ability to do this easily suggests hypermobility (Figure 9-1).
7. To detect curvatures of the spine, bend forward and have a helper check your backbone for straightness. While you are bending forward, have your helper check the curve of your lumbar spine. If it remains flat, this suggests arthritis.

8. To detect degenerative arthritis, bend backward. Arching the back compresses facet joints and causes pain if the joints are arthritic. Arching may also aggravate sciatica caused by a ruptured disc.

9. Sit down. Do you feel pain? Sitting may cause deep buttock pain if you suffer from piriformis (muscle) spasm or bursitis.

10. Now, try to put your right heel onto your left knee or vice versa. This is the Patrick test (Figure 9-10). An inability to perform this motion suggests hip arthritis. (This test can also be performed lying down, as shown.)

11. Try to rise from your seated position without using your hands. If you are unable to do this, you may have hip muscle weakness.

12. While you are seated, have a helper slowly lift each of your legs to straighten the knee. If you have a ruptured disc, pain may occur on the side of the back where the disc is ruptured.

13. Lie on your abdomen with a pillow under your stomach. Raise each of your legs alternately, bending at the knees. Now, lift the whole leg backward, one side at a time. If you have a ruptured disc, back pain may occur on the side of the ruptured disc.

14. Lie on your abdomen with a pillow under your stomach or bend over a table with your knees bent and have a helper perform the percussion (tapping) test (Figure 9-3). Percussion should begin with a very mild thump using a fist, and then increase in force slightly. The helper first thumps down the middle of the back, about as hard as pounding a wad of dough or clay, percussing about every 2 inches. Then he or she moves out 2 inches from the center of the spine and, beginning at the waist level, percusses again down to the beginning of the buttocks; the helper repeats this procedure down the other side of the low back. Pain elicited below the level of the thump may signify disease at that level. Pain that radiates into a leg suggests a ruptured disc. Myofascial pain will feel worse at the site of a trigger point.

15. To check for a tight hamstring, lie on your back and put a 4-foot rope around your foot near the toes. Straighten your leg and pull it overhead, keeping the knee straight. You should be able to pull the leg straight up to 90 degrees (Figure 9-19).

16. Measure and compare the circumference of your thighs and calves. The dominant side (right side if you are right-handed) is usually ⅜- to ⅞-inch larger than the other. If one side is unusually small, this could suggest a weakened muscle or a nerve injury.

17. The Ober test detects overly tight thigh muscles. Lie on your uninvolved (pain-free) side with knees and hips comfortably bent. Wrap a 4-foot rope twice around your ankle, leaving the ends about

(continued)

equally long. With your upper hand holding the rope loosely behind your knee (not yet pulling), move your upper thigh backward to straighten the hip joint; try to get the knee behind the hip. Now slowly pull the rope, and thus the knee, into a tight bend. The Ober test is often used to spot a contracture of the iliotibial band, but it is an excellent test to detect shortening of the thigh muscles. The technique can also be used to lengthen the shortened muscles.

18. To test for a tight fascial band in the thigh, lie on your uninvolved (pain-free) side, close to the edge of a bed (Figure 9-11). Keep the lower leg bent and the upper knee straight. Hang the upper leg out over the side of the bed. Place a sock or purse filled with 3 to 5 pounds of stones or coins over the ankle. If you feel a tightness, pulling, or aching, try the same test with the other leg and compare. Abnormal tightness indicates fascia lata fasciitis, or a tight iliotibial band.

19. While you lie on your back, have a helper compare the lengths of your legs. The helper pulls your legs straight and then compares the locations of the ankle bones and heels. (Although this test is inaccurate, it provides a clue to a possible source of pain.)

Table 9-3
Possible Causes of Low-Back, Pelvis, or Hip Pain

Complaint	Possible Cause
Sudden catch in the back	Mechanical back pain
Back pain worse while performing tasks	Degenerative-disc disease
Stooping posture	Arthritis
Back pain with numbness and weakness in leg	Sciatica; ruptured disc
Back pain with numbness but no weakness	Pseudosciatica
Back pain worse after resting or sitting	Myofascial back pain
Aching back and aching mind	Psychogenic (emotionally induced) back pain
Pubic pain (just above genital area)	Pubic-bone disorders
Tailbone pain	Coccygodynia
Buttock pain with or without numb leg	Piriformis syndrome

Complaint	Possible Cause
Deep pain in the buttock	Weaver's bottom (ischial bursitis)
Pain at the side of the hip	Tendinitis and bursitis
Numbness at the side of the thigh	Neuralgia (meralgia paresthetica)
Pain in the groin, associated with a limp	Arthritis of hip
Clicking hip (painless)	Snapping hip!

Table 9-4

Habits that Aggravate or Cause Persistent Low-Back, Pelvic, or Hip Pain

Complaint	Aggravating Habit
Pain and stiffness, worse in the morning, better with movement	Interspinal bursitis, resulting from working with hands overhead; ankylosing spondylitis, which can involve entire spine; myofascial back pain (trigger points present), often due to improper use, poor posture, prolonged sitting or standing
Pain worse during and after lifting, pushing, reaching overhead	Degenerative-disc disease (may need to use abdominal muscles more often); ruptured disc; osteoarthritis
Pain and limp during walking	Ruptured disc; arthritis of hip
Back pain with numbness in leg but no weakness	Myofascial back pain, or hip bursitis, often due to repeated bending with straight knees during work or when making beds
Back pain with numbness in leg with weakness in leg	Ruptured disc; spinal stenosis; spinal tumor
Crampy pain in buttocks after walking	Spinal stenosis
Tailbone pain	Coccygodynia, often result of prolonged sitting, exercising on the floor; ruptured disc; rectal muscle spasm; pelvic muscle spasm

(continued)

Complaint	Aggravating Habit
Numbness and tingling in the outer thigh area	Neuralgia (meralgia paresthetica), often resulting from a large belt or leaning over a work table
Pain in front of the pelvis	Osteitis pubis, possibly from sports injury, pregnancy, or pelvic organ infection

Table 9-5

What's Harmful, What's Helpful for the Low Back, Pelvis, and Hips

Harmful	Helpful
Having weak abdominal muscles puts a strain on the low back.	If possible, perform exercises that strengthen the abdominal muscles and then *use* these muscles. Try to keep them contracted most of the day.
Shoveling snow, weeding the garden, or lifting heavy objects can cause an acute attack of back pain, often referred to as "a catch in the back."	Lie on the back and elevate the legs with a sofa cushion placed under the ankles, not the knees; place moist heat packs under the back, then do numerous knee-to-chest lifts.
Bending over with the knees locked can injure the back.	Always bend at the knees, not at the waist.
Twisting at the waist while holding large or heavy objects can cause back strain, as can constantly carrying an object, such as a young child, on one side of the body.	Turn or rotate the entire body by moving the feet. Draw the object to the chest, lift it with the arms held stiff, and use the thigh muscles for strength. Hold the object centered in front of you.
Standing for prolonged periods, especially on a concrete surface, rapidly tires the back muscles.	Place one foot atop a 2×4×8-in. wood block for a while and then alternate, thus transferring body weight from one foot to the other. Wear rubber-soled shoes when working or walking on concrete.

Harmful	Helpful
Having one leg that is more than 0.5 in. shorter than the other should not be overlooked as a cause of back pain.	Have shoes built up for the foot of the shorter leg.
Sitting for too long can strain the back.	Sit on a bar stool; doing so is uncomfortable and promotes frequent changes of position. Break up desk work and card games by standing up and moving around every 30 minutes. Use cruise control, if available, when driving long distances.
Doing strenuous physical work or engaging in a sport activity on an occasional or weekend basis can lead to back pain.	Do trunk-stretching warm-up exercises before engaging in any strenuous activity.
Sleeping on the stomach or flat on the back can cause backache.	Sleep on one side or on the back with the knees and feet elevated with a cushion or pillow.
Sitting or falling hard often results in pressure injury to the coccyx, or tailbone.	Protect the point of tenderness at the tip of the coccyx by using a foam-rubber or spongelike cushion that is at least 3 in. thick and the size of a seat cushion. Cut a 3-in. circle out of the center of the cushion with a bread knife. For at least a month following injury, place the cushion under the tailbone whenever seated or doing exercises on the floor.
Bending over with the knees locked is a very common cause of pain in the buttock region. Persons who can touch the floor with their palms are likely to bend improperly.	Always bend at the knees, not at the waist.
Applying pressure to the sciatic nerve, [which occurs with a rup-	Take proper care of the back by strengthening and using the

(continued)

Harmful	Helpful
tured disc, direct injury, constriction of the spinal canal (spinal stenosis), or muscle spasm adjacent to the nerve], can result in sciatica. Sciatica is a symptom complex of pain, numbness, and tingling radiating from a buttock to below the knee. Another cause of sciatica is bursitis at the side of the hip. Here again, bending over with the knees locked is a common cause.	abdominal muscles to support the back, attaining and maintaining ideal weight, avoiding prolonged periods of sitting or standing, wearing rubber-soled shoes when working or walking on concrete, assuming proper rest and sleep positions, and performing trunk-stretching exercises before engaging in strenuous activities.
Carrying a large wallet in a back pocket can cause sciatica. Similarly, wearing a tight belt, leaning over a drafting table, or improperly positioning a seat belt can put pressure on a nerve, causing numbness, tingling, and a burning sensation in the lateral hip and thigh region.	Check for pressure placed on the pelvic bones by a wallet, belt, or workbench and, if present, remedy the situation. Learn to wear seat belts so that pressure on the pelvic bone is avoided (either across the thighs or abdomen is preferable).

Table 9-6
Exercises for the Low Back, Pelvis, and Hips

1. *Abdominal strengthening:* Lie on the floor with your knees bent; place your arms across your chest. Exhale and roll the upper trunk up about 3 to 6 inches but keep your chin and neck straight. (If you have a hiatus hernia, start with pillows under your head and chest.) Now extend your arms forward and above the knees. Hold for 30 seconds and begin breathing while holding the position. Repeat 3 to 10 times (Figure 9-15).

2. *Rotator stretch:* Lie on the floor, knees bent, hands behind your head. Curl upward to sit up and at same time twist your right elbow to your left knee and return to the floor. Repeat with left elbow to right knee.

3. *Pelvic tilt:* Stand against a wall with your back to the wall, or lie on the floor with knees bent. Place your hands behind your back

at the waistline. Squeeze your abdomen and at the same time tighten your buttocks to rock the pelvis forward (like a belly dancer doing a pelvic grind). You should feel the low back flatten backward against your hands. Hold this position for 5 to 20 seconds, repeat for 1 to 2 minutes twice daily (Figure 9-16).

4. *Hip and low-back flex:* Lie on your back with both knees bent. Hook an arm under one leg and draw the knee to your chest; hold 10 seconds; then repeat with the other side; and then pull both knees to your chest at the same time. Repeat the exercise twice daily (Figure 9-17).

5. *Knee-chest flexion exercise:* Lie on your back on a firm surface (on the floor or on a board on top of a bed); draw both knees slowly toward your chest and curl your head and shoulders up toward the knees. Do not bring the head forward first. Bring the head and shoulders up together; otherwise, the front neck muscles will feel a strain. Now rock your buttocks upward. Hold 10 seconds and repeat 10 times. Repeat the exercise twice daily. The knee-to-chest exercise can also be performed while you are seated on a chair with the knees spread apart, feet on the floor. Extend your arms forward and down between the knees toward the floor, with your shoulders and chest approaching the knees until you feel a pull in the buttocks or low-back muscles. Hold this position while breathing for 10 to 20 seconds and repeat six times. Repeat the exercise twice daily (Figure 9-18).

6. *Hamstring stretch:* Lie on your back with the legs bent at the knee, feet to the floor. Raise one leg and loop a 4-foot length of rope under your toes; pull the leg straight up. Slowly increase the pull and direct the leg higher, or toward your head. Hold 1 minute with increased forward pull every 10 seconds. Then repeat with the other leg. Repeat the exercise twice daily (Figure 9-19).

7. *Trunk stretch:* Sit on the floor, legs straight. Keep your knees straight. Exhale and reach forward, grasping your shins; then breathe and pull the trunk forward while bending the elbows outward. Hold for 30 seconds; repeat 3 to 6 times. Repeat the exercise twice daily (Figure 9-20).

8. *Buttocks squeeze:* Pretend you are holding a pencil between the cheeks of the buttocks. Squeeze the buttocks hard; hold 10 seconds. Repeat often throughout the day.

9. *Chinning-bar stretch:* Obtain a chinning bar and fit it into a doorway. Grasp and hang by your hands; draw the knees up toward the chest. Hold as many seconds as possible, let go, and then repeat for 1 to 2 minutes, two or more times a day (Figure 9-21).

(continued)

10. *Back extension:* Lie on your stomach; press the top half of your body upward with your arms as fully extended as possible and with legs and pelvis kept against the floor. Do 10 repetitions, four or five times a day (Figure 9-22).

11. *Upper-back straightening:* Lean across a kitchen table, counter, or ironing board with abdomen, chest, and nose against the surface. Place your hands on your buttocks. Keep your chin neutral. Draw your shoulders back. Raise the head and chest together as a unit about 2 to 4 inches while keeping your abdomen against the table. Hold 10 to 20 seconds; repeat three to five times twice daily (Figure 8-6).

12. *Thigh stretch (Ober test):* Lie with painful side up, knees and hips comfortably bent. Wrap a 4-foot rope twice around your ankle, leaving the ends about equally long. With your upper hand holding the rope loosely (not yet pulling) behind your knee, move your upper thigh backward to straighten the hip joint; try to get the knee behind the hip. Now slowly pull the rope, and thus the knee, into a tight bend. A pulling sensation should be felt in the front of the thigh near the knee. Hold this pull for 60 seconds. Perform the stretch twice daily (Figure 9-7).

13. *Weighted-leg pendulum exercise:* Fill a sock or small bag with 2 to 10 pounds of sand, gravel, or buckshot. Tie the weight with a stocking to the ankle of your involved (painful) side. Now place a low stool near a door jamb so you can hold onto the jamb for balance. Stand on the stool so that your uninvolved leg carries your body weight. Begin to swing your weighted leg front to back by giving it a swing and then passively letting it swing back and forth until it slows down. Give it another active swing. After 1 minute of front-to-back movement, turn your body on the stool so you can push the leg out in front of you and swing it in the same manner from side to side. This may be painful, but try to force sideways movements, also for 1 minute. Perform the exercise twice daily (Figure 9-23).

14. *Weighted-leg thigh exercise:* Fill a sock or purse with 3 to 5 pounds of stones, buckshot, or any substance available. Attach this bag to your involved leg, just above the ankle. You can tie it on with an old stocking. Now lie on your uninvolved (pain-free) side close to the edge of a bed. Keep your lower leg bent and your upper knee straight. Hang your upper leg out over the side of the bed, and let the weight pull the leg toward the floor for 3 minutes. Do this twice daily (Figure 9-11).

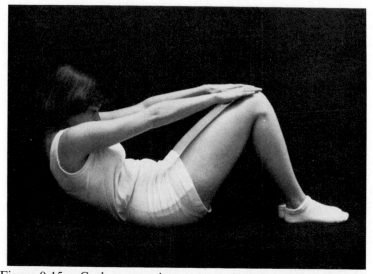

Figure 9-15.   Curl-up exercise to strengthen abdominal muscles.

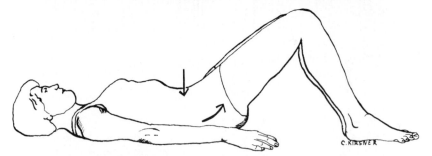

Figure 9-16.   Pelvic tilt to flatten lumbar lordosis.

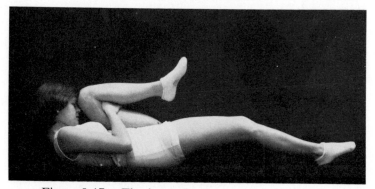

Figure 9-17.   The knee-chest exercise lying down.

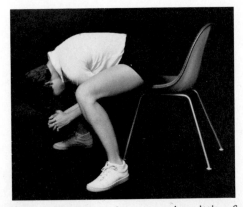

Figure 9-18.　The knee-chest exercise sitting forward.

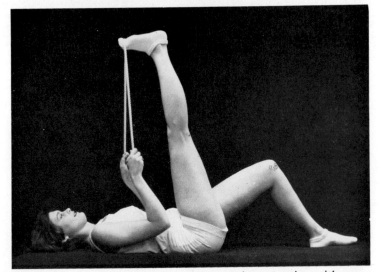

Figure 9-19.　Leg-stretch test and hamstring exercise with rope.

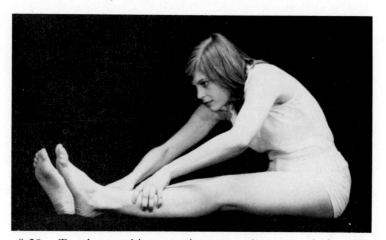

Figure 9-20.   Trunk-stretching exercise—a good warm-up before work or sports.

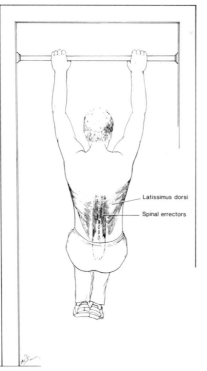

Figure 9-21.   Hanging stretch to help elongate spinal muscles and relieve spinal pressure.

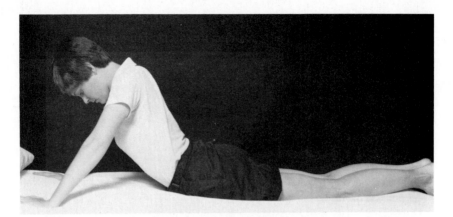

Figure 9-22.   Partial push-up to extend spine (McKenzie exercise).

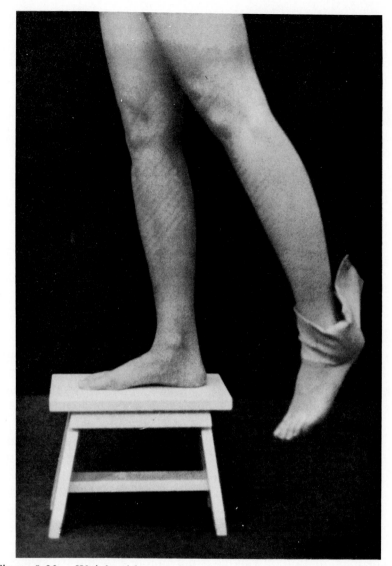

Figure 9-23.   Weighted-leg pendulum exercise to relieve pressure in the hip joint.

CHAPTER 10

The Knee and Thigh

You probably have wondered why so many people have arthritic knees. Physicians, on the other hand, marveling at the complexity of the knee joint, wonder how it manages to do as well as it does! This joint is mechanically very complex, not just a simple hinge. It is made up of five bones: the thigh bone, or *femur*; the kneecap, or *patella*; the two lower leg bones, known as the *tibia* and *fibula*; and the *fabella,* a small bone behind the knee (Figure 10-1). Inside the knee, the femur has two knuckles that fit into the tibia. Two cartilages, which act as rocker panels for these knuckles, are called *menisci.* These tear easily from injury. To answer your question "Why?" you must consider the amazing mechanics of this busy joint, the knee.

The main motion of walking is not simply a to-and-fro swinging hinge. Did you also know that the knee has a sliding and gliding action when you walk? In addition, the knee has a slight circular rotation, called the "screw-home" motion. The upper bone, the femur, rotates on the lower bone (the tibia) as you step forward or upward. So, when you step forward, all of these motions are happening in that one forward step; and you're adding your body weight to the stress of the motion. Now, if you have a fat belly, that puts

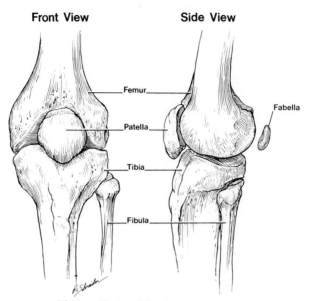

Front View   **Side View**

Femur

Fabella

Patella

Tibia

Fibula

Figure 10-1.   The knee bones.

the weight in front of the knee and aggravates both the "screw-home" twist and the sliding motion. Next, consider that knee getting most of its action while you are walking on a rigid, concrete floor. And imagine the jolt the knee must take with every step you take.

Lastly, think about climbing up a stairway. If you're walking behind the person with those knees, notice their behind and notice how it waddles slightly left and right. That translates into more circular "screw-home" stress on the knee. In addition, during stair-climbing, the body leans forward, putting much stress on the knee-cap and forcing it into the knee joint.

Now do you see why we marvel at such complexity? But this is also why we doctors are not as fast about recommending knee-joint replacement. No man-made knee can possibly put up with the abuse that your own knee manages to sustain day in, day out.

Actually, arthritis in the knee joint may begin by age 20, when shock-absorbing cartilage begins to fragment and split! But nature endows us with so much cartilage that it lasts many more years in most of us. However, there are those of us with small defects in the formation of the knee, with abnormal angles, rotations, or shape. Between 60 to 80 percent of knee arthritis occurs because of slight birth defects, not from injury, and about 15 percent of people are destined to wear out the knee prematurely.

Because of constant motion and wear and tear at some time, most of us will have a painful knee in our lives. Let's consider how a knee heals. As in any other joint, all of the tissues except cartilage can restore themselves. But remember, the knee has two knuckles; and when we wear out the cartilage prematurely, it is almost always just one of the two knuckles. The exception is when rheumatoid arthritis or other inflammatory forms of arthritis afflict the knee.

The most important protector of the knee is the quadriceps muscles that lie in the front of your thigh. These muscles, combined with their partners, the hamstring muscles behind the thigh, provide bracing and stability to the knee joint. When you twist and tear a ligament (a joint hinge), the tearing causes a loose knee joint that can rock from side to side. Nature can repair it if the quadriceps muscle is strong; and the repair will happen, because in your response to the painful stepping you will try to walk with the knee held stiff, avoiding bending of the knee. What you are doing then is contracting the quadriceps, tightening up this internal knee brace; and that allows the ligament or hinge to recover! So, as we begin this chapter, you can see that you may be on the way to "arthritis" of the knee; but if you keep the knee strong, your weight reasonably under control, your muscles strong, and the use of stairs at a minimum, your knee will manage to survive intact. It does in about 80 percent of cases.

We hope that you don't think from the foregoing the knee is made up of just five bones and two hinges. Smooth movement happens because muscles are protected from rubbing against the knee bones and each other by the interposition of small lubricated cushions, or bursas. Bursitis of the knee is probably a more common cause for knee pain than arthritis. These sacs swell whenever pinched or irritated. Figure 10-2 shows the inner view of the knee and some of these bursas. Housemaid's knee, in which bursitis occurs out in front of the kneecap (Figure 10-3), is one of the few forms of bursitis in which you can actually see a swollen bursa.

Knee problems can be divided in a number of ways. If the lining membrane is involved; or if cartilage that lines the knee bones is fragmented and bone is exposed, we call the problem "arthritis." If the to-and-fro movement is impaired by loose fragments of bone or cartilage, the group of problems is known as "internal derange-

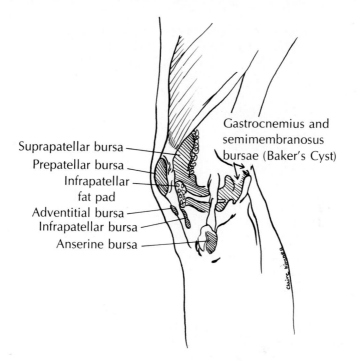

Figure 10-2.   Side view of the knee seen from the inner aspect.

ments." All the other problems, including those in the soft tissues surrounding the knee and also alignment problems, are called "non-articular" or "soft-tissue rheumatism." Arthritic knees can hurt as much if not more, it seems, than any other part of the body. One of our patients says her knees are a better indicator of coming rain than the television weather reporter. When the barometric pressure falls, a sharp ache occurs in her knees that often has her close to tears, she says. Pills do not help, but, fortunately, heat does.

When a knee gives you pain, buckles, gives way, pops, locks up, or swells, you have to decide first how serious it is. Listed at the end of this chapter are tables outlining danger signs for the knee (Table 10-1), self-examination techniques (Table 10-2), possible causes of discomfort and aggravating factors (Tables 10-3 and 10-4), commonsense solutions (Table 10-5), and helpful exercises designed to alleviate pain (Table 10-6). The following discussion will guide you through the maze of knee disorders and help you care for yourself. If you don't have any of the caution signs, chances are

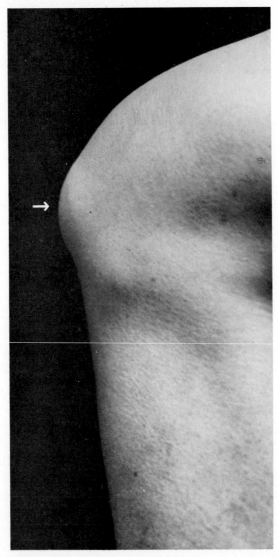

Figure 10-3.   Housemaid's knee (prepatellar bursitis). Note mild bulge of fluid-filled bursa.

good that you can treat the problem yourself. As you will learn, it does help to decide first whether the problem can be located above, in front of, below, or behind the knee. However, when the pain seems to be deep or all over the knee, you probably need profession-al help.

Arthritis of the Knee

So what! Most of us have it or will get it! *But* it doesn't bother 99 percent of the people who have it! The term "arthritis" should be reserved for knees in which cartilage is damaged or the joint membrane is inflamed and swollen. When x-rays show arthritis spurs or if the x-ray taken when standing demonstrates some loss of cartilage, it doesn't necessarily mean that these features of arthritis have anything to do with the pain in your knee. In fact, in one study, 35 percent of patients seen for knee arthritis and showing some x-ray changes of arthritis really had a soft-tissue reason for the pain; the arthritis was not causing symptoms! In fact, x-ray changes might confuse the doctor and lead to inappropriate treatment!

Arthritis is usually painful, and the knee is often tender along the inner joint line. Pain gets worse with walking but is relieved if you lie down. Swelling sometimes can be seen above the kneecap if your leg is not fat. The knee may feel warm to the touch. If it is very painful, get off your feet immediately, and stay off for a day or two. Apply ice to the knee for as long as you can stand it. Repeat the ice applications every few hours for a day or two.

DON Z.: SPORTS ADDICTION

Don Z. is a man in his midforties, an enthusiastic racket-ball player. Told by one of us (R.M.) that he must give up the sport, he refused to listen. Bothered by the intense pain the sport brought on, he then went from clinic to clinic where, much to his anger, he received the same advice. A real diehard, he played on and just blocked out the negative prognosis.

One weekend he went out of town, where he attended a cocktail party. Meeting a physician there, he did as a lot of us do; he couldn't resist asking about his health. For whatever reason (probably from not having all the facts), the doctor told him it was all right to continue racket ball.

The outcome? Knee surgery—much, much sooner than he would have needed it if he could have given up his addiction. We say addiction because participation by a certain type of individual in any of a number of sports can lead to addiction. Running is not the only trouble producer.

Perhaps the moral of Don Z.'s story is that advice obtained at a cocktail party may not be worth the liquid that writes it. Be careful. You may hear what you want to hear.

If you have arthritis, try to suppress the inflammation with anti-inflammatory medication. You can use various kinds of aspirin or ibuprofen products. Acetylsalicylic acid is aspirin. Compounds that contain only acetaminophen will not suppress inflammation but do relieve pain. If you don't tolerate aspirin or ibuprofen, you might try other types of salicylates such as magnesium salicylate or choline salicylates. Your pharmacist can help you choose one of these other salicylates that can help as much as aspirin.

If you are not better, then get crutches; either rent them or borrow a pair from the Arthritis Foundation, a Veterans of Foreign Wars (VFW) post, or elsewhere. To use crutches, place them about 12 inches in front and out to the side of each foot. When you are standing straight, the crutches should be about 2 inches below your armpits. Grip lightly at the handles, and keep the top of the crutch close into your chest. When you step forward with the right foot, get the left crutch out in front; lean on it while stepping forward onto the right foot. Then move the right crutch forward and swing the left leg forward, leaning onto the right crutch. Walk just as a horse does. Keep the involved knee stiff. If you have to use steps, go up with the good leg, then bring the bad leg up to the step, just as a child would climb the step, one at a time. If you don't have a bathroom facility on the first floor, get a portable commode and place it in an inconspicuous place such as a closet, so that you have to use steps only to get to and from bed.

Try to keep your muscles strong by performing exercise 1, Table 10-6. If you and your doctor agree that the problem is truly arthritis then, after the inflammation has subsided, learn all of the joint protection hints provided in Table 10-5 and apply them. Strengthen the leg further using exercise 2, Table 10-6. When strong and free of symptoms, you might keep up the strength by doing the weight lifts every 3 or 4 days, indefinitely. When away from home, you can keep the muscles strong, also. Whenever seated, try exercise 3. If your arthritic knee is unable to fully straighten, add exercise 7. Stretch the leg before getting up for the day and again before retiring. Then later in the morning strengthen one leg, and in the afternoon work the other leg, as discussed above.

If your self-examination reveals bowleg or knock-knee deformity, exercise might help. Some of our patients have had a modest improvement by using the bowleg or knock-knee exercise presented in Table 10-6, exercises 4 and 5. This should be done in addition to exercises 1, 2, and 3. When you exercise an arthritic knee, it will probably make some noise and hurt. As long as pain lasts less than half an hour afterward, you're safe to keep on. But if pain worsens, or if the knee seems stiffer, you should seek professional advice. Many patients ask about stationary-bicycle exercise. The same rules apply. If pain is worse after exercising, or if the knee stiffens, then this exercise isn't for you. Stair-climbing is *never* a good exercise for an arthritic knee. If you have arthritis or if the bulge test (Table 10-2, item 6) is positive, then please also read the last section of this chapter, When to Seek Professional Help.

Internal Knee Derangements

The most widely known internal knee derangement is the *football player's torn cartilage* (meniscus). Any of the internal knee derangements, such as when the "rocker panels" or other internal parts lock up, will interfere with walking. The knee may suddenly buckle or just give way. Or, when you get out of the car, your knee may not straighten. However, after jiggling or kicking, it then straightens. This is called "locking." It is like trying to close a door when a pencil is stuck between the door and the doorway at the hinge. Many other causes for locking or internal derangements are being discovered through *arthroscopy*. This new technique allows the doctor to see inside the knee with a small tubular scope attached to a video camera.

But this procedure should not be the first approach to an internal knee derangement. The procedure has some risks that can be worse than the original problem. If fluid has formed on the knee, then that will probably have to be drawn off and the knee may be injected with a cortisone mixture. The doctor may want to see if bleeding inside the knee has occurred. Bleeding within the knee signifies serious disturbance such as a ligament tear. But that is rarely found. With the same treatment as described here for arthritis, about 80 percent of these internal derangement conditions will resolve themselves.

Only if these conservative measures fail should arthroscopic examination and treatment be carried out. As we stated earlier, some of us think that the arthroscope is being used too often. But it is a major improvement over previous surgical treatments. Before the arthroscope, the knee had to be opened; and when it had healed, motion was often less than normal because of scar tissue. Not so with arthroscopic surgery. If your knee has been buckling or locking and particularly if the bulge test (item 6, Table 10-2) is positive, use crutches and see your doctor. If you are sent to an orthopedist and that physician wants to arthroscope your knee, ask, "What will you recommend if you don't find anything serious?" Then ask what is the harm of doing these measures first. However, if bleeding within the knee has occurred or if a loose bone chip can be seen on x-ray, arthroscopic treatment *should not* be put off.

Soft-Tissue Knee Disorders

Now we come to the largest group of knee problems, those disturbances of the soft tissues that surround the knee. These you can often prevent, and if they do occur, you can perhaps diagnose and treat the condition yourself. Please refer to Tables 10-3 and 10-4 again if your knee is acting up, and you don't seem to fit the symptoms of arthritis or an internal derangement. Here are some features that indicate that your knee problem is arising in the soft tissues:

1. Pain is worse after or during rest. The pain might awaken you from sleep (bursitis). Or the problem is most noticeable after sitting, when you first get up. Then it improves as you walk.
2. Walking helps, at first.
3. The knee looks normal, is not swollen, and has normal skin temperature.
4. An aggravating factor is likely.

The soft-tissue disorders of the knee will be discussed according to the location of knee disturbance.

Mary C.: Tripping the Light Fantastic!

Mary was first seen by one of us (R.P.S.) at age 48. An active woman, she looked and felt much younger. She exercised regularly to keep her slim, trim appearance. When she moved to her new split-level home, she began to use stairs much more frequently. Knitting was her favorite pastime, and she began making things for her grandchildren, often working many hours at a time. One day she noted an aching in the front of her knee and some swelling around it. Stairs had become a definite aggravation. Thinking that arthritis had begun, she sat longer, walked less, and tried to "favor" her knee. However, now both knees not only became painful, they also began to give way.

Mary's self-examination revealed swelling in the soft tissues just below the kneecap. A fat pad at this location can be squeezed by the kneecap during stair climbing or after squatting. This is what must have happened, because Mary had weakened the quadriceps muscle and had allowed it to shorten from sitting for long periods. The result was deterioration in the mechanics of knee movement. Had x-rays been taken, they might have shown some loss of cartilage and slight spur development; both would otherwise have been normal for her age. Simply having her avoid the stairs as much as possible and doing the knee-strengthening exercises proved helpful.

But our story doesn't end there. Eight years later Mary returned with a new problem. Her right knee was painful and awakened her each night. For the past month she had also noted the knee hurt when she began walking. She was now living in a one-floor home and had made certain she limited sitting time to about 30 minutes or less at a time. So, what could be the problem? The pain was along the inner aspect of the knee. No swelling was detected. The stress test (Table 10-2, item 5) suggested an injured medial collateral ligament, a knee "hinge." Mary and her husband had recently taken up square dancing. Although she did not recall a twisting injury, that type of injury can be a cause of her condition. Using a simple elastic support, strengthening the quadriceps muscle (Table 10-6, exercises 1 through 3), and learning to turn with her feet and not twist at the waist proved helpful. Mary recently wrote that she has "beaten" arthritis twice!

Pain at the Front of the Knee

Pain may be sent into the knee from a bad back or hip. A simple test is to lie down and raise the involved leg. Grasp behind the thigh with both hands and hold the thigh still at an approximately 45-degree angle. Now bend and straighten just the knee. If it seems normal, the problem is probably coming into the knee from above the knee. Here are some problems you can diagnose:

Tight thigh muscle or myofascial leg pain, sometimes called "cinema knee," is characterized by pain in front of the lower thigh and knee that is noted when you first arise from sitting. But because this pain gets better as you walk, it cannot be ascribed to arthritis. Rather, a likely cause is thigh and hip muscles tightened from prolonged sitting. It may happen after going on a long trip, playing cards, or after sitting in a movie. Both knees are usually involved. Figure 10-4 shows the location of a trigger point in the thigh muscle that sends a dull aching pain into the front of the knee. The Ober test, described in Table 10-2, item 7, demonstrates the method of reproducing the pain for diagnosis. When you perform this test, first draw the thigh as far backward as you can, then bend the knee as far as you can. You should feel the pain, and the thigh feels tight. Treatment is described in Table 10-6, exercise 6 and Figure 10-5. Make sure you don't sit longer than about 45 minutes. Get up and move about. The exercise should be continued for 2 or 3 weeks and performed whenever you sit for more than an hour.

If *bursitis or housemaid's knee* begins suddenly with redness, swelling, and severe pain, it demands immediate medical attention. An infection in the bursa can get into the underlying bone or can spread into the blood stream. Gout can also strike like this. But other cases of bursitis begin gradually with slight swelling, as can be seen in Figure 10-3. When the swelling occurs without tenderness or redness, you can apply ice overnight and avoid kneeling on your knee

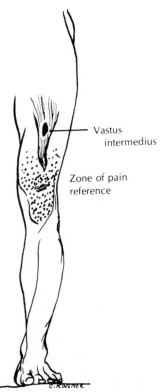

Vastus intermedius

Zone of pain reference

Figure 10-4.   Trigger-point location for myofascial knee pain (tight thigh muscle).

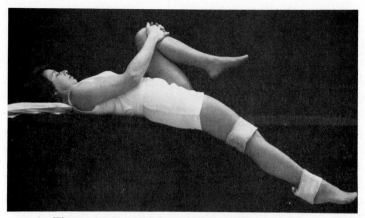

Figure 10-5.   Thigh stretch with leg weights.

caps. If you have a job that requires kneeling, try a kneeling pad. These can be obtained either at stores catering to workers (electricians usually know where to buy them) or at gardening or athletic supply stores. Some workers develop a very thickened and irritated bursa in front of the kneecap and may require surgical removal of the bursal sac.

Dancers and acrobats can so forcefully contract the thigh muscles that some muscle or tendon fibers of the thigh muscle rupture, resulting in a *quadriceps tear*. This causes swelling above the kneecap and loss of the ability to fully straighten the knee. Prompt, expert medical attention is mandatory.

Patellar-alignment problems occur when the kneecap draws sideward instead of forward, resulting in abnormal stress on the knee—particularly during stair-climbing. The test for this is detailed in Table 10-2, item 3. Can you feel the kneecap draw outward during the last part of the movement as the knee straightens? If so, you can sometimes decrease the pain and help your knee by strengthening the thigh muscle using Table 10-6, exercise 3. If that is pain-free, then proceed to exercise 2. But don't lift the weight fully straight. Avoid stairs as much as you can. If your kneecaps point outward as you walk ("grasshopper-eye" kneecaps) and pain persists, see your doctor. An operation can correct this alignment problem.

Other kneecap problems *(patellofemoral pain syndromes)* can begin under the kneecap. Arthritis can begin with irregular cartilage on the underside of the kneecap. Also, folds of the joint membrane *(plicae)* may develop there. When the kneecap is painful and you feel a grating sensation or noise as you arise from sitting, the problem is likely to be under the kneecap. Table 10-2, item 3, shows some of the tests you can do for the kneecap. These will reproduce the pain. Keep the thigh muscle strong by doing exercise 1, Table 10-6, until your doctor tells you it is all right to proceed to the more vigorous weight-lifting exercise (exercise 2). Avoid kneeling. Use a mop for floor scrubbing instead of getting down onto your hands and knees, or use a low mechanic's stool or a milking stool, with your legs apart. Then you can lean forward to scrub the corners or to pull weeds.

Stabbing, burning pain over the kneecap, called *prepatellar neuritis,* can follow an injury to the soft tissues and nerves in front of the kneecap. Ice may help. Most cases will subside in a week or so. If prolonged, see your doctor.

Just below the kneecap lies the patellar ligament that binds the lower end of the kneecap to the tibial bone. Sometimes a fat pad or the tendon becomes irritated, causing *tendinitis of the kneecap.* In track stars, this is known as "jumper's knee." The fat pad may swell along either side of the ligament, and you can feel a rubbery bulge on either side of the patellar ligament just below the kneecap. Pain is aggravated when you rise from a chair, climb steps, or squat. Sometimes walking may be difficult. Ice may help, along with avoiding prolonged sitting, climbing stairs, or squatting. The condition recovers very slowly.

Just below the kneecap is a small bony projection, the tibial tubercle, that can be very painful in children (*Osgood-Schlatter disease*). In adults, bursitis can develop over the tubercle. Apply ice and avoid kneeling if you have this problem. Pain on either side of the tubercle (about 3 inches below the knee, in front of the leg) that is worse when first arising from sitting, and better when walking, may arise from tight hamstrings behind the thigh. See the next section.

We have already mentioned jumper's knee, but pain can result from *overload syndrome,* any excessive load placed upon the knee. Dancing, twisting, pivoting (as in golf), jumping (as in basketball or volleyball or on a trampoline), and running are just some of the causes of knee-joint strain. If you are loose-jointed, as described in Chapter 7, you must maintain very strong thigh muscles to participate in sport activities. Also, if your knees bow backward when you stand "straight," you should slightly bend your knee forward while standing still.

Pain on the Inner Side of the Knee

We have already discussed arthritis and internal-knee derangements that cause pain when you walk. The soft tissues that lie along but to the outside of the knee joint, on the inner side, include the medial collateral ligament, or knee hinge, and the anserine bursa. Many middle-aged women develop a big pad of fat over the inner side of the knee, and this pad may become very painful. Often a bursitis develops within the fat. If you have a painful, fat knee, squeeze the fat pad from front to back, with your thumb at the front of the pad, and your fingers behind the pad. If the squeeze is exquisitely painful, you probably have a bursitis. See discussion of *anserine bursitis* below.

Ligament strain is incurred when the inner knee hinge is stretched. This is often a result of sitting with a leg tucked under your body, sitting cross-legged, or twisting the body to the side instead of turning with the feet. People with loose-jointedness are more prone to this problem. The stress test, as described in Table 10-2, item 5, which draws the foreleg away from the midline, will stretch the ligament and aggravate the pain. Treatment includes wrapping the knee with an elastic bandage or using a tubular elastic knee support and strengthening the thigh muscles as prescribed in Table 10-6, exercises 1 through 3.

When the knee pain awakens you, and it is at the inner aspect of the knee, *anserine bursitis* is a likely cause. Often it is associated with a ligament strain. Treat it as described above for ligament strain. In addition, apply ice several times a day and try aspirin or ibuprofen. Your doctor can try more potent anti-inflammatory drugs or inject the tissue with procaine and long-acting corticosteroid.

Persistent pain at the inner aspect of the knee may be due to arthritis of the hip or to bones rubbing together from arthritis. The Patrick test for hip arthritis should be done (see Chapter 9). If pain does not seem improved and if walking is painful, then your doctor will need an x-ray of the knee or pelvis or both and sometimes even a bone scan of the knee.

Pain Behind the Knee

If the knee won't fully straighten, or if you can feel a swelling the size of an egg behind the knee, you need expert medical attention. Arthritis and a *Baker's cyst* are likely. Figure 10-6 shows Dr. W. M. Baker's original report from 1877. A Baker's cyst can develop from the knee joint and rupture into the tissues behind the knee joint. If

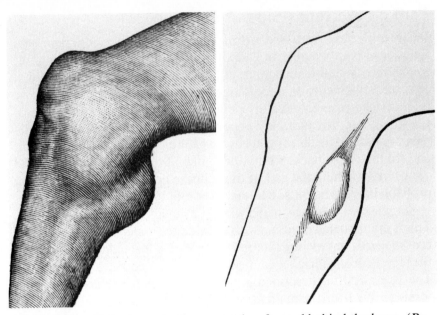

Figure 10-6.   Baker's cyst: a large cyst has formed behind the knee. (*Reprinted from the original report by W. M. Baker, Saint Bartholomew's Hospital Reports, London, 1877.*)

you notice this, avoid squatting, heavy lifting, or climbing steps until you see your doctor. The cyst can rupture further into the lower leg and calf. If it does, the entire lower leg will swell and become inflamed. The problem also occurs in children who suffer a form of childhood arthritis. Sometimes only one knee will be affected. Parents may not notice the problem, or the child simply develops a limp. Suddenly, the leg is feverish and swollen. The knee may no longer be swollen if the cyst ruptures. These children should be considered as having had arthritis because they are at risk of developing a painless inflammation inside the eye that can lead to blindness. Baker's cyst is also a common complication of arthritis in the elderly. Rupture may be mistaken for phlebitis or bad veins.

Inflammation of the tendons behind the lower thigh, called *hamstring tendinitis,* may cause pain behind the knee and also in the front of the upper foreleg. The pain worsens after rest or after sitting. Walking may be a little difficult. The simple test that stretches the hamstrings is detailed in Table 10-2, item 4. As the leg is pulled straight and upward, the hamstrings will feel tight, not normal.

While you are pulling the leg as high up as you can, have a helper poke into the muscles behind the middle-thigh region. Three hamstring muscles lie behind the thigh, and one or more may be very painful. Treatment consists of local heat followed by stretching as presented in Table 10-6, exercise 7. Later, strengthening of the hamstrings can be carried out as detailed in exercise 8.

ROGER R.: AN INCORRECT DIAGNOSIS OF JUVENILE ARTHRITIS

Roger R. was first seen by one of us (R.P.S.) when he was 10 years old and not very happy. Roger had been diagnosed previously as having rheumatoid arthritis. Although there had never been any swelling in his legs, he did have pain in and around the joints. Roger, of course, could not participate in any physical education classes or play at any sports. The previous doctor had further predicted that Roger would be plagued by arthritis all his life.

It did not seem to Dr. S. that this was a true case of arthritis, and he felt it was probable that Roger had shortened hamstrings. Tests proved that this was correct. Together, Roger and the doctor set about stretching those hamstrings. Roger was very diligent in doing his exercises, and he was soon getting around much better, and without pain.

There is a happy postscript to this story. When Roger was 28 he was written up in *Time* for his efforts on behalf of nature conservation; and a recent news photo showed Roger on a water tower, unfurling banners for an organization dedicated to saving the whales and seals.

A major nerve trunk lies behind the knee and can be easily injured by sitting on a sharp-edged counter or tufted chair, resulting in *nerve palsy.* Some cases have resulted from prolonged use of a recliner chair. When the nerve has been damaged, the lower leg becomes partly paralyzed; the foot dangles, and it cannot be raised at the ankle. Pain behind the knee is also common. You should see your doctor if this has happened to you.

Outer-Thigh and Knee Pain

A dense band separates the front thigh muscles from the hamstring and other muscles behind the thigh. This *iliotibial band* and another tissue, the *fascia lata,* can be irritated, scarred, or inflamed (Figure 10-7). Runners commonly develop inflammation that causes pain and a noisy sound along the outer side of the knee during knee movement. The sound is similar to that produced by rubbing a wet finger

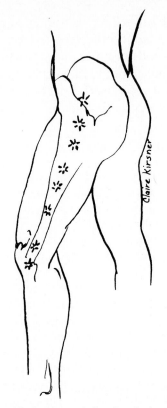

Figure 10-7.   Site of irritation of the fascia lata and iliotibial band.

on a balloon. When these outer-thigh tissues are stretched, a pulling sensation is felt in the band. The treatment includes rest and stretching as described in Table 10-6, exercise 9.

Pain and tenderness over the outer knee joint can result from many disorders. If the tissue is tender to light touch, a *fibular bursitis* may be present. Simply protecting the knee with an elastic tubular splint and walking with a stiff knee may help. Other possibilities include a *sprained ligament* or an *internal knee derangement*.

When to Seek Professional Help

Any feature listed in Table 10-1 should send you right to the doctor; on the other hand, if the problem began slowly and then worsened with painful walking or swelling, you should also get competent medical advice.

When the joint swells, the fluid may have to be removed. Arthritis-joint fluid is loaded with chemicals and enzymes that result in further damage. The fluid should be removed if the knee has remained swollen for a week or longer. But the fluid will return if the inflammation is not suppressed. Nonsteroidal anti-inflammatory drugs can help. If fluid is drained, a shot of cortisone can block the fluid formation for many weeks and allow healing to occur. If you have a shot of cortisone into the joint, don't stress the joint for at least 2 weeks or you can cause *painless damage*! Analysis of the joint fluid is necessary in order to diagnose many kinds of arthritis, particularly gouty arthritis. But, more importantly, if fever or redness is present, the fluid should be analyzed for infection.

Sometimes a diagnosis is not easy, and you may have to visit the doctor during the times when the knee is acting up. A torn cartilage cannot be diagnosed by x-ray unless dye is first instilled. This technique, called *arthrography,* is less risky than arthroscopy, but often arthroscopy will still have to be performed. In rare cases a bone scan will show arthritis that can't be detected by other means.

The problem of a persistently painful knee, with normal x-rays, is not rare. Make sure you are not causing the problem. See Tables 10-3 and 10-4 for possible causes of persistent knee pain.

You may be referred to a physical therapist who can help you get into an exercise program if pain is severe, if weakness is severe, or if a knee is injured. Exercise that is gradually increased and frequently monitored can achieve good results in most cases.

Once you have improved, look over Table 10-5 and make sure you use good body mechanics. Stop pushing yourself up from a chair. Avoid stairs when possible. Reduce your weight if you are significantly overweight. Wear shoes with shock-absorbing soles.

Sylvia K. and Rachel M.: Bad Knees Can Be Like Prison

Sylvia K., 86, is R.M.'s patient. Ordinarily, she is a happy, purposeful, delightful, insightful woman, but she suffers from severe osteoarthritis of the knees. Having gone through all the stages of discomfort that aching arthritic knees can bring, she has become increasingly more limited in her movements and now, in fact, must use a walker.

When she was asked what the pain in her knees was like, she answered so promptly that it was obvious she had been making the comparison for some time, "It's like prison!—just like the concentration camp I was in in Poland. I thought I was free. I have loved my freedom, and now I am in prison again."

There is much poignancy in this woman's story, and her doctor has great feeling for her, but there is little to be done to comfort her, except for strong pain pills and anti-inflammatory agents. Like most of us, she would be much happier if she could be more active. She has always wanted to do all she can—and every day. The only positive factor is that she was in her late seventies before she was so severely limited. You may wonder if her poor knees are the result of conditions in the concentration camp. The doctors think it unlikely, although the cold and deprivation and the poor and inadequate food certainly didn't help. Unfortunately, Sylvia K.'s heart disease prevents her from having knee surgery.

Perhaps while we are on the subject of knees, a word of caution is in order. Those of you who do have bad knees probably have a list of things that intensify the pain. Certainly humidity and barometric pressure can add greatly to your discomfort. So, too, can overuse. One of our patients, Rachel M., learned a very painful lesson several Decembers ago. She is an avid shopper, who has a gift list that reaches from Bloomingdale's to Harrod's and who greatly loves everything about the Christmas season; but she suddenly found herself grounded one Christmas Day. She had spent almost the entire day with a heating pad on her propped-up knees. Now, much wiser, she buys gifts throughout the year and limits her holiday gallivanting to those things which are most meaningful to her and which bring others and herself the most enjoyment.

As we have said before, the knee is a very complicated joint, which can take a lot of punishment. But sometimes enough is enough, and even fantastically constructed mechanisms give way in the face of excessive wear. How fortunate we are that, in most people, parts of the knee can be replaced.

However, if you are one of those who are "born to shop," be sensible. Stop for a cup of tea in the store's restaurant. Or why not plan to interrupt your foray with lunch or a shampoo and set? Remember, too, what we said earlier about people who say they'll finish a task if it kills them. It seems there are also people who will always want—and try—to do one more thing. The Type A person is alive, but perhaps not flourishing.

Table 10-1
Danger Signs in the Knee and Thigh

Warmth and redness
Weight loss, fever, night pain
Regional lymph-gland swelling
Loss of thigh-muscle size above knee
Positive stress test
Excess motion from side to side during stress test
Limb discoloration (dusky blue or pale)
Increasing pain during walking
Locking and buckling while walking or arising from sitting position
Numbness, tingling, and weakness
Swelling of the knee

Table 10-2
Self-Examination of the Knee and Thigh

1. Stand with bare legs about 20 feet from a full-length mirror. Walk slowly forward and look at the appearance of your legs in the mirror. Are they straight? Is the muscle mass of each thigh similar? Watch the kneecaps. Do they point straight forward or tip outward or inward? If they do not point straight ahead, a faulty alignment (torsion) is likely, and predisposes you to arthritis.

2. Stand sideways to the mirror and straighten legs fully. Do your legs arch backward? This indicates loose-jointedness (see Chapter 7).

3. Sit down. Lift one leg from the floor while keeping your fingers on the kneecap as the leg straightens. Is there grating, popping, or deviation of the kneecap to the outside as the leg straightens? Do you feel a rubbery swelling just below the kneecap on each side of the midline? This suggests a swollen fat pad. Repeat the leg lift with more pressure on the kneecap, pressing it into the knee. Does this cause a lot of pain? Now from the sitting position, put your hands on your thighs and stand up. Can you do it or is there significant thigh-muscle weakness? This weakness will lead to worse arthritis pain.

4. Lie on your back and take a 4-foot length of cord or rope. Loop it over your toes and the ball of one foot. Now put your leg straight up, slowly, keeping the other leg slightly bent at the knee. Can you pull the leg straight up overhead? Does this cause numbness and

(continued)

tingling or pain in the kneecap? Can you lift your leg 90 degrees upward? If not, tight hamstrings may be your problem. Repeat with the other leg (Figure 10-8).

5. Have a helper assist you with the stress test. Lie on your back and have the helper place one hand on the outer side of your knee and the other hand on your foreleg. She or he pulls your leg away from the midline while holding the knee stationary (Figure 10-9). Does this cause pain on the inner side or the outer side of the knee? Now place one hand on the inner side of the knee; hold to keep knee from moving and push foreleg toward the midline. Does this cause pain on either side of the knee? Was there any rocking of the foreleg on the thigh, demonstrating looseness of the knee joint? The ligaments may need extra support (gained by doing weighted leg lifts, as in Table 10-6, exercise 2).

6. To perform the bulge test, lie with your leg out straight and have the helper place his or her thumb on the inner side of the kneecap and forefinger on the outer side of the kneecap. Then with the other hand placed just above the kneecap, have your helper press down over the upper knee and feel for bulging along the sides of the kneecap. Any bulging suggests arthritis of the knee.

7. To test for pain in your thighs, lie on your side, both knees drawn up slightly. Grasp the ankle of your upper leg. If you can't reach it, then first make two turns of a 4-foot rope around the ankle and grab hold of both ends with your upper hand. Now, before pulling, move the knee backward, pushing the thigh backward as far as you can, then slowly pull the foreleg, bending the knee (Figure 10-10). The hip should let the thigh travel slightly backward. Does this cause significant pain in the thigh just above the knee? If so, a trigger point in the thigh (myofascial knee pain) may need treatment.

Table 10-3

Possible Causes of Knee and Thigh Pain

Complaint	Possible Cause
Pain above kneecap	Shortened thigh muscles (quadriceps)
Painful kneecap, no swelling	Patellofemoral knee-pain syndrome; overload syndromes
Painful swelling over kneecap	Housemaid's knee
Painful swelling around knee	Arthritis or gout

Complaint	Possible Cause
Pain just below kneecap	Tendinitis
Pain below the knee	Short hamstring
Pain and buckling	Internal derangement of knee
Locking of knee	Torn cartilage
Night pain, inner side of knee	Bursitis
Constant pain on inner side of knee and thigh	Referred pain from a bad hip
Pain only while walking	Arthritis
Pain only when arising from chair or using stairs	Myofascial thigh pain or ligament injury
Swelling behind knee	Baker's cyst
Stinging pain over knee	Neuralgia
Pain on the outer side of knee	Fibular bursitis; iliotibial band friction syndrome; fascia lata fasciitis
Knee won't straighten fully	Arthritis

Table 10-4

Habits That Cause Persistent Knee and Thigh Pain

Complaint	Aggravating Habit
Pain at night in knee	Bursitis or ligament irritation from twisting or sitting cross-legged
Pain when arising but not while walking	Prolonged sitting that allows shortening of thigh muscles
Pain while walking	Decompensated knee arthritis due to pushing off from chairs
Swelling in front of knee	Getting down on hands and knees
Swelling behind knee	Repeated squatting
Neuralgia in front of knee	Falling on kneecap; auto injury in which kneecap struck dashboard
Locking and buckling	Twisting injury to knee
Ligament looseness	Sitting with leg tucked under you

Table 10-5

What's Harmful, What's Helpful for the Knee and Thigh

Harmful	Helpful
Pushing off from chairs with the hands wastes the quadriceps muscle.	Keep the hands in the lap when rising from a sitting position.
Repetitively twisting the knee while dancing or exercising can damage it.	Modify or avoid knee-twisting dance steps and exercises.
For some persons, bicycling can strain the knee.	Pace bicycling if it causes knee pain.
Engaging in sport activities on an occasional or weekend basis without proper conditioning or warm-up is potentially harmful to the knee.	Engage in sport activities regularly to stay in condition. Do warm-up exercises.
Climbing stairs repeatedly is irritating to the knee.	Limit stair climbing. If lack of a toilet on the first floor necessitates stair climbing, one solution is to place a portable commode somewhere on the first floor.
Sitting for prolonged periods allows the muscles behind the knee to tighten up.	Limit sitting to 30 minutes; then move around.
Having certain foot disorders can result in poor alignment of the leg bones, which in turn affects the knee.	Consult a physician.
Wearing shoes having worn-down heels can aggravate knee problems.	Buy shoes with proper heels and check them for signs of excessive wear.
Working on the hands and knees on a hard surface can result in bursitis in the front of the knee. Also known as water on the knee and housemaid's knee, this swelling is visible in front of the kneecap.	Instead of working on the hands and knees, use a mechanic's or milker's stool; either one sits low to the ground. Sit with the legs apart and reach forward to perform, with little effort, such tasks as gardening and washing floors.

Table 10-6
Exercises for the Knee and Thigh

1. *Bed exercise for very debilitated or recently injured person:* Place
    a rolled towel beneath the knee and press your straight leg down
    against the towel, using a maximum quadriceps contraction. Hold
    for 5 seconds; repeat 10 to 100 times. Do one leg at a time.

2. *Knee-strengthening with weights:* Sit on a hard chair or on the
    edge of a firm bed with knees just over the edge and with a firm
    rolled towel under the lower thigh. Add weights to your foreleg
    (beginning with a 1- to 5-pound weight); place a towel over the
    foreleg above the ankle, with weights on top of the towel. You
    can make weights by stuffing a plastic bag into a tube sock, then
    filling it with sand, gravel, or buckshot. Drape the weight over the
    lower leg or ankle. If you are long-legged, stack two telephone
    books (2 inches each) under your heel so your foot is about 4
    inches from the floor. Lift your foot slowly but not as far as to
    straighten it. Hold for a count of five. Repeat for 5 minutes. Begin
    with weights of from 1 to 5 pounds and increase them to 20
    pounds as strength permits (Figure 10-11).

3. *Strengthening exercise for the knee:* Sit on a chair with knees
    bent and with feet resting about 2 feet out from the chair. Cross
    good leg over bad, at the ankle. Now attempt to raise the bad leg
    against the good one. But resist the upward thrusting leg with the
    other leg. No actual motion takes place. Hold for 10 seconds and
    repeat for 5 minutes. If both legs are bad, later in the day you
    should repeat the exercise with the bad leg over the good leg.

4. *Bowleg exercise:* Place a plastic wastebasket between your ankles
    while you are lying down on your back. Squeeze your legs
    together, trying to crush the wastebasket. Hold for 20 seconds;
    repeat 10 times.

5. *Knock-knee exercise:* Make a loop of a 4-inch elastic bandage and
    loop it around your ankles, which should be about 6 inches apart.
    Safety-pin it to make it permanent. While lying flat, draw both
    legs apart against the loop for 10 seconds and then repeat 10 times
    twice daily.

6. *Thigh stretch:* Lie at the edge of a bed and apply 2-pound weights
    just above your knee and at your ankle. Draw the other knee
    toward your chest and hang the weighted leg off one side of the
    bed with the knee straight. Allow the weights to stretch your leg
    for 3 minutes. Repeat twice daily (Figure 10-5).

(continued)

7. *Hamstring and leg stretch:* Lie on your back with the legs bent at the knee, feet to the floor. Raise one leg and loop a 4-foot length of rope under your toes; pull the leg straight up. Slowly increase the pull and direct the leg higher, or toward your head. Hold 1 minute with increased forward pull every 10 seconds. Then repeat with the other leg. Repeat the exercise twice daily (Figure 10-8).

8. *Hamstring strengthening:* Strap 3- to 10-pound weights on your ankles and lie face down with your feet hanging off the end of the bed. Lift a leg, bending the knee. Keep your thigh in contact with the bed. Draw the foreleg back toward 90 degrees and return slowly to straight position. Repeat 30 times; then do the other leg.

9. *Iliotibial band stretch:* Fill a sock or purse with 3 to 5 pounds of stones, buckshot, or any substance available. Attach this bag to your involved leg, just above the ankle. You can tie it on with an old stocking. Now lie on your uninvolved (pain-free) side close to the edge of a bed. Keep your lower leg bent and your upper knee straight. Hang your upper leg out over the side of the bed, and let the weight pull the leg toward the floor for 3 minutes twice daily (Figure 10-12).

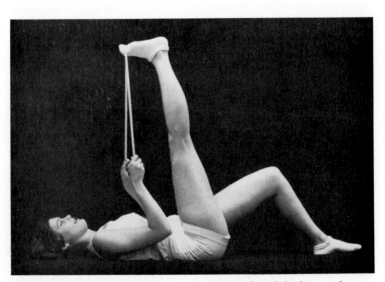

Figure 10-8.   Rope test and treatment for tight hamstring.

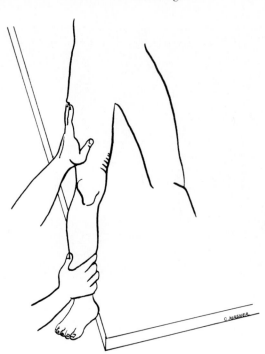

Figure 10-9.　Stress test.

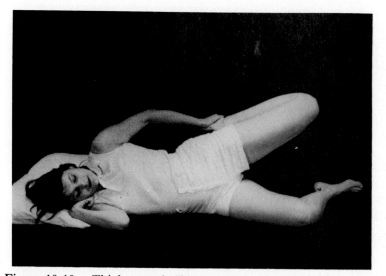

Figure 10-10.　Thigh stretch (Ober test) for tight thigh muscles.

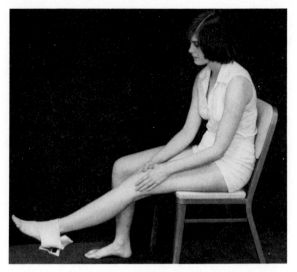

Figure 10-11.   Weight-lifting knee exercise.

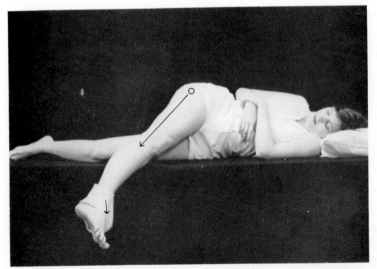

Figure 10-12.   Technique to stretch the fascia lata and iliotibial band.

CHAPTER 11

The Foreleg, Ankle, and Foot

Whether you are into sports activities that produce an impact load onto the foot (such as volleyball or running) or you weigh too much and stand on concrete for long periods of time, the result is *cumulative overload strain*. Then, if you wear worn-down or poorly fitting shoes, foot pain or deformity can and will result. Shoes were meant to cover and protect the foot, not to disturb it. When a woman with bunions and calluses walks into our office in high-heeled and narrow, pointed shoes *and* superfluously says, "My feet are killing me!" we marvel at her debt to vanity. Another example of self-mutilation is the runner or calisthenics addict who has developed serious ankle arthritis and wants it fixed so he can continue exercising!

This chapter will also help those of you with leg cramps, heel pain, burning feet, and other common afflictions of the lower leg and foot. However, curing these examples of overload strain or improper footwear will require behavior modification to protect the feet and not to abuse them. Listed at the end of this chapter are tables outlining danger signs for the foreleg, ankle, and foot (Table 11-1), self-examination techniques (Table 11-2), possible causes of discomfort and aggravating factors (Tables 11-3 and 11-4), commonsense solutions (Table 11-5), helpful exercises (Table 11-6), and shoe modifications (Table 11-7) designed to alleviate pain.

Lower-Leg Problems

Before we jump into your possible problems, a brief review of basics is in order. The shinbone is the *tibia,* and out to the side and deep in the muscles in the outer leg is the *fibula.* The round bone at your outer ankle is the lower end of the fibula. See Plates 11-1 and 11-2 and Figure 11-1.

Most of the leg muscles have tendons that pass downward into the foot. The tendons are easily injured where they pass the ankle. Arthritic conditions of the ankle often afflict tendons as well. Arthritis swelling will be present all the time, particularly troublesome in the morning. If you have swollen ankles only at night and they don't hurt when you walk, that is *not* arthritis. More than likely swelling is due to problems that cause fluid retention. Similarly, arthritis causes pain but *not* numbness and tingling. These result from pinched nerves, although the pinching can also result from swollen tendons, bursitis, or bony enlargement. Bad veins may cause calf pain that occurs when standing or walking but is relieved by resting and elevating the leg. People with bad veins can develop brown, thick skin above the ankle. When a vein clots, thrombophlebitis may result in tenderness and deep calf-muscle pain that increases with walking. See Table 11-1 for danger signs.

Ligaments hold the bones together, and the ligament at the outer ankle is the weakest and most likely injured. Once you have twisted and thus sprained an ankle, further injury is likely, particularly if you are loose-jointed. Beneath the inner ankle ligament lies a tarsal tunnel through which many tendons, blood vessels, and nerves pass into the foot. This tarsal tunnel lies just below the round inner ankle bone. A pinched nerve or nerves in the tunnel results in pain and numbness in the bottom of the foot (Figure 11-2). More about that later. The foot regions to be considered include the hindfoot and heel, the midfoot, the forefoot and metatarsal area, and the toes. The eight bones of the ankle meet the leg bones on top and the five metatarsal foot bones below. The *plantar fascia* is a thick fibrous tissue that runs along the bottom of the foot and attaches to the toes in front and to a broad, spurlike ridge across the heel.

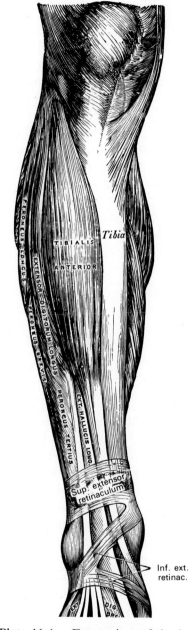

Plate 11-1.   Front view of the leg.

Compartment Syndrome

The muscles of the inner and outer foreleg are encased in snug compartments, with blood flow dependent upon normal pressure within each compartment. When you injure one or another of these compartments, the accumulation of blood and fluid or the resulting swollen muscles will send the compartment pressure shooting up. At a certain point the pressure stops the flow of blood, and the nerves and muscles within the compartment begin to "scream" for help. Similarly, overuse in sports can also lead to muscle swelling that sends the pressure up. The resulting distress is known as a *compartment syndrome*. The main features of this are:

1. *Pain*. This may occur anywhere, but it is usually over the shin bone at either side.
2. *Pallor*. The foot loses some of its blood supply and turns grayish white.
3. *Paralysis*. The foot won't respond well to your attempts to move it.

These serious features may begin within 12 hours after injury or overuse. See Table 11-1 and Chapter 14.

Shin Splints

This term can mean different things to different doctors, but in general shin splints are a painful condition at the inner aspect of the leg below the knee. This pain follows overload from running, jogging, dancing, or carrying heavy packages for long distances without resting. The problem is that the cause can be as minor as muscle strains or as major as a fractured tibia. People with flatfeet (weak arches) tend to get more strain in the foreleg muscles; this can result in shin splints caused by swelling of the membrane where muscles attach to bone. Sometimes people with flatfeet may have no problems. However, when they do, the foreleg muscles can be very sore for long periods of time because of the overwork of the inner foreleg muscles in supporting the long foot arch.

Prolonged standing on a new job can lead to shin splints in a flat-footed person. This is the pain in the anterior tibial compartment. Figure 11-3 shows what flatfeet look like when observed from the back. Untrained and underdeveloped muscles can easily be in-

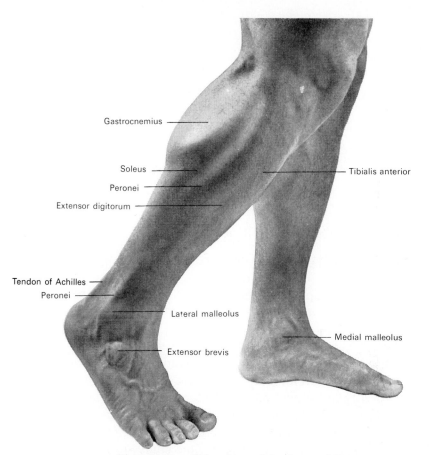

Plate 11-2.   Side view of the leg and foot.

jured by beginning joggers or runners. Shin splints do not lead to a compartment syndrome. The pain should subside with rest, warmth, and massage. The foot color and movement should not be affected. If pain on standing continues, and if tenderness is detected on the tibial bone just below the knee along the inner aspect, you could have a *stress fracture*. These don't show up on x-ray until several weeks after the stress; a bone scan may be necessary. So, foreleg pain that does quiet down with rest is nature's way of telling you to "cool it." If you are into sports or calisthenics or other activities that require much repetitious leg movement during weight bearing, then you will have to exercise and warm up before the activity. Table 11-6, exercise 4, is good for the foreleg. If you work on concrete, be sure to wear shock-absorbing soles with a comfortable arch and

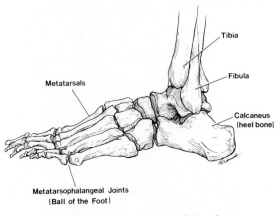

Figure 11-1.   Bones of the foot.

fit. If you are moving to a condo or apartment with a concrete floor, try wearing running shoes in the house. Avoid going barefoot or wearing sandals or slippers. If the pain does not subside promptly, contact your physician.

Leg Cramps

Those of us who are seized with agonizing pain in leg or foot muscles are mostly silent sufferers. Only our spouses know what agony we go through. Muscle cramps can involve large thigh muscles, foreleg muscles, or the very small midfoot muscles. Cases of fractured leg bones resulting from a cramp have been reported! Crampers are either day crampers or night crampers. One study suggests that leg

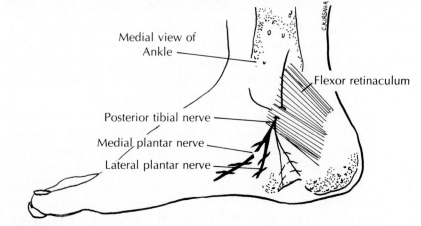

Figure 11-2.   Location of nerve compression for tarsal-tunnel syndrome.

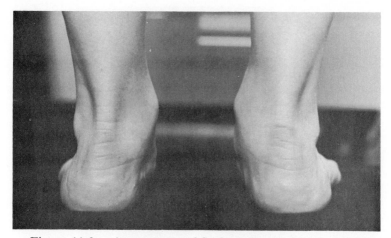

Figure 11-3.   Appearance of flatfeet viewed from behind.

cramp is inherited, and those who cramp in the night tend to have other family members who similarly cramped at night. Also, day crampers tend to come from families who cramped in the daytime. Just what causes cramp and why only some of us are so predisposed is unknown. Some conditions that aggravate cramping include low potassium, calcium, or magnesium; use of diuretics (water pills); and some rare nerve and muscle diseases. Wearing flat slippers may also be at fault. But for most of us there is no simple answer. However, you can often prevent cramp by performing a simple exercise, first described by Dr. H. W. Daniell in California. It is shown in Figure 11-4 and described in Table 11-6, exercise 1. If leg cramps persist, then you can try a number of medicines containing quinine (available by prescription or over-the-counter). Often they need be taken only for a week or so, then saved. Cramps tend to occur in sieges, lasting just a few days followed by long cramp-free intervals.

Growing pains in children are practically never due to growth spurts; they occur more often at times not related to growth. Probably they represent leg cramp. Some are due to juvenile arthritis in which the swollen joints are not always noticed. If your child has leg pain and arises with stiffness or a limp, then please have your doctor carefully examine the child's joints for swelling.

Restless Legs

Do you fall asleep only to have your legs suddenly kick out at your bed partner? This jerking is common after age 50 and is known as

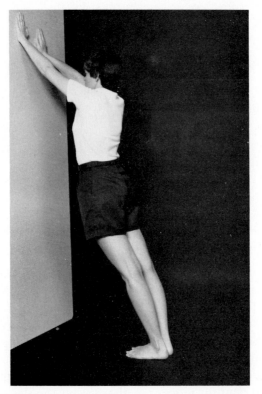

Figure 11-4.   Daniell leg stretch for leg cramp.

myoclonic movement. It is gaining interest among researchers. But more distressing to some people of all ages is painless, uncontrolled leg movements when trying to fall asleep. These restless leg movements get worse the more you try to stop them! Sometimes the cause is caffeine sensitivity, anxiety, fatigue, or medical conditions such as low blood sugar, diabetes, low thyroid, and conditions that result in kidney failure or anemia. Sometimes the leg-stretch exercise will help (Table 11-6, exercises 1 and 2). Try avoiding all dark beverages for several weeks. It may just eliminate those restless legs.

Leg and Ankle Bumps and Nodules

Erythema nodosum or *erythema annulare* are red, painful, nodular swellings in front of cr behind the leg that can result from a wide variety of nonmalignant medical disorders ranging from a strep infection to tuberculosis. The doctor will have to do some extensive investigations, including throat and nose cultures for strep, skin tests, a chest x-ray, and blood tests. These will depend upon where you live. Coccidioidomycosis (desert fever), histoplasmosis, and sarcoidosis occur in certain regions of the country.

Surfer's nodules are painful bumps over the front of the leg and foot. Similar nodules can develop in children who play on hardwood floors with their feet and forelegs resting against the floor while seated with their legs bent underneath.

Pump bumps are hard swellings of the hindfoot just above the heel. If you have a heel bone that has an enlarged angular bony prominence, you are more likely to be bothered. Loafers, moccasins, pumps, or shoes with stiff or high counters (the back wall of the shoe) can induce pressure or friction on the hindfoot at the Achilles tendon. The resulting callus can be very painful. Sometimes, a bursa may form beneath the skin and can become acutely swollen. Treatment includes measures to reduce friction by wearing laced, well-fitting shoes; placing strips of adhesive-backed foam rubber on the shoe counter at each side in order to hold the shoe a bit away from the pressure point or cutting a V-shaped notch at the contact point; and wearing lower-heeled shoes.

Ankle Arthritis and Tendon Injury

Loose-jointedness or previously injured ankles can predispose you to arthritis; if you twist your ankle, take the following precautions. First, if it is swollen, follow the RICE program:

Rest: If necessary, use crutches until walking is not painful.

Ice: Apply ice often until swelling has subsided. Aspirin, ibuprofen, or prescription nonsteroidal anti-inflammatory drugs can help.

Compression: When the swelling has subsided, begin elastic support. A simple tubular ankle elastic support is available from a pharmacy. Some are sewn in a figure-eight style. Choose whichever looks and feels most comfortable.

Elevation: Raise the injured ankle to just above heart level to reduce swelling and improve blood flow.

Begin conditioning the ankle as soon as the swelling has subsided. Try the ankle-rotating exercise shown in Figure 11-5 and described in

Table 11-6, exercise 4. You can do a further exercise by placing a 2-foot board across a rolling pin; step up on this and rock from side to side. One minute for each exercise several times a day should help. As soon as you can walk without the ankle hurting, begin a slow run in 10-foot circles. Before further jogging, perform the test in Table 11-2, item 3. If the injured ankle has more movement than the good ankle, running or contact sports may be hazardous. Consult your physician.

Osteoarthritis rarely afflicts the ankle unless the joint has been seriously injured. Rheumatoid arthritis more often strikes at the tendons than the actual joint. But only a careful examination by an experienced doctor can determine whether it's the joint or tendons that are swollen. Whichever it is, the swelling will be present when you arise after sleep, and the joint will hurt when you first step on it. You can treat it with the RICE routine if it is very painful, at least until you can see your doctor. As treatment takes effect, exercises are important. Begin with Table 11-6, exercises 2 and 4. Your doctor may use a commercial ankle support that laces and can be worn inside a shoe or a custom brace similar to the old polio ankle braces. Sometimes, a custom-fitted shoe insert that supports the foot can provide comfortable walking.

Once an x-ray shows that there is arthritis in the ankle joint,

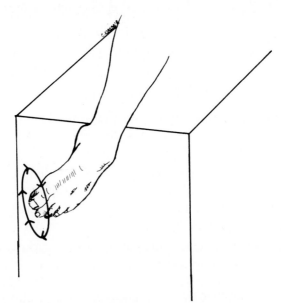

Figure 11-5.   Ankle-rotating exercise.

improvement is not likely. The best thing that you can do is prevent more damage by avoiding cumulative-impact load as in jumping, climbing, or twisting the ankle. This can also happen in square dancing. The use of artificial ankle joints has not proved consistently useful at this time.

Tendinitis in the ankle is marked by friction or inflammation and can result in swelling of the tubular tendon sheaths surrounding the tendons. The ankle feels stiff and a bit painful. Swelling, which can be felt as a sausagelike thickening under the bony prominence of either ankle, may develop. And it may extend part way above the ankle. The first few steps are often painful. You can use the RICE treatment regimen and also deep ice massage. Grasp an ice cube with a towel or make an ice cone using a paper cup filled with water, pinched at the top, and then frozen. Apply the corner of the ice to the tendon area and deeply rub over the tendon for several minutes; repeat the treatment four or more times daily for a few days.

Any failure of this treatment is a sign of possible serious ankle problems. An experienced physician should be consulted (Table 11-1).

The heel cord, or Achilles tendon, has a tendency to strain and rupture, resulting in *Achilles tendinitis*. If you cannot stand on your toes, see your doctor immediately. If the tendon is swollen but seems intact, try the RICE treatment and use several heel pads in your shoes to elevate the involved heel at least 1/4 inch. Later, try Table 11-6, exercise 3.

Heel Pain

Pain behind the heel or around the back edge of the heel results from problems in the lower leg or tendon structures, whereas pain at the bottom of the heel often comes from foot strain. Inflammatory arthritis disorders often involve the soft tissue behind and along the sides of the heel. Arthritis rarely strikes the underside of the heel. Also, arthritis will cause stiffness when you first begin to walk. When the heel pain lies behind and along the sides of the heel, tests for ankylosing spondylitis or the spondyloarthropathies (those inflammatory forms of arthritis that are associated with inflammation of the sacroiliac joints and with a positive HLA B27 genetic determination) should be performed by your doctor. If tests show inflammation, back stiffness, or limited back movement, there may be ankylosing spondylitis (inflammatory arthritis of the spine). Your doctor can prescribe a nonsteroidal anti-inflammatory medication. If the pain persists for some months, an x-ray may show a fluffy calcium deposit where the tendons attach behind or at the bottom of the heel bone. The inflammation does ultimately subside without persistent pain.

The worst affliction of the heel and ankle area can result from diabetes and syphilis. A total crumbling of the heel and ankle bones is a rare and dreaded complication of these diseases. People with diabetes should take special care of their feet. They should wash and thoroughly dry their feet every day. Open shoes should not be worn. Any injuries should be taken care of immediately.

Pain at the bottom of the heel is much more common. It can result from bursitis or from small strains within the plantar fascia. The *plantar fascia* is a thick sheet of dense fibrous tissue radiating from the toes to the heel spur on the underside of the foot.

Bursitis of the Heel

Bursitis on the back of the heel under a pump bump has been mentioned earlier. More commonly, a bursitis can occur under the heel and cause pain when you walk and also when you aren't walking. The pain is in the center of the bottom of the heel. If you press deeply into this point there will be severe pain. On rare occasions the heel will feel swollen, but the overlying skin and tissue are so thick that visible swelling is unusual. The bursa forms here as a result of the hard heel striking down and then becoming inflamed during walking or running. Also, if you walk on concrete with bare feet you may get bursitis.

Amelia Y. and Her Trampoline

One active woman in her late sixties, Amelia Y., visited her doctor's office three times complaining of sore heels. Did she jog? No, but she walked a lot. The doctor was puzzled. Not until the third visit did she reveal that, yes, she had a trampoline, and she just had to exercise on it three times each day if she were to have a firm, trim derriere. "Vanity, vanity..."? No, not really. Just keeping one's investment current. Finally, she came to her senses and stopped that form of heel strike; then she improved.

Treatment includes placing a pad in the shoe under the heel. A 1/2-inch foam-rubber pad can be obtained from most shoe-repair or athletic stores. Cut a hole, 1 inch in diameter or about the size of a quarter, in the center of the pad. Wear the pad in your shoe at all times for a month. If a shoe is particularly hard underneath the heel, dig a hole into the heel of the shoe just under the pad.

Aspirin or ibuprofen (Chapter 15) may help. If this doesn't solve the problem, a shot of a cortisone medication will get rid of it in nearly every case. People who are significantly overweight may suffer prolonged bouts and recurrences of heel bursitis.

Plantar Fasciitis

The fibers of the plantar fascia that attach to the heel can be injured simply during prolonged standing if you have flatfeet. Recently, one of our patients was treated for bursitis caused by walking barefoot on the concrete floor of his new condominium. Examination of the plantar fascia as detailed in Table 11-2, item 5, will reveal tightness, tautness, and tenderness in the plantar fascia along the bottom of the foot. The tenderness increases as you press toward the heel. Pain deep in the heel that worsens as you walk is common. Treatment consists of stretching the leg and foot with a rope draped over the toes. See Table 11-6, exercise 2. Try wearing a neutral shoe in which the heel and sole lie at nearly the same level (Figure 11-6). At first this may be uncomfortable, but gradually the fascia will stretch and pain may subside. If you have very flat feet, a long-counter shoe may be necessary. This "orthopedic" shoe has the hard heel counter extended almost to the lacing area along the inner wall of the shoe.

Arthritis of the Midfoot

Beginning about an inch in front of the ankle, the bones may become arthritic. Pain at the junction of the ankle bones and the first metatarsal, on the inner aspect of the foot, is usually due to spur formation. As the spur enlarges, you can detect a marble-sized bump on top of the foot at this location. At first, you may only be able to feel it. Tight lacing above the tendon can cause injury to the tendon by squeezing it against the spur. Toe movement may then become painful, and for treatment you must create a bridge for the tongue of the shoe. Because arthritis may also occur in the ball of the foot, you need a laced shoe if you have pain. You can construct the bridge by building up strips of adhesive-backed foam rubber applied to the underside of the tongue. To locate the position of the spur, rub lipstick

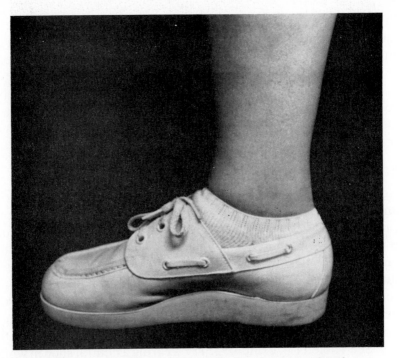

Figure 11-6.   Neutral shoe. Heel and sole are level.

onto the spur or involved tendon site, slip the shoe on, lace, and tie it. When you take off the shoe, the lipstick will mark the spur location on the tongue. Now place the foam strips along either side. Voilà! a bridge! Also, use elastic shoelaces to ease the pressure from lacing. A good arch will prevent progression of the arthritis.

Pain in the Forefoot

The common foot problems in the forefoot include *metatarsalgia* and *neuroma* (benign growth on a nerve between the bones of the foot).

Metatarsalgia is characterized by pain in the ball of the foot that may result from bursitis between the metatarsal bones, arthritis of the first toe joints in the ball of the foot, calluses, ligament strain, or a plantar wart. Look at the area under the ball of the foot. If you see a penny-sized hard callus, squeeze the edges toward each other.

If that increases the pain, chances are you have a plantar wart, a chronic condition that is usually resistant to simple treatment. Removal may require freezing or surgery.

If a callus is present but not very tender, press deeply and see if an arthritis-enlarged joint has developed. See Table 11-2, item 8. Sometimes the two bones get jammed one over the other. This, too, may require surgery. If not, application of a medicated patch for treatment of calluses may help. But a change in shoe style is also necessary. A neutral shoe may provide comfort. Note that the heel is at the same level as the forefoot.

Ligament strain results in a flattened metatarsal arch (across the ball of the foot). Often, this results from obesity, wearing high-heeled shoes, prolonged standing, wearing overly flexible shoes, and from cumulative overload as in dancing, jumping, or running. Special shoes, padding, and exercise all help. Also Table 11-6, exercise 5, may help, especially gathering the towel or newspaper with your toes. Laced shoes with rigid toe portion can help.

Bursitis and *neuromas* are hard to distinguish from each other. If the metatarsal bones have enlarged and the ends have become squared, bursitis between the bones may occur. The swollen bursa then squeezes the nerve traveling out to the toes. Much less common is a *neuroma,* a bulbous swelling on the nerve between these bone ends, usually affecting the third and fourth toes. (The big toe is number one.) Neuroma pain is very sharp. Women notice that it hurts especially when they wear high heels. Too often the first treatment for foot pain is surgery for a "neuroma," but neuromas are uncommon. If item 7 in Table 11-2 causes pain, bursitis is a more likely cause of the pain. Treatment should consist of relieving pressure on the metatarsal region either with a neutral shoe, a running shoe, or the placement of metatarsal bars under the shoe behind the metatarsal heads (Figures 11-7 and 11-8).

A *stress fracture* (also called a *fatigue fracture* or *march fracture*) can cause pain and swelling in the ball of the foot, usually of the metatarsal bones, and can result from a long walk, shopping, or running. The cumulative impact results in bone stress and fracture. The hairline fracture may not show on an x-ray, but often when an x-ray is taken a month later, the healing fracture is evident. Your physician may provide treatment with metatarsal bars; this will usually provide pain relief and assure satisfactory healing.

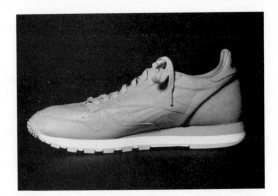

Figure 11-7.   Running shoe with microcellular-foam sole.

Toe Problems

Many toe problems are congenital or come from wearing narrow, pointed shoes. Many people have a family history of bunions, hammertoes, unusually long toes, or short toes. Sometimes people are born with six toes, but this may not cause a problem.

A *bunion* can occur when the big toe turns toward the other toes. In many cases this results from an inherited short first metatarsal

Metatarsal bar   Thomas heel

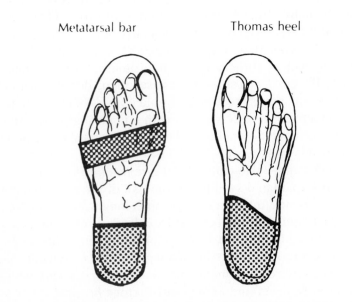

Figure 11-8.   Metatarsal bars are located behind the metatarsal heads.

bone. It may also occur if the bone spreads outward, causing the big joint at the ball of the foot to rub against the shoe and inflame a bursa. This can become thick, swollen, or even infected. Placing a foam insert between the toes can help prevent the bursitis, but the best treatment is using a shoe with a broad or box toe. If the bunion is inflamed, the first thing you must do is rule out gout because gouty arthritis (discussed below) is more painful than any other foot problem. In fact, the pain of the swollen, inflamed joint is so intense that the patient can't even tolerate a sheet touching the skin. If the bunion is irritated, use an old shoe, cut out the area surrounding the bunion, and don't wear any other shoe until the inflammation has subsided.

Surgery for bunions is not always the answer. About 15 percent of cases are not helped by surgery. According to one estimate 15,000 people a year are worse after bunion surgery. Proper shoes and other conservative measures (Table 11-7) should be used before considering surgery.

Gout is an accumulation of uric acid in the blood and tissues to such a degree that microscopic needlelike crystals form and attack the joint. Gout comes on suddenly, often overnight. Although the great toe is the usual site for gouty arthritis, other joints can be involved including the joints of the ankle, knee, elbow, wrist, and finger. The shoulder, back, and hip are rarely attacked. The attack gradually subsides after a week. If you don't treat the gout, you may have another attack in a matter of months or years. Also, if the uric-acid salt concentration in the tissues increases, heart disease or kidney failure can occur. Gout may result from kidney disease or use of moonshine whiskey (as a result of lead contamination) or diuretics (water pills). Most often, it is inherited. Colchicine or nonsteroidal anti-inflammatory drugs can treat or prevent the attacks. But the eventual primary treatment is to lower the uric-acid level to less than 6 milligrams per 100 milliliters of blood. Probenecid and allopurinol are the most commonly prescribed drugs that lower uric acid. The medicine must be lifelong, particularly in the case of inherited types of gout. In the opinion of most experts, high uric acid levels in the blood without the presence of gouty arthritis do not require treatment. Only those who have arthritis run the risk of further trouble. Gout can also cause kidney stones, in which case the patient will benefit from persistent use of drugs that lower the uric-acid level in the blood (see Chapter 15).

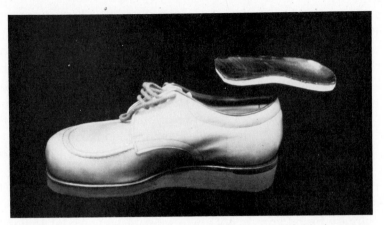

Figure 11-9.   Extra-depth shoe with heat-moldable insert.

Any of the second to fourth toes may become angled upward at the middle joint. If one does, a corn will develop on top of the up-lifted joint. This is known as a *hammertoe*. Sometimes padding or an extra-depth shoe will provide relief (Figure 11-9).

In *arthritis* of the toes, the big-toe joint may enlarge and form a spur across the top of the joint. It feels like a sharp lip on top of the first joint at the ball of the foot. See Table 11-2, item 6. If you wear flexible shoes, they will allow the toe to extend during walking, and then the tendons may become injured as they cross this ridge. Acute pain that lasts longer than a week may result. Also, flexible shoes may lead to further enlargement of the joint and loss of joint motion. See if you can bend the big toe downward as you can the other toes. If you can't bend it downward, then treatment may not help as much. People who have arthritis in the end joints of their fingers or at the base of the thumb are likely to get the arthritis in the big-toe joint. Also, arthritis may follow an injury in which a heavy object has fallen onto the joint. Ballet dancers get a variety of big-toe problems. Toe exercises can help. See Table 11-6, exercise 5.

Tarsal-Tunnel Syndrome

Injury to the nerves under the ligament at the inner aspect of the ankle may cause a burning, throbbing, painful foot condition. The pain almost always awakens the person from sleep. In fact, any foot pain that is worse after you have gone to sleep should suggest a tarsal-tunnel syndrome. In addition to injury, other causes include inflammation of the tendons, arthritis of the ankle, and strain when a flat-footed person goes barefoot for prolonged periods. The test is presented in Table 11-2, item 9. If you suspect a tarsal-tunnel syndrome, see your doctor. He might advise an injection with a local anesthetic and corticosteroid beneath the ligament and recommend arch support shoes or running shoes.

What to Do about Shoes

Table 11-7 provides some shoe advice for various foot problems. To begin with, check your shoe size by having your foot measured while you are standing up. Next, buy shoes that feel good. Third, use running shoes for trips to stores that have concrete or tile floors. Also use them at home if your floor is concrete. The running shoe absorbs the impact of concrete and makes the wearer use the entire foot when walking.

We recommend that people with recurring problems or painful flatfeet try the following order of treatment measures:

1. Buy proper shoes of the correct size and fit. Shoes vary as to length, width, depth, and shape. The shoe last is the form around which the shoe is made and may be long and narrow or short and broad. Tie shoes are always preferred because they lock the heel back in the shoe and prevent forward shift and friction during walking. Cushioned soles are essential for walking or working on concrete. A long-counter oxford may help you if you have painful flatfeet.

2. Try shoe adaptations of felt, foam, or moldable inlays. Also, wedging, lifts, or bars may be added.

3. Use soft, pliable inserts in preference to rigid inlays.

4. Try rigid molded-plastic inlays if pliable inserts fail. The rigid inlays are expensive and need adjustment frequently. They have a useful life of about 3 years.

5. If all else fails, molded shoes may be helpful. But they are the most expensive solution.

When to Seek Professional Help

When should you see a podiatrist or an orthopedist? The best answer will come from your family doctor.

If you note any of the caution signs, you should see a competent medical doctor first. Infections, gout, other systemic diseases, circulation problems, or nerve problems should be considered. If the problem is a local disorder and you have tried the measures detailed here, the doctor may try an oral medication (such as a nonsteroidal anti-inflammatory agent) or a local injection of a corticosteroid and suggest that you wear protective shoes.

Table 11-1
Danger Signs in the Foreleg, Ankle, and Foot

Discoloration of the leg and foot (blue, red, or white)
Swelling, warmth, redness of limb
Swollen glands in the groin
Crampy pain during walking
Pain of increasing intensity while jogging
Pain in the heel cord; inability to stand up on toes
Night pain
Numbness and tingling in the lower leg, aggravated by coughing
Weakness or loss of sensation in the leg or foot

Table 11-2
Self-Examination of the Foreleg, Ankle, and Foot

1. Standing straight with feet together, observe yourself in a full-length mirror. Do the toes point straight ahead? Are the ankles turned inward? Have a helper look at your heel cords. Do they travel straight down or do they angle outward? Is the skin color normal? Is there swelling?
2. If swelling is present, press deeply over the shinbones. Does the skin stay indented, showing fluid retention? If so, kidney, heart, or vein problems may be complicating the problem.
3. Sit on a chair, cross your leg, and place your ankle over your other knee. Grasp the heel and turn the ankle inward and outward. Is there excessive movement or pain? Is the pain in front, all over, or below the ankle in the ligaments? Loose ligaments may indicate the hypermobility syndrome (Chapter 7).

4. If the heel is painful, press deeply into the center of the bottom of the heel. Is it severely tender? This would indicate bursitis. If moderately tender, test for plantar fasciitis.

5. To test for plantar fasciitis, sit with the right foot resting on the other knee. Grasp the toes with your right hand and draw them toward your shin. This will stretch the bands along the bottom of the foot. With the other hand use your thumb and press deeply about every inch from the ball of the foot (metatarsal area) back to the heel (Figure 11-10). Is this moderately tender? Do the bands feel harder than the tip of your nose?

6. Examine your big toe by grasping the base of it and feeling for a sharp bony ridge on top of the joint. Test the downward motion of the big toe. Does it move about 60 to 90 degrees? Is the movement painful? The presence of a ridge or painful downward motion suggests arthritis.

7. To test for intermetatarsal bursitis, press just above the webs of the toes, between the bones at the end of the foot, just before the toes join the foot. Is there tenderness? This would suggest bursitis. Now, with one hand, grasp the toe joint just above the web of the second toe and, with the other, grasp just above the web of the third toe; rub these together with an up-and-down motion. Try this with other adjacent toes. Does this send pain out to the toes? If so, either bursitis or a neuroma is likely.

8. To test for metatarsal-joint arthritis, press down right over each of the metatarsal joints. Does this cause pain or feel swollen or both?

9. To test for a tarsal-tunnel syndrome, press deeply into the soft tissue about 1 inch below the round ankle bone at the inner aspect of the ankle. Press and rub downward and backward toward the heel. Does this create or accentuate tingling in the bottom of the foot?

Table 11-3

Possible Causes of Foreleg, Ankle, and Foot Pain

Complaint	Possible Cause
Night cramps in leg or foot	Unknown; aggravated by diuretics, poor nutrition, inactivity before bedtime, prolonged squatting

(continued)

Complaint	Possible Cause
Easily twisted ankle	Hypermobility syndrome; previous injury
Swollen ankles, morning or night	Arthritis
Swollen ankles in the evening, not present in the morning	Edema (fluid retention)
Bumps above or behind ankle	Erythema nodosum (painful red nodules); painter's bosses; arthritis; pump bumps
Pain at inner ankle or in front of ankle	Arthritis; tendinitis
Ankle pain when walking or standing	Arthritis; tendinitis; ligament strain
Painful heel	Plantar fasciitis; arthritis; flatfeet; heel spur
Bumps on instep in front of ankle	Arthritis
Pain under forefoot	Metatarsalgia; bursitis; plantar wart; stress fracture (march fracture)
Pain in forefoot with burning in toes	Intermetatarsal bursitis; neuroma; diabetes; vascular disease
Pain and numbness at night in foot	Tarsal-tunnel syndrome; neuralgia
Aching feet when standing; dark skin over lower leg	Vein problems
Big toe deviated away from midline	Bunion
Red, swollen big toe, not hot	Bursitis over bunion; tendinitis
Red, swollen big toe, hot and exquisitely painful	Gout; arthritis; infection
Painful bump over bent toe (second or third toe)	Hammertoe

Table 11-4

Habits That Cause Persistent Ankle and Foot Pain

Complaint	Aggravating Habit
Swollen ankles morning, day, and night	Too much standing and walking; too much salt in diet; possible heart, liver, kidney disease
Pump bumps	Shoes that have too high or hard a counter or that slip on the heel
Heel pain	Going around barefoot when your feet are flat; new job with more standing; shoes without much arch support; obesity; walking with a pounding heel strike
Metatarsalgia	Wearing high-heeled shoes; soles too soft; shoes too narrow or too large; prolonged standing
Painful bunions	Shoes too narrow or too loose
Burning feet	Walking barefoot with flatfeet; diabetes; vascular disease; metatarsal bursitis

Table 11-5

What's Harmful, What's Helpful for the Foreleg, Ankle, and Foot

Harmful	Helpful
Some forms of leg cramps appear to be inherited. Persons who have nocturnal leg cramps tend to have similarly afflicted family members, as do those with daytime leg cramps. The precipitating mechanism is not clearly understood.	Stretch the calf muscles by performing the following maneuver. Stand 3 feet from a wall and lean forward, placing the hands on the wall. Keep the bare feet flat on the floor; do *not* allow the heels to rise. With the outstretched arms touching the wall, walk the palms upward on the wall as if

(continued)

Harmful	Helpful
	climbing the rungs of a ladder. Reach as high as possible, until the heel cords are stretched to the maximum. Maintain this position for 30 seconds, then walk the palms down the wall. Perform this maneuver three times each after supper, midway between supper and bedtime, and at bedtime for 1 week. Doing so often prevents nocturnal leg cramps. To alleviate a cramp in progress, apply ice or a hot shower spray to the most tender muscle.
Being loose-jointed may provoke repeated ankle injury, with the ligaments at the outside of the ankle giving way and tearing.	Wear low-heeled shoes that tie up close to the ankle; high-necked shoes that tie above the ankle may give less support to the ankle. Good walking shoes have rubber soles and stiff heel counters.
Having flat arches, a condition common in loose-jointed persons, may cause joint and muscle fatigue. Working on a hard surface, standing in one position for prolonged periods, or being overweight compounds the problem.	Use arch supports if deemed necessary by a physician. Many loose-jointed, flat-footed persons have no ankle problems and thus do not need to wear arch-preserving shoes.
Wearing shoes with crepe soles, many of which are too flexible to support the metatarsal area, can be injurious.	Invest in a pair of running shoes. One of the best-designed types of shoes available, they are cushioned, have a moderate arch, and shift body weight back toward the ankle and away from the metatarsal arch, or ball of the foot.

Harmful	Helpful
Wearing slippers or moccasins or going barefoot aggravates metatarsal and toe pain.	Try running shoes for everyday use. Always wear shoes that shift body weight behind the metatarsal arch and that tie or buckle to keep the feet from slipping forward.
Walking or standing on concrete (which we all are doing increasingly) promotes joint and muscle fatigue. This is true even when the concrete is covered with carpeting.	Select shoes with rubber soles, which act as shock absorbers.
Squeezing the forefoot, which tends to widen with age, into too narrow a shoe may cause nerves to be pinched between the bones of the toes. Having bunions can also be problematic. Neuralgia, with a burning sensation and aching pain in the forefoot radiating to the toes (usually the third and fourth), is symptomatic of improper shoe fit.	Ensure that shoes fit properly. Sometimes, use of an external metatarsal bar helps to spread the toe bones. Wear shoes with enlarged toe boxes to accommodate troublesome bunions. Fortunately, today's specialty shoe stores usually stock shoes having extra depth and enlarged toe boxes.
Having burning pain in the feet at night suggests a pinched nerve at the ankle or neuritis caused by diabetes or a nutritional deficiency.	Consult a physician.

Table 11-6

Exercises for the Foreleg, Ankle, and Foot

1. *Daniell leg cramp exercise:* Face a wall in bare feet; stand an arm's length away. Reach your palms to the wall and "walk" your palms up the wall slowly until the maximum stretch is felt at the heels of your feet, but don't let the heels raise up from floor. Now push your pelvis forward to increase the stretch, hold for 10 seconds, and repeat three times. Perform the three stretches, four times a day. Continue for at least a week (Figure 11-4).

2. *Leg stretch:* Lie on your back with the legs bent at the knee, feet to the floor. Loop a 4-foot length of rope across the ball of one foot; draw this leg straight in the air while the other leg is bent. The ankle should be at a right angle with the leg. Pull gently and, with increasing force, stretch the muscles behind the thigh, knee, and calf. Hold 1 minute, then stretch the other leg. Repeat the exercise twice daily (Figure 11-11).

3. *Calf stretch:* Stand with both feet on one step of a stairway; hold onto the handrail. Keep your heels hanging off the step; just the ball of foot should be on the step. Raise up onto your toes; then drop down, letting the heels drop below the forefoot. Return to starting, neutral position. Repeat, and gradually shift your weight to the involved leg. Repeat the exercise twice daily.

4. *Ankle-rotation exercise:* While barefoot, curl your toes and keep your foot in a cupped shape. Now rotate the forefoot with the great toe making a circle clockwise for 1 minute, then repeat counterclockwise. Repeat the exercise twice daily (Figure 11-5).

5. *Toe exercise:* Stand on a telephone book and curl your toes over the edge for 1 minute. Place a towel on the floor in front of a chair. While sitting, repeatedly try to gather the towel with your toes. Place a page of a newspaper on the floor and crumple it with your toes. Repeat the exercise twice daily.

Table 11-7
Helpful Shoe Modifications

Problem Area	Possible Shoe Modification
Great toe	Broad toe box; shoe cut out around bunion; vinyl patch to enlarge toe box; thicker or more rigid sole; broad external rocker bar; felt ring
Other toes	X incision above toe; wider shoe size; metatarsal pads; extra-depth shoes
Metatarsal area	Pads; excavation of innersole beneath lesion; closed-cell foam pad (Spenco); molded flexible insert with open-cell foam (Plastizote); short external metatarsal bar (1 inch wide); longer external rocker bar; vinyl covering to widen toe box; anterior-placed heel
Plantar region of midfoot, flexible flatfoot, plantar fasciitis	Long-counter shoe; Thomas heel; scaphoid pad; flexible arch support; cut out under heel spur; 3/16-inch foam medial arch insert; wedging of the medial sole
Dorsal midfoot	Strips of foam rubber cemented to inner tongue to lift tongue off lesion; elastic shoe laces
Heel	Heel lift; heel pad; cutout heel pad; excavation of innersole beneath heel spur or lesion; plastic heel cup; V incision into rim of counter

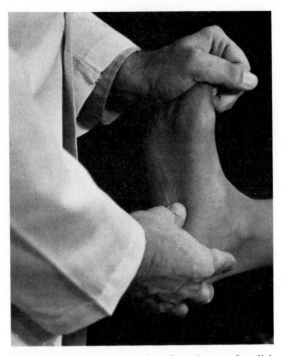

Figure 11-10.   Examination for plantar fasciitis.

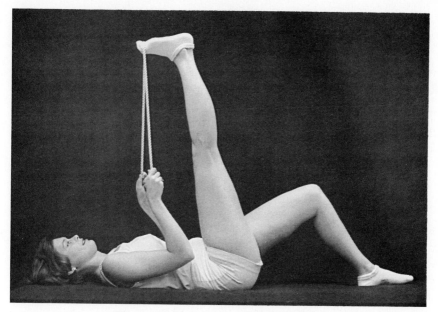

Figure 11-11.   Leg and foot stretch.

CHAPTER 12

When You Hurt All Over

If your arthritis tends to jump around—in your shoulders for a time, then your back or hips, hands or legs, and this is added to a background of allover pain when you awaken, you are probably suffering from fibrositis. *Fibrositis* is a condition with widespread aching and fatigue and the presence of tender points at specific locations; it involves many soft tissues but does not cause damage. This nondeforming disorder must be distinguished from the ones that can cripple or have other serious consequences. This chapter will help you sort out these conditions.

The "allovers" can result from acute illness, chronic debilitating illness, psychologic illness, or stress. The condition may start as a local problem such as a headache or backache that gradually becomes a widespread problem.

This chapter will help you work with your physician and will emphasize the steps you can take to help in diagnosis and treatment. In most instances the conditions to be considered will have lasted 3 months or longer. By that time easily diagnosed conditions will already have been excluded. Listed at the end of this chapter are tables outlining danger signs (Table 12-1), self-examination techniques (Table 12-2), possible causes of allover pain (Table 12-3), aggravating factors (Table 12-4), commonsense solutions (Table 12-5), and exercises for posture and conditioning (Table 12-6).

Please keep in mind that more than 100 rheumatic diseases are diagnostic potentials. In addition, a huge number of other medical problems can give rise to a sense of general illness and pain. These include blood and marrow disorders, infections, tumors, endocrine and metabolism problems, allergic reactions, and even psychologic or mental illnesses. If you haven't yet seen your physician, here are some questions that you can ask yourself to prepare for what may be a very detailed examination:

1. What is the history of the pain?

    a. Location of the pains.

    b. Duration and severity of pain.

    c. Its relation to rest or movement.

    d. The type of pain (such as, burning, aching, throbbing, intermittent, constant).

    e. What has helped? What has made it worse? How did it begin?

2. What is the possible relation of pain to other factors?

    a. Current medications.

    b. Occupation, hobbies, or sports.

    c. Life stresses, depression, need for alcohol or drugs.

Drugs that can cause allover aching include clofibrate, diuretics, cimetidine, lithium, cancer drugs, alcohol, and amphetamines. Rarely are food allergies a contributing factor. Sugar substitutes or caffeine sometimes can be contributors to pain. Mental stress can play havoc with the nerves and muscles.

Be honest in your answers. If you are up against a "brick wall," such as a bad relationship, an uncompromising in-law or boss, or a tragedy, be "up front" with the information.

1. What information do you have about a known illness?

    a. The head and neck.

    b. Digestion.

   c.   Breathing or heart problems.

   d.   Liver diseases.

   e.   Kidney or bladder problems.

   f.   Genital or sexual problems.

Take a look at Table 12-2. A self-examination may provide some clues to your problem. Item 1 considers visible and measurable abnormality that can arise from systemic conditions that affect the nerves and circulation or conditions that cause a rise in body temperature. Items 2, 4, and 5 may lead you to consider the various types of arthritis and connective-tissue diseases. Items 3 and 6 test nerve function for conditions within the brain, spinal cord, or such disorders as neuritis or Parkinson's disease. Abnormalities discovered during the examination should be listed for your doctor's consideration.

We can tell you about the rheumatic conditions that cause widespread illness or disability. But more importantly, we want you to take steps to prevent further disability and to improve the quality of your life. This chapter will provide you with some well-accepted self-help methods and goals.

Delays in diagnosis can result in terrible social consequences. Recently, a 39-year-old woman reported that 8 years ago her husband, a construction worker, left her and their five children. She went to school and, with much effort, received a degree in business and found a job managing a small trucking company. Then 2 years ago, fatigue, hair loss, and joint pains began. In failing health and with the strain of work and child raising, she moved to the small town where she grew up. She no longer knew anyone there, she had no family left in the community, but she sought peace. She had taken a medical leave from work, had exhausted all of her funds, and had suffered the indignity of going on public assistance. When a diagnosis of lupus was made, treatment was begun; but still she had severe back and chest pain. Further examination revealed fibrositis, with disturbed sleep, morning fatigue, and tender points that reproduced her pain. Although she has just begun treatment of the fibrositis, the diagnosis has been a victory for the patient. This wasn't a mental condition or stress-related pain. When she works out this condition, we believe she will pick up her career and fulfill her ambitions. The lupus has already remitted from treatment.

Rheumatic Diseases

Any discussion of the rheumatic diseases must be broken down into those conditions that are inflammatory and involve many organs and body systems and those that are degenerative, structural, or caused by local injury.

Inflammatory Connective-Tissue Disorders

The connective-tissue diseases include rheumatoid arthritis, systemic lupus erythematosus, systemic sclerosis (scleroderma), dermatomyositis, polymyositis, and mixed connective-tissue disease. Other inflammatory rheumatic diseases include polymyalgia rheumatica, giant-cell arteritis, and the spondyloarthropathies. In addition, systemic vasculitis of various types is a rare cause of widespread tissue damage. These disorders can be diagnosed only with analysis of the history, physical findings, and laboratory-test abnormality. Because the causes of these disorders are unknown, we have no specific test that is 100 percent reliable. Some normal people can have a positive test for rheumatoid arthritis or a positive antinuclear antibody test and yet have no evidence of a connective-tissue disease. These false-positive tests can result from a previous viral infection, liver disease, or simply from aging. On the other hand, 18 percent of patients with definite rheumatoid arthritis have normal tests! The next few pages contain a brief description of these diseases and will help you recognise them *early*. We hope reading these descriptions will get you under proper treatment.

Rheumatoid arthritis can begin with generalized aching, but the main feature to watch for is stiffness in the finger joints that lasts for more than half an hour after you have arisen. Stiffness may begin in any joint area but should affect both sides equally. Joint tenderness occurs early, and the tissue between joints is not nearly as tender. Joint swelling due to rheumatoid arthritis will last at least overnight, with the swelling worse upon arising. This is the opposite of fluid retention in which the swelling increases as the day goes on. Blood tests that help include the Westergren sedimentation rate, the latex RA test, and a sheep-cell agglutination test. X-rays are not helpful until the joints have been involved for several months. We hold off taking x-rays for 6 months in many cases.

At one time, because of psychologic-test results, rheumatoid arthritis was thought to be an emotional illness. However, when psychiatrists studied the manifestations of the disease and eliminated questions that were inappropriate for these patients, the tests showed normal results.

LOWELL G.: A FIREMAN OF COURAGE AND PERSISTENCE

One of the most interesting persons to visit one of our offices was Lowell G., a young fireman who, at 35, had contracted rheumatoid arthritis. Lowell was courageous not only on the job but also at home, where he built a complete gym in his basement in order to carry out the exercise regimen necessary for him to remain active in his job. He loved his work and would perform any exercise and other therapy suggested to him. Because of his diligence and persistence, Lowell worked as a fireman until he was 55, extending his worthwhile career by 15 years.

Systemic lupus erythematosus (SLE) can appear as a sudden and severe illness; as a blood disorder with low platelets, low white-blood-cell count, or an anemia; or as rheumatoid arthritis. Additional key features that start early include hair loss, Raynaud's phenomenon (described below and in Chapter 7), allergy to the sun, and recurring sores in the mouth.

Systemic sclerosis, or *scleroderma,* begins with Raynaud's phenomenon in most cases, and then a stiffening of the skin around the fingers, arms, face, and neck. Tiny red spots (telangiectasis) may be seen in these areas that fade if you press them with an eyeglass or any translucent object.

Dermatomyositis and polymyositis are rare connective-tissue diseases that damage the muscles that support the head, move the limbs, and sometimes even those that move the eyeballs. Weakness is the major complaint, sometimes to the point that the patient can't raise his or her head up from the pillow. Blood tests are helpful, but a muscle biopsy is needed to confirm the diagnosis. About 6 percent of the patients with dermatomyositis have an underlying cancerous condition. Patients with a purplish color change of the upper eyelids or rose-colored skin over the knuckles may have dermatomyositis.

Mixed connective-tissue disease combines features of scleroderma, lupus erythematosus, rheumatoid arthritis, and polymyositis. These features don't occur all at once, but change with time from one presentation (such as arthritis or lupus) to another (such as scleroderma). Symptoms begin slowly and are mild; the diagnosis is suspected when an antinuclear antibody test demonstrates a speck-led pattern. Young women are most commonly affected.

Systemic vasculitis is a term for a number of severe illnesses in which the blood vessels become inflamed, with microscopic abscesses within the vessel walls. For example, the patient may come with a sinus infection, pneumonia, and kidney damage (Wegener's granulomatosis). Or, another vasculitis, *polyarteritis nodosa*, may present with painful pea-sized lumps along the arms or legs, numbness and weakness, and high blood pressure. These conditions are usually severe, with features of limb pain, fever, skin reddening, and weight loss. If chills occur, infection should be suspected and blood cultures should be obtained before a diagnosis of vasculitis is considered.

Polymyalgia rheumatica has not yet been fully established as a disease entity. The main features, the sudden onset of stiffness and severe aching in the shoulders or hips, or both, can result from many diseases. Two major features are an elevated red-blood-cell (Westergren) sedimentation rate and a dramatic response to prednisone treatment, with all features returning to normal within 2 weeks. Sometimes polymyalgia will abruptly stop; if so, no treatment is needed. Mild symptoms don't always need prednisone. Nonsteroidal anti-inflammatory drugs will often help.

Giant-cell arteritis, or *temporal arteritis,* can begin with similar complaints. Both polymyalgia rheumatica and giant-cell arteritis strike persons past 50 years of age. Giant-cell arteritis usually has a few other features such as headache, eyeball pain, dimming vision, or jaw fatigue with chewing. Anemia, neuritis, and arthritis can occur. A biopsy of the vessels along the scalp in front of the ear can determine the diagnosis, but this requires painstaking examination of a suitably long artery segment. If untreated, the arteritis can close off a major blood vessel leading to blindness, heart attack, or stroke. Often giant-cell arteritis is very, very painful.

Spondyloarthropathies include ankylosing spondylitis, Reiter's syndrome, psoriatic arthritis, and the arthritis associated with both Crohn's disease and ulcerative colitis. The features include stiffness and pain in the low back, stiffening of the spine, swelling of lower limb joints, an inflammation of the eye, and separation of the nails from the nail bed. These disorders are genetically linked by the HLA B27 gene. The sacroiliac joints are the main targets for inflammation. Loss of spinal movement is common and can be determined by performing the test in Table 12-2, item 4. Diagnosis and treatment include use of the nonsteroidal anti-inflammatory drugs and exercises as described in Chapters 8 and 9. The patient's sleep position, with the neck and back flat on the bed, and the appropriate treatment when psoriasis or intestinal inflammation has been discovered are important.

In summary, the key features of connective-tissue diseases include morning stiffness of the small joints of the hands and feet that persists for at least 30 minutes; small-joint tenderness during movement; any joint swelling that is visible and lasts more than 24 hours and is present upon arising; swelling of a second joint within 3 months; sunlight sensitivity with rash or fever; or cold sensitivity with blue, white, and red discoloration of the hands. (This latter symptom is called Raynaud's phenomenon and may also occur during stress. See also Chapter 7.)

Degenerative Disorders

The degenerative or structural rheumatic problems leading to widespread aching include osteoarthritis, a short leg, body asymmetry where half the body is slightly smaller, malformations of the vertebrae, or loss of muscle tone from unusually sedentary habits or occupations.

Osteoarthritis is not simply the arthritis you get from age or injury. We are learning that osteoarthritis is a group of disorders with a variety of causes. The end result is the premature breakdown in the shock-absorbing cartilage that lines the ends of bones in the joints. When this cartilage becomes pitted, thin, and worn, then bone-against-bone action during use will lead to enlargement of the bone ends, cysts within the bone, stiffness, and sometimes redness and swelling with the accumulation of excessive amounts of joint fluid. The joint fluid may contain enzymes and acids that can cause further damage. Swollen end joints of the fingers, a disorder called Heberden's nodes, may occur as an inherited arthritis or may result from injury. Osteoarthritis rarely affects the first knuckles that lie above the crease of the palm. Also, osteoarthritis rarely affects the ankle despite the tremendous amount of weight and strain borne by that joint during your lifetime! Using joint-protection advice can lead to longer-wearing and more comfortable joints. See Table 12-5. Osteoarthritis of the small joints of the back can lead to widespread aching and loss of spinal movement. Treatment is discussed in Chapter 9.

Arthritis Treatment

Helpful treatment measures for arthritis begin with a satisfactory diagnosis and treatment program. You must understand why you take medication and the importance of taking it regularly. For example, when aspirin products are used for rheumatoid arthritis, the anti-inflammatory benefit can occur only if the tissue level of the aspirin is adequate; this is much more than the amount needed for reducing pain or fever. If you go longer than 8 hours between doses, or if you miss a dose, the body will have washed out much of the tissue level of aspirin.

Next you should pay attention to what your body is telling you. Fatigue and pain must be respected. They are nature's way of saying, "Not today!" Study Table 12-5 and reduce joint stress. On bad days, expend much less effort. Get more rest. You might just take a rest by lying flat on your back on the floor with your limbs all lined up. And if exercises have been prescribed, do them in small batches.

Keep life and death in perspective. Are your symptoms just in the nuisance range or are they possibly life-threatening? Let the molehills be! You may be disappointed that you can't get the day's tasks done; but if you magnify the problem, and keep on, you may be fighting your illness inappropriately and causing even more fatigue and damage.

Try to get into an appropriate conditioning program. Will your doctor permit you to get into the Arthritis Water Exercise program (sponsored by your local Arthritis Foundation)? For persons less ill, water aerobics, dance exercise, exercise machines, brisk walking, swimming, bicycling, jogging, or even playing racket-ball sports may be appropriate.

Remember that work tasks bend joints. But it is the muscles straightening joints that need the conditioning of exercise to protect the joint, to prevent deformities. Most prescribed exercises are for strengthening the extensor (straightener) muscles, but conditioning programs also improve circulation, tone, and endurance. In addition, they can provide mood elevation. We like to have all our patients with a connective-tissue disease keep good posture. Pain causes *reflex-guarding postures* that lead to fatigue and this results in poor posture, weak muscles, more pain. Therefore, we urge patients to perform some of the helpful exercises detailed in Table 12-6.

Lastly, consider your attitude. You didn't ask for this disease, and your doctor didn't give it to you. Try to approach it as objectively as you can. If you are depressed, if your family is not supportive, if you have special needs that you can't afford, talk to your physician, minister, church-related or public social-service agency, the Arthritis Foundation, the Society for the Handicapped, the Bureau of Vocational Rehabilitation, Mental Health Clinic, or your best friend! Don't give up without investigating these very effective support groups and individuals.

Fibrositis

Fibrositis, also known as fibromyalgia, is a current label for a rather specific disorder that has five features:

1. Morning stiffness and aching of at least 3 months' duration
2. Fatigue, often with no apparent cause
3. Poor sleep, after which you awaken feeling more tired than when you went to bed; or unsettled sleep in which you wander all over the bed
4. The presence of four or more tender points at typical tender-point locations. (See Figure 12-1 for the location of tender points.)
5. Absence of any other disorder explainable by appropriate test method

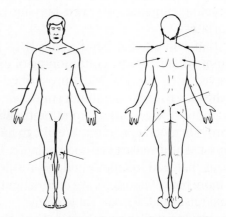

Figure 12-1.   Tender-point locations for fibrositis.

Other features that can develop include tension or migrainelike headaches, mucous colitis or spastic colon, numbness and tingling (usually brief and following sitting or sleeping or while on the toilet), mottled skin, cold hands or feet, a compulsive nature, and a compulsiveness to be on time. Women are afflicted nine times as often as men.

Researchers at the University of Toronto have suggested that sleep disturbance is a prominent component of fibrositis. They believe there may be a chemical upset that either causes the sleep disturbance or results from it. This then sets up an abnormality in the nervous system and in the blood vessels supplying the muscular tissue. At present, these studies and many others suggest that the problem does not lie exclusively within the muscles. Muscle biopsy is being performed for research purposes, but is not presently of diagnostic value; it can result in a new source of pain and spasm!

Fibrositis may begin very gradually or follow a stressful event or accident. The tender points appear to correlate with acupuncture points, and the persistence of these points suggests a vicious pain-spasm-pain cycle. The brain, upon receiving the pain impulses, sends back signals that result in muscle or blood-vessel spasm and the resulting ache keeps the cycle going. The 1969 discovery of an *antipain* center in the brain has set off a great deal of research on pain. At McGill University, experts proposed a "gate theory" for pain transmission along the nervous system, and theorized that there are gates along the nerve pathways carrying pain messages. At every gate are antipain message centers that can interrupt the transmission of the pain message. Endorphins are the antipain substances that are under investigation. An entirely new chemistry for diminishing pain is expected to result from this research. Fibrositis might result from an imbalance in this antipain system.

Several researchers have studied the muscle chemistry in fibrositis. The tender points have substances that produce much lower energy when compared with non–tender-point tissue or with normal muscle tissue. These findings have been noted in studies of muscles that had poor circulation. The pain-spasm-pain cycle may lead to muscle fatigue and loss of blood circulation.

Psychologically, patients with arthritis and fibrositis are no different from others who suffer pain. Tests show that they behave as any other human being experiencing pain does. Chronic pain leads to depression, hostility, and other defensive responses; but these disappear when pain decreases. Pain is affected by mood, stress, fatigue, depression, and climate. A low-pressure weather system moving toward you often causes more aching and pain. Similarly, rising humidity can worsen arthritis. But weather doesn't *cause* or *prolong* these diseases. Moving to a warm climate may provide more comfort, but it is not likely that the disease will go away. Needless to say, stress always has a big part to play when pain is present for any period of time.

Management of fibrositis begins with a careful history and physical examination by a competent physician. Appropriate tests are necessary in order to rule out other possible causes.

Next, medication that induces more restful sleep should be used. Meprobamate or tricyclic compounds such as amitriptyline, nortriptyline, protriptyline, or doxepin should be tried. Often very small doses are helpful and have few side effects. A few people are stimulated by the tricyclics and experience palpitations and nervousness; they should try a number of these preparations or some combinations with chlordiazepoxide. We have used these drugs for nearly 25 years without a single serious reaction! Sometimes the improvement in sleep will markedly reduce the tender points. Many patients will overcome the sleep disturbance and require no medication for long periods of time.

Acute, painful episodes can be treated with cyclobenzaprine or other muscle relaxants. Some patients have additional localized pain with a trigger point in an injured muscle. Throughout the chapters on each body region we have indicated myofascial trigger-point locations. A trigger point differs from a tender point in that the trigger point causes pain at a distance from itself, as presented in Figures 12-2 and 12-3. These may be treated with ice massage, a pressurized coolant spray-and-stretch regimen (described in the chapters treating individual areas of the body), or with an intralesional injection of a local anesthetic with or without a crystalline corticosteroid preparation. Often one or two such treatments of any of these may eradicate the painful trigger point.

Pain medications are of little help, and oral corticosteroids are of no benefit. The nonsteroidal anti-inflammatory drugs are often helpful in reducing the rheumatic pain of fibrositis (see Chapter 15).

Exercise can help the fatigue, poor posture, and tight musculature. Studies suggest that gradual aerobic exercises are more helpful than stretching ones. We prescribe the exercises in Table 12-6,

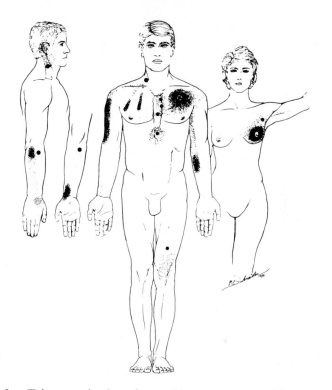

Figure 12-2.   Trigger-point locations with zones of pain reference, front view.

and we encourage use of an aerobic program. If the low-back or lower-limb joints are painful, an aerobic program in a swimming pool can be helpful. Such programs are available at the YMCA and YWCA and at private health facilities.

The tight muscles are more easily injured. We think that if you have fibrositis you are more prone to tendinitis and bursitis, and it is therefore important that you review the harmful practices listed in Table 12-5. These may help you avoid additional pain and disability.

When tender points are found, you can be reasonably assured that the pain disorder is *not* of psychologic origin. Many of our patients come to us thinking the problem must be imaginary because nothing has been found, even after several visits to their own physician. Also, their friends and family have grown tired of their long-standing complaints of fatigue and pain and perhaps have even suggested that the problem was imaginary. What a victory it is for these

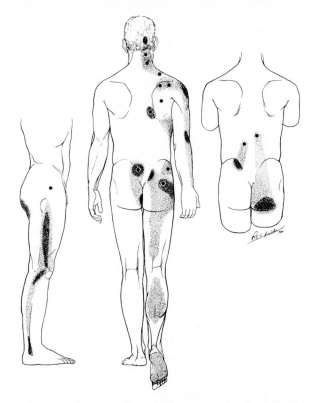

Figure 12-3.   Trigger-point locations with zones of pain reference, back view.

patients when a correct and treatable diagnosis is found! In one study, the rate of hospitalization in patients with fibrositis was cut fivefold once the diagnosis had been made.

Pain of Psychological Origin

Psychogenic rheumatism is an ache in the body from an ache in the mind. The conditions described here are often treated by psychologists and psychiatrists, whose success is variable. A lot depends on the patient's ability to change mental and physical behavior. Psychogenic conditions differ from those of fibrositis in several ways. First, when these patients are well, they are very well. Fibrositis patients do get better, but seldom are they completely well. Second, as we have mentioned, patients with psychogenic rheumatism do not have the tender points that are present in fibrositis; rather, they may have the touch-me-not syndrome described later. Third, psychogenic-rheumatism patients also do not function well: often their entire life is centered around their symptoms. Fibrositis patients usually "keep going."

The most seriously psychologically ill patients are those with true psychosis with "somatic delusions." These patients interpret reality inappropriately. They "see" nonexistent visions or "smell" nonexistent odors. In addition, these patients may believe they are being harmed by people around them, and they feel pain or experience paralysis that is nonexistent. Often, they fear harm is imminent. The next group in the psychologic category is the neuroses, which are less serious. Although they are largely imaginary, these are very persistent because they have a central core of fear or anxiety. These patients too are very apprehensive. Health may be their main focus, and minor symptoms may become greatly exaggerated or given undue consideration. Hypochondriasis is one feature of neurosis; often the patients have complaints that include many functions of the body—vision, digestion, sex, locomotion, etc.

Some patients with mitral-valve prolapse have chest pain, but they are so nervous and upset that their condition cannot be attributed solely to the valve problem. Many investigators even feel the symptoms bear no relation to the prolapse but rather are a neurotic manifestation. During World War I many soldiers had similar symptoms when facing combat. During polio epidemics, many who feared polio became incapacitated with a weakness and fatigue called *neurasthenia*. In the past, fear has even brought on epidemics of neurasthenia and "soldier's heart."

Some patients have a personality disorder that leads them to use pain as a weapon. Doctors refer to this as "assertive pain" because these persons use the pain to satisfy a need to control the behavior of others.

Another problem is the patient with a "pain-prone disorder." Doctors Dietrich Blumer and Mary Heilbronn of the Henry Ford Hospital Department of Psychiatry described this patient as usually the strongest personality within the family or work group. Suddenly, this person develops a complaint that rarely, if ever, improves, and he or she can no longer function. A comprehensive investigation reveals that the pain is of obscure origin, the patient has many other health concerns, and (inappropriately) wants surgery. Always denying any conflicts, the patient states that his or her family is "just fine" and fiercely claims to have always been a "workaholic." In fact, the patient frequently has features of depression, alcoholism, and loss of self-motivation. Other family members also may suffer from depression or alcoholism, a crippling illness, or chronic pain. Also, spousal abuse is common. The pain-prone patient's condition is thought to arise from a conflict in which a rigidly maintained ego desires to be independent and to care for others, while the patient's emotional needs seek to be dependent and passive.

The *touch-me-not syndrome* is also commonly encountered. Stress may result in such overwhelming pain that the patient cannot be touched. All parts of the body hurt. Even the face and forehead cannot tolerate light stroking. This pain problem usually indicates a serious emotional disturbance and psychological evaluation should be undertaken.

The above-mentioned disorders require psychotherapy that may range from finding better ways for the patient to cope with stress to putting the life situation into a better perspective by seeking formal inpatient treatment at a psychiatric institution.

When to Seek Professional Help

If you have difficulty coping with stress, perhaps you can benefit from a relaxation program. Have you ever used yoga or meditation? Yoga breathing is easily learned. You can get a book or videotape on yoga from the library and practice this method of breathing before you have to undertake a stressful task. Or you might seek a psychologist skilled in teaching a self-hypnosis program. Biofeedback should really be restricted to those who are deemed suitable for it after psychologic interview. Many also deal with stress by participating in aerobic exercise, jogging, racket sports, or dancing.

Your physician can help by giving you a thorough checkup because reassurance is one form of treatment. Antidepressant medication also can be effective for chronic-pain relief even if depression is not present. We mentioned medication for help in sleeping. Sedatives, however, do not help fibrositis. Pain pills are often depressants and are of little value. Muscle relaxants and nonsteroidal anti-inflammatory agents do seem helpful to many with fibrositis (see Chapter 15). Your physician or minister may help solve social problems that are common sources of stress. And be sure to look over Table 12-4 for possible causes of persisting generalized pain.

Dr. David Neustadt of Louisville suggests you consider four R's for coping with stress:

Roles: The ability to carry on relationships as parent, spouse, student, or breadwinner. Look for loss of self-esteem.

Reactions: Your emotional response to your disorder—anger, hostility, anxiety, discouragement, or defeat.

Relationships: Insurmountable problems at work, in the family, in school, or with friendships may create "brick walls," for which you need an outsider's help. Just discovering or considering what a normal person should be expected to do under the circumstance may reduce your stress.

Resources: Are you able to find help in community programs, from counselors, or from a minister or priest?

If you are referred to an occupational therapist, she or he may help solve a mechanical body-stress problem. The therapist looks at the "joint work" needed in everyday tasks. Some rearrangement of your kitchen, home, or job may be effective in reducing pain and disability.

A physical therapist, upon referral, may recognize a minor structural disorder that can be improved through exercise.

Any chronic rheumatic-pain disorder can be frustrating; but if you live your life in a manner that allows you to achieve your goals without compromising your health, you can look back and say, "I have been a successful human being." Patients with persistent rheumatoid arthritis who can adapt their living habits successfully are true heroes. Similarly, many a patient with fibrositis can continue gainful employment and care for the family if pain and fatigue are respected. Thus, on good days, do more; on bad days, do less.

Pain clinics can provide a multidisciplined approach to pain. The more successful clinics focus on behavior during pain rather than the pain itself. Graduates from these programs usually find their pain the same, but they say they tolerate it better, more effectively. The programs must include psychology, orthopedics, physical medicine, and other disciplines. They often can treat even patients addicted to narcotics.

Table 12-1
Danger Signs When You Hurt All Over

Fever, chills, weight loss, swollen glands
Joint swelling
Inability to move joints fully
Weakness
Numbness or tingling
Bluish or whitish discoloration of limbs
Change in bowel or bladder habits
Shortness of breath
Pain that changes character (daytime to nighttime)
Pale color in nail beds

Table 12-2
Self-Examination When You Hurt All Over

1. Has your appearance changed? Look into your eyes for yellow jaundice, look at your nails for pale color. Look at your muscles for loss of your usual appearance. Weigh yourself daily. Record any loss. Take your afternoon and evening temperature. If greater than 100.5°F, report it to your physician. Examine your bowel movement for a black or tarry appearance.
2. Check your joint motion and appearance. Move all four limbs, one at a time, and note the range of movement. Was any movement painful? Pinch each joint between two fingers or with both hands on bigger joints. Are they more tender than you think they should be? Are the joints swollen in the morning? (Ankles may swell at night from fluid retention, rather than arthritis.)
3. To test your strength, step up one step of a stairway with each foot; if normal, then with someone's assistance, step up onto a chair; test each leg. Lift arms overhead, one at a time. Sit in a chair and then rise without using your hands. These tests should all be accomplished without difficulty.
4. Have a helper watch your low back as you bend over. It should curve upward, not stay flat. Have your chest circumference measured at the nipple line while you are breathing out, then again while breathing in. Your chest should expand at least 2 inches.

5. Have a helper examine you for tender points as shown in Figure 12-1 and trigger points shown in Figures 12-2 and 12-3. Begin the test with moderate pressure on the middle of the thigh, where tender points are not usually present. Then use similar pressure at the side of the neck, behind the neck, and downward into the muscles above, within, and on the inner aspect of the shoulder blade. The helper continues the test farther on down on each side of the backbone while you are bending forward, while you are seated, and also while you are leaning forward. Have the helper press along each side of the breastbone beginning just below the collarbone.

6. To test your nerve function, hold a teaspoon and slowly bring it toward your lips. Does the movement occur smoothly, or with a ratcheting motion (a possible sign of Parkinson's disease). Stand up on your toes, then on your heels. It should be easy. Try to walk along a seam of carpet or linoleum.

Table 12-3
Possible Causes of Allover Pain

Complaint	Cause*
Upon awakening, joints feel stiff and sore but are not swollen; trunk worse than limbs; no weakness	Fibrositis/fibromyalgia; rheumatoid arthritis (early); spondyloarthropathies
Weakness; soreness all day	Polymyositis; neuritis; rheumatoid arthritis; drug reactions
The above symptoms plus sunlight sensitivity	Lupus erythematosus
The above symptoms plus cold-induced bluish, whitish hand discoloration	Systemic sclerosis (scleroderma); mixed connective-tissue disease
Pain to the touch anywhere on your body	Touch-me-not syndrome

* In addition, diabetes, thyroid disorders, parathyroid disorders, infections, anemias, malignancies, and allergies are some of the other medical problems to be considered and excluded.

Table 12-4

Possible Aggravating Habits in Allover-Pain Syndromes

Complaint	Aggravation
Neck and trunk pain; trunk stiffness, aching	Prolonged sitting or standing; improper sleep position; hidden chest or lung condition; inadequate treatment for sleep disorder
Generalized pain in trunk and limbs	Diabetes; hyperthyroidism; sensitivity to medications, licorice, or caffeine; diuretics; rheumatoid arthritis; infection; depression; tumor
Weakness	Nerve or muscle disorders; low potassium; other diseases
Weakness; numbness; tingling	Diseases that injure the nervous system such as diabetes or cancer; improper diet; alcohol

Table 12-5

What's Harmful, What's Helpful for Allover Pain (Joint-Protection Principles)

Harmful	Helpful
Head and neck	
Prolonged sedentary postures; tilting the head down or backward; lying with the head propped up on the arm of a sofa; sleeping with a thick pillow or with the head propped up on several pillows	Keep the neck straight. Eye-to-work distance should be about 16 in. Elevate handwork by placing it on a lap pillow. Video display terminals should be at eye level; work to be copied can be placed on an elbow-jointed easel. At a desk, use an adjustable chair that allows you to change the chair's height. In bed, use a thin, small pillow. If head elevation is necessary, raise the mattress by inserting a rolled blanket between the mattress and springs.
Shoulder	
Repetitive movements, such as vacuuming, push-ups, or sports in which the arm moves like a piston; prolonged work with your arms over your head	To avoid an overuse injury, pace any activity in which repetitive movements are necessary. Thoracic-outlet syndrome in women may be alleviated by the use of a support brassiere. When writing, hold the painful shoulder backward and upward.
Elbow	
Using your arms to push yourself out of chairs; repetitive and rotating motions; fist clenching	Pace harmful motions. To avoid tennis elbow, practice rising from chairs without using your arms. Reduce grip pressure by using pipe insulation on tool handles.

(continued)

Harmful	Helpful
Wrist and hand Repetitive motions; prolonged handwork; an I'm-going-to-finish-this-even-if-it-kills-me attitude; clenched fists at night (indicative of a state of tension)	Use larger muscles when possible. Pace repetitive activities. Use a plastic pencil holder during prolonged writing. Use nylon spandex gloves (turned with the seams out) during sleep. Use pipe insulation on tool handles.
Low back Prolonged standing or sitting; improper lifting, i.e., bending with straight knees or at the waist; turning the body by twisting the torso	Lift with the thighs, and bend at the knee. When prolonged standing is necessary (e.g., while working in the kitchen or at a machine or cash register), use a wood block 2 inches × 4 inches × 8 inches and step up on it with one foot for a few minutes, then change to the other foot. When carrying a heavy object, carry the item in front of you and turn with your feet. Use cushion-soled shoes when standing or walking on concrete.
Knee Using your hands to push yourself out of chairs; prolonged sitting; twisting the torso while turning; stair climbing	Maintain good alignment and quadriceps (muscles of the thigh and calf) strength. Use the quadriceps to lift yourself out of chairs. Turn your body with your feet. If your house lacks a first-floor toilet, place a portable toilet on the first floor.
Foot Prolonged standing or squatting (may result in plantar fasciitis); wearing flat shoes or slippers if you are flat-footed (may result in leg cramp)	Shoes were meant to cover and to protect the feet, not to compress them. Aging feet sometimes enlarge or toes spread: have your shoe size measured while you are standing.

Table 12-6
Exercises for Posture and Conditioning

1. *Trunk stretch:* Sit on the floor with legs out straight; reach up overhead, exhale, and bend forward, grasping your legs, ankles, or toes depending on your flexibility. Begin breathing while you continue to hold and draw your elbows outward; pull your head and trunk toward your feet. Hold for 20 seconds, repeat three times, twice a day.

2. *Posture and neck exercise:* Stand up against a wall with your feet about 6 inches away from the wall but with your buttocks, shoulders, head touching the wall. Place your hands between your head and the wall to act as a cushion. Push your head backward into the wall while keeping the chin tucked in, like a soldier. Hold for 10 seconds; repeat six times twice daily.

3. *Shoulder shrug:* Grasp two 5- to 10-pound weights and, while seated with arms at your sides, shrug your shoulders slowly upward, backward, then slowly downward; repeat in a slow, continuous motion for 1 to 2 minutes. Repeat twice daily.

4. *Abdominal tuck:* Suck in your stomach or flatten it, as if someone were about to punch you. Get it flat. Now keep it flattened and breathe with your chest, lifting the chest to inhale. Now hold that stomach flat all day!

5. *Overall conditioning:* If you are out of condition, begin with an aerobic water exercise or group exercise structured for beginners; then progress to walking briskly, mild jogging (less than 20 miles a week), swimming, bicycling, or rowing. Avoid jumping activities, such as using a trampoline.

CHAPTER 13

But the Very Best Is to Run[1]

I was stunned and infuriated to find that my friend Mary G., now 77 years old, the most "up" person I know, whose thoughts and acts were always in the stars, who loved life as do few people I know, now faces the ground when she walks. I suddenly realized that although we had talked on the phone almost every week, I had had no idea how much her arthritis had taken over and now hampered her movements. When she answers the phone, the lilt in her voice would make any one think she is fine, and about 36 years old.

As I helped her from her house into my car, the lines from a book of Mother Teresa's prayers drummed against my brain, wasting what Mary was saying. In reply to a suffering woman who couldn't understand why she had to suffer so, Teresa had quoted this:

> *My God, my God, what is a heart*
> *That thou should'st so eye and woo,*
> *Pouring upon it all thy heart*
> *As if thou hadst nothing else to do?*[2]

---

1. This chapter was written by Betty Hueter. It describes how one severely arthritic person copes—beautifully.

2. Mother Teresa, *A Gift for God*, Fount Paperbacks, London 1986, p. 23.

How right Teresa was when she had said that these lines filled her and also emptied her. God certainly does move in on people—on both those who patiently wait and those who impatiently watch. I made an effort to listen to what Mary was saying as we tried to get her into the car.

"This is an awful nuisance for you. And a nuisance for me, too, I might add."

I said, "Don't give it a thought. I don't mind, and we have plenty of time to get there." As we pushed and pulled and tugged to get her into the seat, we were both a bit frazzled; but then we laughed together, realizing that both of us had been too dumb to move the seat back. That done, getting her in was easy.

On the way to the luncheon, I listened intently to her story of how and when her life had changed so drastically. From the way she walked, I assumed the arthritis had now invaded almost every part of her body. "That's true," she replied. She had both rheumatoid arthritis and osteoarthritis and also osteoporosis. This means, of course, that she has both inflammation and bone crumbling. Her hips, knees, hands, feet, shoulders, and back all were involved. Oh, yes, and one elbow was terribly sore. Fortunately it was her left one, so it did not interfere with her studying or household tasks. I asked her to tell me how bad it was, and her voice broke and tears came to her eyes.

"It's awful, just awful, so frustrating! I get so angry, but then that only seems to make it worse. I guess I'll just have to learn to live with it."

"Is there any chance of your having a hip replacement?"

"Nooo." (She has an interesting way of prolonging "yes" and "no," and with a tone that says, "Imagine that!" It's quite attractive.) "I asked about that. But it can't be done. The rest of my body wouldn't allow it. It's a crazy kind of disease, you know, Betty. You don't dare give in to it. And yet you have to go along with it. You have to quit before you have so much pain that there's no hope of putting a lid on it. And also before you get so stiff you can hardly move. Does that make sense to you, that you have to go along with it; but that you can't let it manage you? You have to keep moving—but not move *too* much."

I said that indeed it did. "You have to function within the limits of your pain and stiffness and the other ways in which it hampers you, I suppose, don't you?"

"That's right, I have to be in charge of my life. I can't let it get the upper hand—the better of me. And yet it could so easily control my life—my every hour if I would let it."

"Are you ever without pain, Mary?"

"No, but sometimes it's a lot worse. On days before it rains, when it's getting ready for a real downpour, I'm in deep misery."

"How do you handle that?"

"Whyyy, I cry. Sometimes. Do you think that's awful?"

"Not unless you let the tears dissolve you, wash you out. I think a good cry is a good catharsis."

I think that made her feel better because she said, "And everybody needs a good catharsis now and then, don't you think?"

"You bet. Periodically."

I have known Mary for many years, and I remember how her arthritis first gained on her. The first trouble she had with the disease was when her knees and hips gave her trouble when she walked. Although she was always positive and cheerful and happy, you had only to watch her walk to know she hurt. But she put up with this for many years, rarely missing a day at the very large Toledo high school, where she was chairman of the English department. This is where I knew her. She retired because of the pain, and because she could no longer walk up the stairs to her classroom. It was I who tried to fill her shoes.

I had long been aware what an excellent teacher she was, but through the years I discovered ever so many more positive things about this woman. She had never missed a major game at the school, had headed a girl's group, had been adviser for the yearbook and the senior class, had been in charge of magazine drives, had been the only woman on the athletic committee, etc. After she had retired, it often seemed that half the children she had taught came back looking for her. As one of the men said, "All the kids who came back always came to see Mary." And only then did we learn how very much of her time and thought went to the students. She did everything from attending Chrysanthemum's wedding to knitting booties for the children of the children she had taught.

Today she returns to the school each spring to present ten citizenship awards named for her, two gold and eight silver. The medals are greatly prized. They mean as much, if not more, than any office or recognition at the school.

Although Mary taught English and French and loved all things cultural, she was that rare woman who keeps tabs on the world of sports too. It was in sports that she and her twin sister, Grace (her identical twin with almost identical arthritis problems), excelled when they went to high school and college. Even to this day she follows the football games (major, minor, and sometimes little league), golf and tennis matches, skiing, soccer, hockey, and so on.

"I told Grace, 'Now that the Detroit team is on the west coast, we go to bed every night with the Tigers.'" She's a great Detroit fan.

She tells how she and Grace spent every afternoon of both school and college participating in intramural activities. They did everything—soccer, basketball, track, baseball—whatever was offered, and they earned letters in everything but tennis and archery. Their father, a prominent dentist, often told them, "If you had spent as much time on your studies as you had on sports, you would have been graduated summa cum laude." As it was, they earned only A's and B's. Oh, and they were life guards at the YWCA.

They had boundless energy, according to Mary, and loved being outdoors. Their mother said many times in their later life that when they were children, they often told her, "But the very best is to run!" Mary is convinced that the pounding their legs took was partly responsible for their bad knees, hips, and feet. She has maintained this belief for some time, even when doctors said it wasn't likely. Now it looks as if the world may be catching up to her thinking. Had she known what the medical profession now knows about too-strenuous exercise and the relation of arthritis to heredity, she might have prevented some of her discomfort. We know now that when arthritis is a built-in possibility, it requires an outside factor to initiate it. As yet we don't know what the factor is. In the August 11, 1986, edition of *U.S. News & World Report* in an article entitled "Easy Does It! The New Rules of Exercise," Art Levine and others write, "The fitness motto that flashes today: 'Walk. Don't run.'" And they go on to say:

Standards of exercise are changing. Too much physical activity may be hazardous to your health. A moderate amount of exercise may be enough to help you live longer. Overdoing it is out; underdoing it is in.

Whatever the causes of her arthritis, Mary is in just about as bad shape as she could be. But she is mostly undaunted. She says, "At least I can live independently," and she is very proud of that fact. And her house has two stories. By pacing herself, Mary maintains her circulation and also saves her joints.

One of Mary's favorite expressions is, "I have to keep moving." She told me she often feels "like ol' Black Joe—I's acomin'. I's acomin'." Although it is difficult for her, she thinks coming down stairs and going back up is good for her, but she does limit it to once a day.[3] She walks with a walker or a cane and manages quite well, although walking is laborious.

She also keeps busy. She is a member of three American Association of University Women (AAUW) groups: one in Great Books, another literary group, and the third in music. A member of one of these groups says, "Mary huffs and puffs up the steps, eventually arrives, sits down, and gives the best report of the year."

She says she loves to do these papers for the groups, and she will spend as long as 3 months reading, writing, and then studying her report. Word has gotten around how very good at this she is, and she is often asked to give her papers for other groups.

She donates the money she receives from these lectures to a charity such as the United Way or a man who runs a soup kitchen in downtown Toledo. "I do the reports because it's good for me." Recently when I talked with her, she was busy on Mad Anthony Wayne. I can't remember what prompted it, but she said to me, "Do you know what happened to Mad Anthony Wayne after he died?" I confessed that I didn't, even though I am from Defiance, where Mad Anthony had roamed around the library grounds.

"Well!" she said, "they boiled him."

"Boiled?" I asked in amazement.

"Yesss! He was buried around here you know; and not too long after he died, his son Isaac arrived in a sulky to take his body back home to Pennsylvania. When they dug him up, the doctor who was assisting Isaac found that Mad Anthony was in almost perfect condition, but he wouldn't fit in or on the sulky. So, the doctor got permission from someone, found another doctor, and together they dismembered him, boiled him, trimmed off the flesh and reburied it. Then they put the bones in a bag for Isaac and wished him *bon voyage*. How do you like that?"

---

3. Although Mary thinks the stairs are good for her, the doctors of this book are not as certain.

I said it reminded me of the time that I had taken botany to be free of animals and such things as dissections, but that all winter in the botany lab they had boiled a monkey to get the skeleton clean. I also thought the doctor that Isaac chose was maybe a bit strange.

Is it any wonder her groups love her talks?

The other day Isabella H., who taught at our school and was there when first Mary came, said that she remembered Mary's arrival very well. "She was so young and enthusiastic and had a lot of fresh new ideas—about a lot of things besides English, too. It was interesting to watch her hold her own against the older teachers.

"She would present her ideas, but without antagonizing anyone. And everyone liked her. She just exuded self-confidence, but not in an offensive way. She had such a quick mind. And she loved to study. Can't you just imagine the rich feast of learning she spread before her students?"

Although her pain can reduce her to tears and occasionally depression, when I asked Mary which was worse, the pain or the constraints that arthritis has put on her life, she said, "The constraints. I was so used to doing what I wanted to do, going where I wanted to go. Did you know that almost every spring I would go to Cleveland and stay a few weeks just to go to the opera? I went alone, and I had a marvelous time."

I asked whether music had always been important to her. "Oh, yesss. Mother took singing lessons all her life, and we were taken along when she went for the lessons. But we had to stay in the hall. Then one day one of the teachers there said, 'Why don't we start them on piano lessons?' They did. We were 5 years old. I forgot to tell you that we also sang a duet at our baptism when we were 10." (By now Mary was well aware that I thought her life was unusual, and she was laying it on—completely forgetting that she didn't like to talk about herself.)

"Why were you being baptized at 10?"

"Well, mama and papa wanted us to know what we were doing. And we weren't named until we were 5 months old. We were the first twins ever in our parents' families and I guess they didn't want to get it wrong."

Even though as adults each went her own way, Mary and Grace were as close as matches in a book when they were children. Even at a very young age, they shared an uncanny empathy.

"When Grace had a mastoid operation, my ear hurt terribly, but after the operation neither of us ever had another earache. And we had had some bad ones!"

They looked exactly alike and talked exactly alike. (They still do.) A lot of people couldn't (and can't) distinguish them.

"Just before Grace had her tonsils out, my throat was more sore than it's ever been since. After they were out, it got better immediately.

"In first grade, when Grace broke her arm on the playground, the teacher sent me home too. When mama saw us coming down the street, crying so hard, she asked us which one was hurt.

"We were so close sometimes we got into double trouble. One day we were visiting grandfather. He was a strict person and wouldn't allow any cards in the house. We spent a whole day making a deck out of paper. He didn't catch us then, but he did the day we were practicing communion with the church wine and the wafers, both of which he and grandmother made and furnished for their church. Ohh! Was he mad! But he loved us. He and grandmother weren't much given to hugging, but we knew they would always be there when we needed them. My parents too. They were pretty modern, as I think back. They told us there wasn't any Santa Claus. The only tears ever shed in the house were ours because they never quarreled. Mama said, 'We never have any fights because John won't fight.' He also wouldn't gossip. We used to announce things like, 'Jane's going to have a baby!' and he would say, 'Oh, I've known that for a long time.' We could get exasperated with him, but he was so fair and so intelligent. He was out of Ohio State and practicing dentistry by the time he was 21. We loved him very much."

I asked her about Grace's marriage, knowing she had married an older man.

"Oh, yes, Jim was a year older than father. Grace was 31, and Jim's daughter was a year younger and his two sons were older than we. We didn't think her marriage was such a good idea because there could have been family problems. Papa, though, said it was her life, and we shouldn't interfere. And father knew best, of course. Their marriage was very happy. Unfortunately Jim lived only 10 years after they had been married, but Grace and his children and relatives are still close. Those were 10 wonderful years.

"And of course that's why there is Jenny, without whom I couldn't manage." Jenny is Grace and Jim's only child.

Invariably, whenever I call, Jenny has just done something nice for Mary or for Grace. More often than not, for both of them.

Jenny, who teaches English, is married to George, and she loves everything about housekeeping from cooking to refinishing antiques. Whenever Mary tells me about her, it's difficult to believe Jenny is only one person. She shops for both of them, freezes, cans, pickles—does whatever can be done to food. One day when I was at Mary's, Jenny came in with six stuffed peppers, six cabbage rolls, and two jars of spaghetti sauce for the freezer. Sometimes she'll buy half a bushel of tomatoes, which Grace will help her peel. Jenny also has a dozen small tins in which she bakes pies for their freezers.

Because Mary is too bent over to be able to fling the sheets out when changing the bed, Jenny has taken over. Apparently, too, she has a sense of humor much like Mary and Grace's. Not long ago Jenny said, "You're both great if you don't stand up."

Mary told me, "Jenny sees all kinds of things that we like and surprises us with them."

Because of Jenny's shopping forays, Mary is able to eat a good, well-balanced meal each day. "I don't eat a lot of meat, but I do have chicken or fish or a casserole each night. And I make a pretty salad, which I love. Even though it's sometimes a bother, I stick to my schedule. I need to do that balanced meal to keep well. And I eat at 5:30 every night."

It was Jenny and George who rescued Mary last year when she fell down the steps at 2 A.M. and lay on the floor for 3 hours before she could summon help.

"How did it happen?" I asked.

"Well, I got up to get a glass of water and a pain pill from the bathroom, which is across the hall from my room. On my way from my room, I turned on the light above the dresser. I guess it was so bright it disoriented me for a minute. I must have been confused. Instead of putting my walker on the floor, I set it over the steps and pitched down them head first. Later we found a pool of blood on the landing. Although I don't remember much of it, I must have bumped down those four steps on my right side, scraping everything I own. I was on the floor of the upstairs hall when I came to. I evidently had got my bearings sometime and somehow made it up the four steps to the top. How I did it I don't know. I could never have sat on the step and gone up one at a time. And with my knees I never could have crawled. But I suppose I must have. I don't remember any of it. I could feel the blood on my face and on the floor. My right eye, the only one I can see out of, was swollen shut. Everything was dark. I couldn't see anything unless I lifted my eyelid. I sat there until I could see it was daylight. I would push the eyelid up, crawl a little, push the eyelid up, and so on. The hall light was too high for me to reach.

"Anyway, after sitting there awhile, I finally managed to inch into my room, where I tried to pull myself up by hanging onto a chair, then the dresser, and then the bed. None of these worked. The mattress on my bed is a little smaller than the frame, so there is a little metal ledge between. That had needed dusting for a long time, so I ran my finger across it and ended with a pile of dust at the end of the frame. But there was nowhere to put it, so I spread it out again.

"I was there 2 hours. I could tell by the programs on the radio, which was still on.

"Finally it was five o'clock, and I felt it wasn't too early to call Jenny. She and George came right away, dressed me, and took me to the hospital, where they told me I had a concussion. They put a long bag of ice on my face, and it began to hurt a little less. My head ached terribly."

"Weren't you wearing your medical-alert signal?" I asked.

"Yes, but if they had come, they would have had to break the door down. I didn't want that."

"How long were you in the hospital?"

"A week."

"Could this happen again?"

"No, now my neighbor has a key, and the security people know it."

"Have you changed anything else?"

"Yes, there is a night light in the hall now."

"And the aftermath?"

"Well, I tire more easily, and I've never gotten my strength back."

So, that is Mary to date. I think she manages very, very well— all things considered. It isn't rosy always, but she is able to keep her perspective most of the time. She and Grace talk several times a day and still have tremendous love and support for one another. And there is still the bond of the extreme empathy or extrasensory perception. Call it what you will. It is as strong as it has always been: They always check on each other in the morning, but at least several times a week when Mary calls her, Grace's line is busy—calling you know who.

Last year, after falling down the basement steps, Grace had to have a hip replaced. The day she had the operation, Mary's hip ached worse than it ever had. At the exact time the operation ended, so did Mary's pain.

They no longer give each other birthday presents because year after year they ended up with a duplicate of what they had given.

At least once a week Grace picks up Mary to go to have their hair done. Afterwards they go to one of the several restaurants that are favorites, where they are given deluxe treatment. The other day, a Saturday, Mary called Grace and said, "Let's struggle ourselves out of here tomorrow and go out for dinner."

When she returns from being out, Mary always takes two aspirin or perhaps a pain pill for the pain her trip has brought on. Other days she will get by on three ibuprofen-400 tablets and perhaps two aspirin or a pain pill. In the past, she has taken ibuprofen 800, "but it did not sit well."

Mary tries to stick to her regular schedule. "Things just go better when I stay on it."

She usually gets up at 8 A.M. and is downstairs by 9 A.M. It takes her 2 or 3 minutes to go down those 10 stairs. About half way down the steps, Chester, her big gray Persian cat, begins howling for her to let him out of the kitchen. "I's acomin', Chester," she tells him. Once she is downstairs, she sits and rests for 2 or 3 minutes.

Her days, aside from her chores, are spent reading, working on her reports, doing the paperwork that her arthritis and other things involve, and keeping up with her sports. On Saturdays she can usually be found with both the radio and the television on, listening to two games—or more, if she switches back and forth.

The other day when I called, Mary's tears were very close to the surface. The lilt in her voice was missing.

"What's wrong?" I asked.

"I've..." It was hard for her to say it, but I waited and she told me she had decided to give up her car.

"That would make you sad, I know."

I recalled that, years ago, I interviewed a 93-year-old artist who had once driven her little coupe the wrong way down a one-way street. A young policeman had been watching, and he asked her to please not drive. She handed him her license. "A car makes you free," the woman told me. After that interview, I drove away in my little Simca feeling sad and unnecessarily privileged.

But Mary is a survivor. And members of her family have lived to 93 and older. She tells me, "Sometimes with all the pain and discomfort, my mind becomes like a bird trapped in a shut room. Sometimes at times like that it seems unbearable. But then my mind quiets, and the pain settles down to a dull, persistent ache—one with which I can live. Do you remember that Robert Louis Stevenson said, 'A generous prayer is never in vain'?"

I say I do indeed and that I think I have a pretty direct line sometimes. And furthermore, if she can fit her excursions around my bothersome angina pains, I think I can find her a driver.

What follows are 28 steps which ease Mary through her days. Perhaps you will find some of them helpful.

Mary's 28 Steps

1. **The Escalator Step: Keep Moving.**
   Try to avoid sitting in one position for more than half an hour. Move around if you can. If you can't walk, move your legs if you can. It helps circulation and prevents stiffness.

2. **Strip Your Life of the Nonessentials.**
   Mary says she now drinks ice water instead of tea or coffee. She says it doesn't make that much difference to her. "I try to simplify my life."

3. **Manage Your Pain. Don't Let It Control You.**
   How much pain can you stand? Do you quit tasks before the pain becomes unmanageable? Set goals within your pain-free or low-pain times. Pace your activities. Learn from your pain. Don't be a martyr. If you have pills which will eliminate or dull your pain, take them. Don't, however, take more than you need. Try to avoid pain-spasm-pain cycles.

   Pain is subjective. It's different for everyone. You perhaps have heard stories such as that of the hockey player who played an entire half with four broken ribs, or ballet stars who won't quit even though they have sprained an ankle. A soldier in battle may not acknowledge pain until after throwing the grenade into the enemy's machine-gun nest.

The threshold of pain is different not only for each individual but also at different times for each person. You have to learn how to manage your pain, to set your goals within the range of your pain. Sometimes people do not wish to take pain medication. Mary doesn't like to feel dopey; she would rather have her mind clear.

Perhaps you can be like the Oriental and put your pain in a box in your mind and keep it there. This seems to work for other problems too.

4. **A Cluttered and Dusty House May Be a Problem Only for the Person Who Doesn't Live There.**
Mary says that selective seeing really does work, and I can vouch for it. Besides, every time she or I pick up a copy of *Architectural Digest* and see the books not only knee-high on the coffee table, but under it, too, we know we're in style.

5. **Don't Make Any Promises or Commitments You Might Not Be Able to Keep.**
Mary plans her talks for her clubs so she can give them in the late spring and fall when the weather is fair. In this way, the chance of foul weather interrupting her schedule is reduced.

6. **Keep in Touch with Friends.**
By phone if there is no other way. Keep up your correspondence with friends. You know how good you feel when a letter comes. If your hands don't let you write or type, perhaps you can put your message on tape. Most people have access to an inexpensive tape recorder.

7. **Practice Relaxation.**
Try meditation or some other techniques with the mental exercises of your choice. Yoga, Zen, etc., can all be of benefit to anyone with a problem, and pain is definitely a

problem. Incidentally, biofeedback has proved very successful for some in diminishing and eliminating severe pain.

8. **Flow with Your Feelings.**
As Mary says, "When you feel like crying, cry." She
doesn't mean, though, that you should wallow in self-pity
or run amok, telling the world to go to hell.

9. **Consider Getting a Pet.**
However, not one that might cause you to fall. A pet can
take you out of yourself. When dogs were taken to visit
residents in a rest home, the people were delighted. Several
people who hadn't spoken in a long, long time talked to the
dogs.

10. **Have Faith in Something Bigger Than Yourself.**
If you don't believe in a divine being, there are a lot of other
options. You might believe in nature's process of healing.
Unfortunately nature takes longer to heal a body than it
does to destroy it or wreak havoc with disease, but often
medicine and other treatment can accelerate healing.

11. **Be Positive. No One Likes a Whiner.**
Several times while we were doing this chapter, Mary said
something like this, "My land! I've told you more about
myself than I've ever told anyone else. It always bores me
to talk about myself. Usually when people say, 'How do
you feel?' I say that I'm fine and move right on to another
topic. But you say this information will help other people,
so I don't mind."
   "I'm grateful," I tell her, thinking that sometimes attitude
is everything.

12. **Work Out Short Cuts. Think Up Ways to Manage with Less
Effort.**
Practice whatever time-, labor-, or energy-saving tricks you
can. Mary stacks things on a stool and pushes the stool
from the table to the refrigerator. And to the counter where
the sink is. She keeps items from a low cupboard shelf on

the counter. It isn't pretty, and she says she shouldn't do it; but as her next-door neighbor says, "Why not?"

13. **Learn to Accept Your Condition.**
As Mary says, "There's always someone struggling just as hard as I am. And there are a lot of people worse off."
I think this means that most of the time she accepts her problems, but occasionally, her logical mind rebels.

14. **Do Things Vicariously.**
If you can't actually do all the things your mind wishes you could, try doing them vicariously. Certainly Mary's programs on the cable sports station must be a vicarious game for her. Vicarious, too, are other things such as her Paris report to the club.

15. **Practice Mind Over Matter.**
When I ask Mary, in wonderment, how she manages, she says, "It's mind over matter, Betty. It's all in the mind. You see in my mind, I still wear pretty shoes and can run. In my mind, I don't have to walk so slowly. I still stand tall and can take the steps two at a time if I like." And then, with a tear, "I'm constantly astounded that my legs won't do what my mind still thinks I can. Yes, and because I was a person who always did things quickly and easily, I am chagrined and then angered that my body won't carry out my wishes. In my mind, I never get tired."

16. **Realize that You Can Think of Only One Thing at a Time.**
When something sad happens, for a while afterward whenever you think about it, quickly think of something else. Eventually you'll be able to think about it comfortably.

17. **Keep Up with Current Events and National and International Happenings.**
Mary subscribes to several cable stations and loves them. "It's marvelous!" she says. "They have nothing but news all day and night."

18.   Try to See Any Humor There Might Be in a Situation.

One day Mary and I were talking about sports. I told her that I really missed playing tennis, and she said, "I loved hockey too, but I wouldn't be much good on a team today, would I?"

"Probably not," I said, "but I'll bet you could play a mean game of croquet."

She laughed and said, "I could really get an eye on the ball, couldn't I?"

"But talk about a sense of humor," said Mary. "When Grace fell down the basement steps before she had her hip replaced, she picked herself up and said to herself, 'Well, I guess I didn't break anything. I might as well do the washing while I'm down here.' And she did. She hates stairs as much as I do."

19.   Take Advantage of Any Services Your Town Provides. Don't Be Afraid to Ask People for Help.

In most communities, the library will bring books you wish to read to your home.

The visiting nurses will come by for a fee that isn't huge.

Don't be afraid to ask neighbors, friends, and especially children whom you know. Most people truly enjoy helping others. It makes them feel good.

Mary said she now doesn't hesitate to ask people to do things like open doors. Only once was anyone rude. A woman at the drugstore opened the door for her but said, "What are you doing out alone? You should be home."

"She must have had a bad day."

"She certainly looked like it. A bad month too."

20.   Sometimes Living Alone Can Be Heaven.

You can take a shower or play records at midnight. You can run around all day in your socks if you want to. You may be locked out of a few things, but on the other hand, you're not locked into anything. When you have arthritis, living alone can spell INDEPENDENCE.

21.   Have an Interest in Something. Be an Authority.

Mary's interest is sports, but the number of things to be

intrigued by is as wide as a set of *The Encyclopaedia Britannica*. Pick a subject and go for it. Remember, the library will probably deliver. I have a friend who reads eight times as many books as I do. The only difference is she's blind and does hers with free talking books.

22. Be Good to Yourself.
Have your hair done if you can manage it. Eat out once a week even if it's an effort. If you can, order a pretty plant, or a pizza, or a box of beautiful grapefruit or oranges. Maybe you could send a cab to bring a friend for a visit. I have a homebound friend whose children sent a childhood friend of hers a plane ticket to visit their mother. It was a lovely birthday surprise.

23. Don't Give In to Self-Pity.
It's one way to depression. Mary says you can't dwell on your problems unless you're working on something that will better your condition or your attitude or your well-being.

24. Take One Day at a Time.
"Be glad when you've been able to complete the day without a major mishap," Mary says. "I used to get so impatient because I couldn't do things, but now I'm used to it. But even though I'm more patient now, I still get frustrated."

I said, "I imagine that given who you are and with all you once did, you will always find that true. Maybe it's just a given you'll have to work with."

25. Be a Listener.
When there's nothing for you to do, give someone a call and really listen to what that person is saying. Or invite someone over. Don't be a passive listener. Practice making helpful comments. Practice asking questions. Listen to Barbara Walters or Ted Koppel. It's a skill you can learn.

26. Expand Your Self-Image.
A self-image, you know, isn't a steady thing. In the best of us, it waxes and wanes just like the moon or the tide. But you can do a great deal to enhance your self-image. *Read-*

er's Digest once put out an interesting little book called *Giving Yourself Away.* There were all kinds of lovely and interesting tales of people who gave part of themselves. Mary shares *Sports Illustrated* with the young man next door, who keeps things repaired around her house and handles her trash.

For me, Mary does two things. I'd hate to live without either of them. Whenever the Book-of-the-Month Club puts out a dividend catalog, she gives me about 50 dividends, and I go on a buying spree and order beautiful $20 and $25 books at ridiculously low prices. How about a $50 art or literary book for $2.00? She also is always there when I need help with grammar. Once in a very great while (like once a year), she is baffled. But we always can work it out together. I'd be a lot more ignorant without her.

27.   Problems Are Often Solvable If You Educate Yourself.
This is one of Mary's most important rules. Because she refuses to be overpowered by anything, she finds out all she can about things. I think she's the kind of person Henry Peter Brougham was thinking of when he wrote:

> Education makes people easy to lead, but
> difficult to drive; easy to govern, but
> impossible to enslave.

Mary is a free spirit if I've ever known one. She has arthritis; it does not have her. And the only person she might ever be said to be a slave of is Chester, her 16-pound, 1 1/2-foot-wide, gray Persian cat, because Chester is in charge. "I live with Chester," says Mary.

28.   Make Use of Memories.
When you want to give up, try reliving some of your best times. The quotation "God gave us memories so we would have roses in December" has great merit.

I hope these suggestions will help you improve the quality of your life. As the doctors say in this book:

Any chronic rheumatic-pain disorder can be frustrating; butif you live your life in a manner that allows you to achieve your goals without compromising your health, you can look back and say, 'I have been a successful human being.' Any patient with persistent rheumatoid arthritis is a true hero if he can adapt his living habits successfully.

I can't say it any better than that.

CHAPTER 14

Sports and Conditioning Activities

Your Body May Be Willing, But...

"The greatest number of sports-related injuries in North America are now incurred by amateur athletes." That is the word from Dr. Lyle J. Michell, writing in the February 1986 issue of *The Journal of Musculoskeletal Medicine*. In addition to being director of the division of sports medicine at Children's Hospital Center in Boston, Dr. Michell is physician for the Boston Ballet and the Boston Marathon.

The new word in fitness may be "Easy does it!" but there are millions out there jogging, jumping, climbing, sliding, etc., and far too many of these millions are unaware that trouble may be waiting for them. They simply aren't in condition. Sports do put you in condition, it's true; but if you are to avoid aching and injuring, you must warm up before a sport, and cool down after it. Some warm-up exercises are outlined in Table 14-1 at the end of this chapter.

Without the warm-up, you can be put out of commission before you really get a running start. The warm-up is the most important preventive measure in any sport. First you should use appropriate stretching exercises that improve flexibility. After that, begin to participate *gradually* in your sports activity. This is especially true if you are over 35.

In addition to the warm-up exercises given in Table 14-1, other preventive measures are listed for many popular sports in Tables 14-2 through 14-8. Follow the directives in these in order to safely participate in sports.

Have a general physical examination. Your doctor will, we hope, ask specific questions about any physical abnormalities you may have and explain how they relate to the activity you wish to pursue. Be sure to check Figure 14-1 for some common ways of looking at yourself to detect any structural abnormalities. For example, specific imbalances of the legs, such as flatfeet, can create the milieu for injuries. A physician spotting such a problem would probably

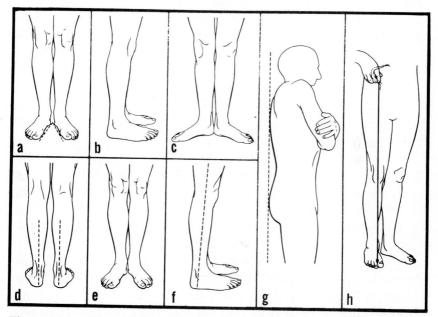

Figure 14-1.   If you follow this alignment chart you can see such simple but important abnormalities as curvature of the spine, unequal leg length, flatfeet, and kneecap alterations. Also look at yourself in a mirror and note leg straightness. How do you stand in the fitness game? (*a*) Feet should point away at about a 30-degree angle. (*b*) Toes should be flat on the floor. (*c*) Arches should be slightly raised (feet are separated to show this). (*d*) Heel cords should be perfectly vertical. (*e*) Ankles and knees should touch. (*f*) Knees should be straight and not bend forward or back. (*g*) Small of back should be slightly curved. (*h*) A weight suspended from a string at the iliac crest (dotted lines) should touch the second toe.

recommend a simple shoe insert to prevent an injury. Other structural abnormalities should be identified and compensated for with appropriate choice of equipment and sports activity. Patients with mild arthritis should avoid impact-type activities such as jogging. Swimming and bicycling may be advantageous.

During this past decade the number of sport participants has brought a large increase in sports-related injuries, and the greatest number of these have been found in amateur sports. Although all these people are active in sports and/or conditioning programs, their overall fitness is less than that of a professional athlete. Lacking fitness, they are prone to strains from overusing tendons and muscles.

One of the body components most apt to be damaged is the ligaments, bands of strong tissue that connect bones and provide stability for our joints. When a joint is unnaturally forced, ligament tissue is damaged. An injury of this type is called a *sprain*. Twisting and wrenching often damage ligaments and their adjacent blood vessels.

Muscles consist of fibers attached to bone by tendons. Muscles are the pulling strength that moves joints and propels us forward. Each muscle has a maximal level of stress; if this level is exceeded by overstretching during a violent movement, muscle fibers tear. This injury is known as *strain*.

Tendons, the bands of dense fibrous tissue connecting the muscles to bone, transmit the muscle force to move our joints. Tendons in the shoulder, knee, elbow, and heel are most prone to injury because they are more exposed and more frequently used. Their injury results in inflammation, swelling, redness, and heat within the tissue. All this brings pain, the warning signal. The reddening and heat are caused by blood rushing to the tendon area to help heal the injury. The inflammation results in swelling. With healing, inflammation and pain subside; function returns.

In addition to ligaments, muscles, and tendons, *bursas* also become easily inflamed. These are sacs of fluid that reduce friction between tendons, muscles, and bone. Inflammation of bursal sacs results in bursitis, a condition with characteristics pretty much identical to the previously noted inflammations.

Sports for Women

The number of women athletes has increased dramatically, bringing with this increase even more injuries from poor physical conditioning. As with men, the results are muscle strains, ankle sprains, and low-back injuries. In general, women have more delicate tissue structure; smaller, shorter bones; a wider pelvis; joints that are more lax; and a lower center of gravity, which produces excellent balance. Finally, women have more extensibility between the femur (thigh bone) and the tibia (shinbone). Despite the extra motion this provides, the resultant relative loose-jointedness tends to increase knee problems.

Women also have a greater tendency toward flatfeet. They have less muscle mass and therefore less power and speed. Additionally, they have a higher proportion of body fat, providing them with better energy use. Because of this metabolic efficiency, they excel in long-distance sports. However, women are prone to iron-deficiency anemia as well as to smaller oxygen capacity, both of which demand greater training to reach maximum effort. Women suffer injuries similar to those of men, but women also have injuries that are due to sex differences.

Vaginal lacerations are a possibility, and some women may experience an early cessation of menstrual periods and other gynecologic problems. In fact, at the 1986 meeting of the American College of Obstetricians and Gynecologists (ACOG) after a discussion of exercise- and sports-related injuries, ACOG's conclusion was that when it comes to high-energy activities the risk of injury easily "rises out of proportion to the actual benefits." [1]

Moderate exercises include racket sports, swimming, and jogging. But the best exercise is walking—it improves both mind and body. Osteoporosis, so devastating to the older woman, may be prevented, at least in part, by walking for one-half hour three days a week.

Preventing Injuries

The best treatment for sports-related injuries in amateurs will always be their prevention. Such prevention ranges from using proper equipment to practicing conditioning that improves body flexibility and stamina. It also must include appropriate strengthening exercises. Your performance goals should be based on your skill and

---

1. Myron Benton, "The Fitness Craze," *Cosmopolitan*, Nov. 1986, pp. 277–279.

capability; that is, be realistic and don't overextend your objectives. You are more likely to suffer an injury when you are tired, tense, or out of shape. Therefore, maintaining a good level of fitness is important. Find your level and exercise at this level regularly. Appropriate protective devices, such as eye guards for racket sports, are critical.

Appropriate shoes also help prevent injuries. At the end of this chapter you will find tables of ideas for preventing injuries in a variety of sports.

If you do receive an injury, should you see a doctor? If the simple first-aid remedies—ice, compression (elastic bandage), elevation—do not rapidly reduce swelling and inflammation, you should find professional help. Pain signals *caution*. If it persists, it signals *danger*! Prolonged inability to use an extremity is also an important red flag. In general, if you are unsure about an injury or its healing, it pays to call a doctor.

When you begin to exercise, avoid *abrupt* changes in the intensity, duration, and frequency of training. Slowly building to your level of training and activity will prevent many of the injuries we often see. Matching strength and flexibility of muscles to your sports activity is important. An example would be appropriate strength-training of the forearm muscles for tennis. Improper footwear causes many overuse injuries, so be sure your shoes fit, have enough impact absorption, and have a flexible sole with sufficient heel support. As we age, our muscles and bones absorb impact shocks less efficiently. Therefore, we should consider the surface on which we play. Especially, runners should avoid concrete and confine their jogging to tracks, grass, or asphalt.

In any sport, equipment should be appropriate if you are to prevent injuries and get maximum enjoyment from the activity. Home-exercise regalia for conditioning really is not necessary, and it may be very expensive. Simple equipment that builds endurance and cardiovascular strength can be very inexpensive: a $3 jump rope will develop endurance as effectively as a $5,000 electronic treadmill, and a $10 three-pound dumbbell can develop upper body strength just as effectively as $30 weighted-pulley equipment.

Eating habits too are important if you are to maintain overall physical fitness. Fad diets, such as carbohydrate-loading before running, should be discussed with a physician or nutritionist. A well-balanced daily diet of proteins, carbohydrates, and fats is best. Before sports participation, fluid should be ingested. Too often, a tennis player in a match on a hot day concentrates so hard on winning that she or he forgets to drink appropriate fluids. Water itself does not contain the chemical balance necessary to maintain our body fluid. Salt tablets and better balanced fluid, such as Gatorade, can be used.

Burning Up Calories

If you want to lose weight, you must burn more calories than you consume. If you multiply your weight by 10, you get your baseline calorie burn—the number of calories you use without moving about. If you are a housekeeper or office worker, add another 20 percent. Factory workers must add 30 percent. Multiply the figure by 7 to get your calorie burn per week. For example, if you are a 150-pound office worker, you probably burn 12,600 calories per week.

	Sedentary Worker	Factory Worker
Present weight	150	235
Baseline calorie burn	1,500	2,350
Additional activity burn	300	705
Daily calorie burn	1,800	3,055
Weekly calorie burn	12,600	21,385

Suppose you decide to consume 1400 calories per day, that is, 9800 calories per week. Figure the calories you will lose per week:

Weekly calorie burn	12,600	21,385
Weekly calorie intake	9,800	9,800
Calories lost	2,800	11,585

Burning up 3600 calories is approximately equal to burning up a pound of body fat. Therefore, you will lose 0.8 pounds per week if you are a relatively sedentary worker and 3.2 pounds per week if you work in a factory.

To lose 2 pounds per week, you must burn 7200 calories more than you consume. As a sedentary worker, you will not attain your goal unless you increase your caloric burn rate by 4400 per week. This is equivalent to about 625 calories, or 2 hours of exercise, per day. However, some activities burn more calories than others. Here are some approximate calories expended per hour for various exercises:

Activity	Calories per hour
Bicycling	180–300
Volleyball	180–600
Golf	200–300
Walking	200–300
Tennis (doubles)	300–350
Aerobic dancing	300–360
Ballroom dancing	300–400
Swimming	300–600
Skating	350–400
Tennis (singles)	400–500
Jogging	500–600
Squash	500–600
Handball	600–660
Cross-country skiing	600–900
Downhill skiing	900
Running (10 mph)	1100–1200

How to Treat an Injury

Although we physicians want to prevent overuse syndromes in amateur athletes, it is just as important to manage acute injuries properly. The RICE program described earlier consists of:

Rest: Although the runner who suffers a contusion (bruised muscle) must stop running, he or she can swim to maintain fitness. Rest of the specific injury site is important, but you still can perform other exercises to maintain strength in other body areas.

Ice: During the first 24 to 48 hours after injury, applying ice is helpful. Apply immediately after injury and for as long as tolerated; then use intermittently. Consider *ice massage* if the skin is intact. This increases deep circulation and healing. Make a cone of ice by filling a paper cup with water, pinching the top together with staples or a paper clip, and then freezing. Remove the ice, hold the larger end with a towel, and rub the narrow end back and forth along the injured tissue. Rub deeply and slowly for 2 to 5 minutes; then return the ice to the freezer for a later application.

Compression: Bandaging the injured part is important for early injury management. Remove bandage intermittently (depending upon comfort) and reapply with equal and gentle pressure.

Elevation: Raise the injured limb to just above *heart level* to reduce swelling and improve blood flow.

Finally, when is it safe to return to play? Some general guidelines include:

Waiting until full motion of the injured joint returns.

Waiting until about 90 percent of the normal strength of the injured extremity returns. (Compare with the opposite side.) Many health facilities in your area will have equipment to measure the specific strength.

Waiting until flexibility has been attained.

Are you unsure whether the stressful demands of the activity will aggravate your injury? Better err on the conservative side or seek professional advice. Any injury that does not seem to be healing should send you to a professional. This is obvious in acute injuries but perhaps not so apparent in chronic overuse injuries.

The following diagnoses and treatment of injuries have been discussed in previous chapters. Specific information related to sporting activities is presented here, but we recommend that you also read other chapters for more information about these injuries and their treatment.

Home-Exercise Programs

The home-exercise program you choose should depend on whether your goal is aerobic conditioning. This increases the efficiency of the heart, muscle development, weight control, flexibility, and release of muscular tension. You need to match your goal with a particular program. All of these goals, however, are important in an overall training program.

Aerobic exercise must be continued and maintained for at least 20 minutes. This type of exercise usually uses the long muscles of the body. You should be able to attain a heart-work capacity of 80 percent; this capacity can be calculated approximately by subtracting your age from 220, and multiplying the result by 0.8. Aerobic equipment includes rowing machines, exercise bikes, machines that simulate cross-country skiing, treadmills, and jump ropes. As we mentioned, less expensive exercise equipment can be suitable.

You can obtain *muscular development* by lifting weights against resistance, for example with dumbbells. In earlier chapters we have already described many more of these exercises for stretching and toning your muscles.

Table 14-2 presents important ideas you should consider before undertaking a home-exercise program. Patients with either back or joint problems should modify the use of exercise equipment and also review that exercise with their physician after a physical examination. Prior to purchasing any exercise equipment try it out in a health club or a store. Generally, a sure way to create an overstrain problem is to participate at a strenuous level with new equipment. Instead, start with a slow exercise program on a regular basis and *gradually* build to your maximum efficiency.

If you wish to release muscular tension and achieve relaxation, use *passive measures,* such as a hot bath. Or you might hang from a chinning bar. Yoga, meditation, and biofeedback are also very helpful.

Racket Sports

We'll use tennis as our illustrative sport because most of the problems of other racket sports occur in tennis and because it is one of the most popular sports.

Two types of injury occur in tennis:

1. *Acute injuries:* Usually of the lower extremities; problems comprise strains of the calf muscles, ruptures of the Achilles tendon, and ankle and knee sprains.

2. *Minor and more common injuries:* Overstrain due to improper stroke or poor conditioning of the upper extremity.

Tennis Elbow

Tennis elbow is a problem of overuse or improper stroke execution. With tennis shoulder (discussed below), it remains the most common problem of both amateur and professional players and usually results from incorrect forearm movements and a too-firm grip. Tennis elbow may occur in other activities that require movements similar to those in tennis, leading to overstrain with tears in the extensor tendons (those that move the wrist joint in an upward direction). These microscopic tears result in inflammation, swelling, and pain. The same problem afflicts the muscles and tendons on the inner aspect of the arm, which flex the wrist downward. Commonly known as tennis elbow or golfer's elbow, the medical term is *lateral epicondylitis* when it occurs on the outer side of the elbow and *medial epicondylitis* when it occurs on the inner aspect of the elbow. These problems relate directly to the frequency of play and age of participant; they are usually the result of an improper backhand.

If there is pain over the outer aspect of the elbow and if it is tender when you press it, you probably have tennis elbow. Pain usually increases if you raise the back of your hand bringing the wrist upward against your other hand. Pain on the inner aspect of the elbow with local tenderness and discomfort suggests medial epicondylitis. The pain is noted when you lower the involved hand (making a downward movement of the wrist) against your other hand.

Treatment of *acute* tennis elbow is less successful than it is for many other chronic problems. You should first eliminate the activity causing the pain and then rest the arm. Stretching, ice, and compression (elastic bandage) should be used for half an hour after the injury and intermittently, several hours a day, until the pain severity and other local symptoms have subsided. Rest is important. Also use stretching exercises and then gradually strengthen the involved muscle groups described in Chapter 6. Institute these early. If pain continues with normal activities or if swelling or redness appears 48 to 72 hours later, use simple first-aid treatment and seek help from a professional.

The physician may use nonsteroidal anti-inflammatory drugs such as ibuprofen or indomethecin for the inflammation and provide appropriate splints. If the condition is prolonged she or he might inject with a cortisone preparation. Limit injections to two or three to avoid tissue injury from the cortisone. As in any injury, healing is complete when pain subsides and motion, strength, and endurance return. It is critical that recreational athletes with tennis elbow participate in regular and consistent isometric (without motion) and isotonic (with motion) exercises for the principal forearm muscles.

These exercises should be under the guidance of a physical therapist or sports physiologist. Your physician can refer you to these people, who are in private practice or with a local health spa.

Treatment for chronic tennis elbow is similar to that for acute tennis elbow. Rest and gradual resumption of use help. The most important treatment of all is appropriate stretching and strengthening exercises. Ice for half an hour after the athletic activity and an elastic compression bandage both help to eliminate pain. A tennis-elbow band just below the elbow can be a great aid in treating, even preventing, this chronic ailment (see Chapter 6). Additional therapeutics include intermittent heat, ultrasound, and friction massage. Again, doctors will use cortisone injections only in persistently intractable cases. Additionally, if immobilization is used, it should be only in conjunction with a stretching and strengthening exercise program. These overall considerations are similar to those for other racket sports.

As before, the primary concept is still prevention. Read and review Table 14-3 before you begin a racket sport. Also, general prevention techniques such as proper equipment, good training, and good judgment are critical. Appropriate shoes for racket sports need a relatively wide toe and excellent support features. Improper equipment, which causes overload patterns (particularly twisting motions), is also a causative factor in tennis elbow. You will obtain better racket control by purchasing a racket with the largest handle you can grip. Use moderate (approximately 55-pound) string tension. A Velcro brace around the upper forearm, just below the elbow, will take care of any worries you have about weakness of the forearm muscles, those affected by tennis elbow. This reduces muscular overload and may also help prevent tennis elbow.

When a player exceeds his muscle capacity, the condition is known as an *overload force*. The most important factor in preventing and avoiding overload forces is the development of a proper tennis stroke. Proper body-weight transfer and strong shoulder-muscle groupings determine the energy you have for hitting a tennis or other racket ball. Most amateur racket-sport enthusiasts find their primary problem is their backhand. If your backhand is correct, the front of the shoulder is depressed, the elbow fixed, tip of the elbow pointing toward the ground, and arm away and with the palm slightly upward. Improperly executed backhand will result from your elbow pointing to the net and your shoulder elevated. To hit the ball with any power, you need a sudden straightening of the elbow and snapping of the wrist, which creates a twisting force at the elbow. If the snap is not strong enough, you can cause microscopic tears of the tendons. Prevention is easy if you will obtain appropriate instruction and use a proper stroke.

Tennis Shoulder

Like tennis elbow, tennis shoulder is a problem of overuse or improper stroke execution. Sport activities requiring repetitive overhand arm use (tennis, squash, etc.) may give you a painful shoulder. The shoulder-joint's anatomy makes it very susceptible to problems such as inflammation of tendons or bursas because the shoulder area, in overhead activities, has inadequate space in which to accommodate the tendons. Plate 5-2 shows the problem: Note the joint at the top of the shoulder where the collarbone meets the acromion, below and to the front of which is another projection of the shoulder bones (the coracoid process). To compound the problem, a sharp ligament runs between the collarbone and the acromion, which can act as a knife during shoulder movements. The area under the acromion process is extremely tight, and in overhead activities the tendons or the rotator cuff are compressed against the bone. After repetitive movements, you probably will end up with small tears and inflammation of the adjacent tendons. With ever more overuse there may, in fact, be rotator cuff tears and degeneration of the area.

Your physician can treat tendinitis successfully if both of you recognize it early. Known as the *impingement syndrome,* this tendinitis has a sequence of problems. In the first stage (usually in younger athletes) the tendon may become pinched. If it does, it results in mild tendinitis manifested by swelling. Pain may occur only during the elevation arc at a straight-out position. Pain is localized and will usually stop when you restrict harmful activity. The second stage (usually in athletes in the 25- to 40-year-old group) brings a more chronic lesion—with scar tissue. Your pain may be worse not only while performing the activity but also while resting. You will note tenderness just in front of the point of the shoulder. More information about the impingement syndrome is in Chapter 5.

At this point in the sequence giving up the activity does not often cure the problem of painful shoulder motion. If it doesn't, more aggressive treatment must be instituted. In the older athlete, aging problems (such as degeneration) may add to the inflammatory process throughout the entire tendon attachments known as the *shoulder cuff*. Weakness, tears, and stiffness compound the problem, and small spurs may develop. Usually you will have pain during both activity and rest. Treatment in this stage can be successful, but it takes a long time.

Treatment for a younger patient with acute problems is similar to any initial conservative program. The patient should rest the shoulder by switching to another sport, but not to swimming. Using ice with an anti-inflammatory medication such as aspirin often works well. If the pain persists or is severe or if there is swelling, a physician should be consulted. Using other physical therapy such as ultrasound and diathermy may help relieve the acute symptoms. Although a conservative treatment program (rest, exercise, non-steroidal anti-inflammatory drugs, and local cortisone shots, as described in Chapter 5) is helpful in some cases, surgery may have to be considered. Because the impingement of the tendons has been caused by the too-small space, the surgeon will increase the space by removing part of the bone. Hopefully, such an operation will return the athlete to a high level of efficiency and enjoyment.

If your problem is so severe that you seek medical care, your physician will probably order shoulder x-rays and may also order special tests. Two of these are an ultrasound test, which bounces sound waves off a tissue to create an image of the tissue, and an arthrogram, in which a dye is injected that shows on x-ray.

Prevention still remains the best, most efficacious treatment for tennis shoulder. Amateur athletes should be more diligent in performing careful warm-up exercises, including stretching of the upper and lower extremities as outlined in this book. Injuries are more likely to occur when the player is tired, tense, or underconditioned. Both isometric exercises (without motion) and kinetic exercises (against a weighted machine) should be used to build strength and endurance of the shoulder and arm. Referral to a physical therapist may be made. Because improper technique is again the cause of these overstrain problems, modifying the serve by softening it or turning the body to avoid the impingement may prevent or alleviate the symptoms.

Tennis Leg

Injuries to the calf muscles generally result from overuse, and they are very common in tennis and other racket sports. Such calf-muscle injuries can occur immediately after sharp twisting or jumping movements, and they usually occur when the player pushes off with the knee straight. Almost all middle-aged racket-sport players have some degree of muscle fatigue. Also, they have degenerative soft-tissue (such as tendon or ligament) changes, which are susceptible to rapid and elevated forces in muscles during play.

Typically, a player experiences a sudden sharp calf pain while running or reaching. The pain is similar to that which results when you are hit in the back of the calf with a tennis ball or racket. There is tenderness over the calf behind the knee and in the middle of the calf muscle. You may see immediate swelling followed by black-and-blue bruises, and any attempt to squat or bring the foot up or both is painful and restricted. Commonly, rupture of some small, thin tendons occurs but without permanent functional loss. You should treat this acute strain by applying ice immediately and intermittently during the next 2 days; you should also apply a compression bandage. Generally rest and elevation of the leg also help. Try to move your ankle and knee as soon as possible. Because symptoms do not quickly subside, you will probably want to seek professional help. When the initial soreness abates, a small heel lift placed in your shoe may aid walking; if so, it should be used for a few weeks. After the acute symptoms do subside, a muscle-strengthening exercise program should be instituted. This should include strengthening the muscles in front of the leg as well as the entire leg musculature. See Table 11-6, exercises 3 and 4. Also, stretching exercises for the calf muscles should be started within a few weeks. Return to play only after you attain your normal leg strength and flexibility.

The key, however, to calf injuries is prevention, and prevention should be routine. In addition, it must include stretching exercises of the calf muscles. There are many techniques for accomplishing this, including wall stretching (Table 11-6, exercise 1) and the preventive measures listed in Table 11-5.

Achilles-Tendon Rupture

The large tendon that attaches the heel to the calf muscle and allows us to raise our heel from the ground is known as the *Achilles tendon*. Rupture or inflammation here occurs frequently and appears to be from repetitive trauma in the area that causes small tears, chronic inflammation, and ultimate scarring. A healthy tendon does not rupture without a great deal of trauma. Again, poorly conditioned and aggressive athletes who are middle-aged are most prone to this injury.

A forced overstrain of the tendon in pushing off with the knee straight may result in *rupture* of the Achilles tendon. Pain is instantaneous. So, too, is swelling in the calf, an indenting in the back of the ankle, bruising of the skin, and an inability to walk. In general, the symptoms and signs are so severe that professional help is almost always sought. It should be sought immediately after the injury! Surgery, which repairs the tendon, is usually indicated. However, nonsurgical treatment may be used. Such treatment requires immobilization in a cast for a prolonged time. Sadly, patients generally do not have the same athletic performance level at the conclusion of the healing period as they did before the injury. Surgical treatment is definitely indicated for most younger patients with the problem.

No matter what the treatment, the rehabilitation program of from 6 to 12 months is critical. After an initial period of from 1 to 3 months of immobilization, a rehabilitation program should be started. Basically, such a program involves a course of exercises, to strengthen the calf muscles, and a gradual stretching program. Most athletes need a full year to return to a reasonable level of activity.

Again, prevention is of great importance. It should involve general conditioning and strengthening, as well as stretching exercises for the calf muscles.

Ankle Sprains

Because of the large, side-to-side forces that the ankle must withstand in the twisting and jumping in tennis, ankle sprains are very common. Generally, these sprains just stretch the ligaments. They do not completely tear them. With rest, mild sprains heal in a few days.

However, if damage is extensive and there is swelling and pain, you should seek professional help. Symptoms, in addition to the swelling and immediate pain, include a loss of the ability to walk. Immediate first-aid measures consist of immobilization (splinting and crutches), compression (elastic bandage), and elevation of the leg. If healing is to take place, casting to immobilize the ligaments may be necessary for a period of 6 to 8 weeks.

During the immobile period you should have a gradually progressive exercise program to maintain the physical status of the rest of your body, especially the other foot and the arms. In all probability you will want a professional (physician or therapist) to institute the therapy.

Again, only when the leg has reached 90 percent of the strength of the other leg and only when it has normal flexibility should you return to activities.

The therapist may suggest inserting ankle supports to help prevent further injury. Preventive measures should be reviewed.

Knee Injuries

Knee problems are also very common among racket-sport enthusiasts. The major problems with the knee are acute injuries to the ligaments and tendons because these are the tissues that must withstand a great deal of the force resulting from the sudden shifts in body direction. However, there may be some chronic problems that only manifest themselves in pain. These include *chondromalacia patellae,* which is a softening of the cartilage, the covering of the patella, injury to the menisci (the cushion between the bones), and tendinitis. The most common knee injury in tennis is the *ligamentous sprain* (tearing of the knee hinge), which may be mild, with the ligament merely stretched, or severe, with tearing of the fibers. Most cases bring immediate pain, swelling, and loss of function. In general, any injury around the knee that causes swelling and pain should be treated by a physician. However, chronic symptoms usually can be treated by general home remedies—rest, ice after exercise, compression, and elevation of the leg. Treatment may also consist of immobilization of the knee until the ligaments heal or the surgery accomplishes its purpose.

For the last few years physicians have been using a small tube (arthroscope) introduced into the knee, usually under local anesthesia, to assess knee injuries. This device has been a great help in more accurate identification of the injury and in appropriate prescription for treatment. Arthroscopic surgery may allow rehabilitation to begin immediately, and thus the patient may retain body tone and flexibility.

After a period of rest, usually from 8 to 12 weeks depending upon circumstances and severity of injury, the patient begins an exercise program involving strengthening the muscles in both the front and back of the knee. Gradual range-of-motion and flexibility exercises should also be instituted by a professional. The aim of these isokinetic (against a weighted machine) and isometric (without motion) exercises is to improve leg stability. Both strength and flexibility must have returned to normal in the leg when compared with the other leg. Only then can the amateur or professional athlete resume a sports activity. Prevention, again, should be given an essential role.

Summary

When an injury occurs, you should stop all activities and immediately institute a first-aid regimen. If the pain or swelling is severe or if symptoms persist, call a physician. Even if you didn't do them before, begin appropriate stretching and strengthening exercises to maintain the flexibility and strength of the appropriate muscles. Good equipment as well as appropriate technique is essential. With common sense and these general concepts, the instances of overuse syndromes will be reduced.

Jogging

Although there are fewer joggers now than there were several years ago, the explosion in the number of Americans interested in physical fitness has led to approximately 30 million North Americans participating in some form of running as a major health-maintenance program. These runners range from the occasional jogger to the world-class marathoner. Each has his or her own peculiarities as far as possible injuries are concerned. And injuries do occur all too frequently. However, the majority of the injuries appear to be related to training errors—including excessive mileage, intense workouts, rapid changes in training techniques, and running on surfaces such as hills or hard surfaces. The most common injuries involve the lower extremities, where the usual complaints are knee problems, shin splints, Achilles tendinitis, plantar fasciitis, stress fractures, and iliotibial-band tendinitis. These conditions and other facts important to joggers are discussed in Chapters 10 and 11.

The many related causes of these lower-extremity injuries come from improperly fitted shoes, usually with both inadequate heel support and too little shock absorption. Heels should be somewhat higher than the sole to save the Achilles tendon, and the sole should be thick enough to take the punishment of the pounding. You should match the sole to the surface on which you are running. Poor running technique and overuse of unconditioned muscles frequently cause these injuries (Table 14-4).

We also need to emphasize certain anatomic factors that would not ordinarily be the cause of a problem but might, with the extreme stress of long-distance running, compound overstrain problems. (In one recent survey more than one-third of persons in a 10-kilometer road race sustained, in the year after the race, a musculoskeletal injury of some sort.) Some severe injuries require specific professional attention. However, most of the common problems (mild strains and sprains) are amenable to home remedies and patience. But if the pain persists or if it is intense, you should seek medical care. This is also true if there is swelling or a malfunction of the extremity.

However, in general, correct shoes, appropriate muscle-strengthening, physical fitness, appropriate stretching and warm-up exercises, and a jogging program that gradually increases the running will go a long way in preventing injuries. It almost goes without saying that the program should be tailored to the participant's capabilities.

In summary, causes of injury include a rapid increase in intensity or level of training, anatomic abnormalities such as flatfeet, rapid change from a hard to a soft surface or terrain (such as running on a flat terrain and then running up and down hills), incorrect shoes, premature resumption of running after injury, and finally psychologic problems that lead to running addiction. All of these can raise the incidence of jogging problems.

Ankle Strains and Sprains

As noted previously, a sprain is a ligament injury whether it be merely a stretch or a complete interruption of the fibrous-tissue bands. Strains involve an injury to or a stretching or tearing of a muscle. Usually a sprain in the ankle occurs when one falls or trips on an irregular surface. The most often sprained ligament is the one on the outer side of the ankle. Treatment of this acute injury consists of the usual first-aid sequence of rest, ice, compression, and elevation. If the sprain is mild, pain will not be severe, and swelling will be minimal. Most of these problems usually resolve themselves within the first week. Healing is later enhanced by heat, massage, and early range-of-motion exercise, as well as muscle-strengthening ones. If the injury is more severe, the pain and swelling will be moderate to severe, and there may be a significant loss of function, particularly in bearing weight. Under these circumstances it is usually safer to seek medical care. Treatment of these injuries usually consists of conservative measures and immobilization (casting) for approximately 6 weeks. Gradually the physician will prescribe a rehabilitation program consisting of range-of-motion exercises and (later) isometric and isokinetic exercises against weights to strengthen the ankle. For a very helpful form of therapy, sew the ends of a broad elastic rubber band (ACE bandage) together to form a 12- to 15-inch loop. Hold your feet about 6 inches apart and slip the loop over them—it will act as a resistive force against which to exercise—forcing the feet outward against the band. Premature resumption of running before full strength and mobility have returned may exacerbate the injury. Rarely is surgical repair indicated.

Plantar Fasciitis

The plantar fascia is a fibrous, stringy tissue that covers the sole of the foot. Runners who have a high arch and relative tightness of the Achilles tendon usually produce an increased force on this tissue with each step. Because of the chronic overstrain syndrome, the plantar fascia usually becomes inflamed and results in pain in the heel as well as along the entire sole when weight is put on the foot. Most of the time the symptoms can be treated with rest and exercises that emphasize stretching the muscles on the outer aspect of the heel as well as the heel cord (Achilles tendon) itself (Table 11-6, exercises 2 to 4). Again, prevention is the best form of treatment and usually consists of appropriate stretching and warming up prior to activity and wearing appropriate running shoes (Table 14-4).

To prevent ankle strains, you must maintain good overall muscle strength in the leg and foot. Also, you should wear running shoes with a heel that is slightly raised and has good support, a cushion under the ball of the sole, and a good arch support. With a shoe of this type, proper ankle support is assured.

Tendinitis

The heel cord, which attaches the calf muscles to the heel and moves the foot in a downward direction, often sustains inflammation or an incomplete rupture. Usually these problems are seen in recreational joggers who are physically unfit, more than 35 years old, and negligent about adequately stretching calf muscles before running. Generally the first signs of injury are worsening pain in the calf where the tendon attaches to the heel. Treatment consists of appropriate stretching exercises, rest, and the use of a one-quarter-inch heel pad in the shoe for a few weeks if it is necessary. Most patients rapidly become asymptomatic with this kind of treatment, but some individuals require the use of oral anti-inflammatory drugs and complete rest. Prevention includes wearing appropriate shoes and doing stretching exercises.

Hamstring injuries also are very common in runners who increase their mileage rapidly or change their training habits. These injuries occur when the foot hits the ground and immediately is stopped or when sudden forward movement occurs, as in the beginning of a race. Again the problem is a strain of the hamstring muscle with minor tears or stretches. Occasionally, a tendon injury is also involved. Acute injuries should be managed by rest, immobilization, compression, and elevation. Before returning to any activity you should be absolutely free from pain and have returned to full strength. You should decrease mileage and try to prevent this type of injury. You can do it by appropriate stretching prior to running or any other activities. Also strengthen the hamstring by pressing the knee flat against the floor or using appropriate equipment under supervision. In addition, the exercises well-outlined in previous chapters will be helpful (Tables 9-6, 10-6, and 11-6).

Shin Splints

When we speak of shin splints, we refer to any pain or discomfort in the inner aspect of the leg that results from repetitive running. The pain is most related to a degree of overuse in an individual with underdeveloped muscles who is also poorly prepared for the rigors of long-distance running. It usually results from small tears in the muscle of the inner aspect of the leg. This muscle, the posterior tibialis, moves the foot in an inward direction. Small tears are usually present at the origin of the muscle on the shin bone and the tibia.

Generally, after a period of rest, your symptoms will be relieved. However, stretching exercises with particular emphasis on the front and back muscles of the leg are important for preventing damage. Avoiding hard surfaces and using shock-absorbing shoes also help this problem. You should undertake strengthening exercises with particular emphasis on muscles in the front of the leg. Many times ice and compression help acute symptoms. If you experience any severe pain that progresses despite rest or if any other symptoms such as tingling or loss of movement of the foot occur, you should immediately consult your doctor—you may be getting a compartment syndrome, with compression of vessels and nerves (see Chapter 11).

Stress Fractures

Another problem that can occur in runners who excessively increase their mileage is a condition known as *stress fractures*. In this condition, the runner experiences pain on the inner aspect of the shin that increases with activity but lets up with rest. Other areas in which stress fractures occur are the metatarsals, the small bones of the foot, and the pelvic bones. Most of the problems involve novice runners or advanced runners who have changed their training program. Usually there is an area of mild swelling, pain, and tenderness on palpation along the affected bone. A physician can diagnose most problems with x-rays, but many problems can be solved simply by rest, even if it is forced by a cast put on the leg.

You can prevent stress fractures by exercising correctly and strengthening muscles. Stretching exercises, proper equipment, and shoes are absolutely essential. So, too, is running only on appropriate surfaces. This is real prevention. It is also important to seek your physician's advice for any pain that does not improve rapidly with rest.

Knee Pain

One of the most common problems afflicting runners is knee pain, and its major causes are chondromalacia patellae, injuries to the cartilage, tendinitis, bursitis, shifting (subluxing) kneecaps, and iliotibial-band syndrome.

Chondromalacia patellae is a softening of the cartilage of the kneecap (patella). The undersurface of the cap is covered with a smooth spongy tissue called cartilage, which becomes softened with overuse. Runners who usually experience pain in the region around the kneecap, particularly while running down hills or on uneven surfaces, may have chondromalacia patellae—subluxing kneecaps are a common predisposing cause. At times there may be swelling about the knee as well as a clicking sensation. Generally by resting and using ice and aspirin, runners can return to full activity in a short period of time. You should use specific stretching exercises with emphasis on the quadriceps (thigh) muscles (Table 9-6, exercise 14), and you should also use isometric and isokinetic techniques (under supervision in a gym or spa).

Additional exercises should emphasize the entire musculature of the lower extremities. Sometimes it helps to use knee braces with foam pads on the outer side of the patella to counteract the strong tendency of every thigh muscle to pull the kneecap to the outside (subluxing kneecap) when you are running. It is important to realize that exercises should be done only in the last few degrees of straightening the knee if you are to prevent any overstress on the kneecap. If pain continues and these simple methods do not work, you should seek medical advice before running any more. Prevention is best accomplished by appropriate stretching and by avoiding overstraining. Keep an even exercise program and don't increase your mileage beyond your running capabilities.

Injuries to the cartilage are another common source of joggers' knee pain. The knee is a complex joint composed primarily of the femur and tibia bones, which are interconnected by strong ligaments and separated by two types of cartilage. One type is smooth and extremely thin, covers the end of the bone, and allows the bone to glide. The other acts as a cushion. This cushion separates the two bone edges and provides some degree of stability. It is these latter cartilages, called *menisci,* that can be involved in running injuries. However, it is definitely more common to find that menisci previously injured may become painful from the overstrain of running. Patients will usually have pain on either the inner or outer aspect of the knee; it is worse with running and improved with rest. Again, first-aid measures such as rest, ice, compression, and elevation tend to reduce swelling; but if swelling or pain persist, the runner should seek medical help. Although treatment may include the use of exercises and extended periods of rest, many times a torn cartilage may be treated with the use of the arthroscope. (See Chapter 10 for a description of this procedure.) Microsurgery via the arthroscope is becoming ever more valuable in treating bad knees.

Tendinitis and bursitis of the knee can also cause problems for joggers. Around the knee there are tendons that may become inflamed from overuse, particularly with downhill running. A bursa on the inner aspect of the knee just below the joint is called the *pes anserine* (or *anserine bursa*). Pain in this area is very often confused with cartilage tears. Most of the time these problems can be corrected by simple procedures such as rest and aspirin. Stretching and using shock-absorbing equipment on appropriate surfaces go a long way in preventing this problem. Again, any persistent problem should be a warning sign that a physician is needed.

Iliotibial-band syndrome is particularly common among runners who run long distances and do interval training. The iliotibial band is a tight, fibrous structure that runs from the hip to the knee on the outer side of the thigh. Movement of this band across the knee joint during running can cause an inflammation and pain during activities. Treatment consists of rest, ice, and anti-inflammatory agents such as aspirin. The problem can best be prevented by appropriate stretching of the band, as shown in Table 10-6, exercise 6, and following the advice detailed in Table 14-4.

Back Pain

Back pain is very uncommon in runners, and serious back pain is present in only about 10 percent of the injuries we see. Patients usually have well-localized problems in the lower back, often with the pain radiating into the back of the leg. Any persistent pain or change in sciatic symptoms with tingling and numbness in the foot or loss of leg power should send you for medical help. Pain that continues after rest is a warning sign. Treatment usually consists of rest and anti-inflammatory medicines such as aspirin. Appropriate stretching exercises during warm-up and the use of proper equipment are important here too in preventing damage and pain. Most runners return to activity very quickly; however, if the symptoms remain severe, you should seek medical help.

Summary

Running has become one of the greatest pastimes in our culture. It is appropriate to note that the symptoms of overstrain are best demonstrated by runners. The injury rate for runners who do more than 35 miles per week is highly significant; 60 percent of individuals training for long-distance running over a year's time develop some level of injury. The injury rate for runners participating in 35 miles or less is not as high. For most of these runners an injury (if it is minimal) can heal quickly, allowing them to resume their level of activity. Simple measures, as outlined in this chapter, are the key. In general, the best treatment is still making sure you do everything you can to escape injury.

Swimming

As a group, swimmers have a lower incidence of injury than either runners or cyclists. Many times swimming can be an interim form of exercise for those with injuries sustained during running or other activities that involve overstrain of the lower extremities. On the other hand, some problems are peculiar to the swimmer. Approximately 10 percent of swimmers during their lifetime suffer shoulder problems. Although other injuries can occur, swimmer's shoulder pain is the most common. Chapter 5 dealt with the problem, and we have mentioned the peculiar anatomy of the shoulder. This peculiarity (a too-small area for the tendons) predisposes the swimmer to the development of tendinitis and tears of the rotator cuff. Still, the incidence of shoulder injury for the average swimmer is very low.

Among *competitive* swimmers, however, 60 percent of the participants had shoulder problems. Again, the swimmer can manage most problems by resting, using appropriate stretching, and gradually exercising with strengthening exercises to make the rotator cuff strong and durable. A change in technique may help a swimmer avoid injuries. Anti-inflammatory drugs may also be helpful, but if pain and loss of function continue, the swimmer should seek medical care. However, most cases of swimmer's shoulder may be prevented by appropriate shoulder strengthening exercises. (See Chapter 5 or consult a professional.) Just as important is warming up slowly. In addition, a swimmer should keep mileage within his or her capability. It is most important to understand one's own capabilities in athletics if injuries are to be prevented! See Table 14-5.

Bicycling

The big increase in bicycling is largely due to the interest in aerobic exercises for cardiovascular conditioning. Bicycling is also pleasurable, and it does provide transportation. It also ranks among activities consuming a lot of calories, and it can be an important exercise program for losing weight. Any individual can participate in cycling without enduring the repetitive-impact force to the lower extremities. At times, athletes who have been injured can substitute bicycling as a means of exercise. They can still maintain their overall fitness and strength level while allowing their injuries to heal. Although the frequency of bicycle injuries is low, they do occur. These injuries include fractures, sprains, and contusions (muscle bruises). Additionally, knee pain and other problems can result from overzealousness. Most cycling injuries occur during accidents, mostly from falls. Overuse also causes problems—usually sprains and knee pain. Patellofemoral-area syndromes (kneecap disturbances) usually come from inadequate training, overuse, or poor use of equipment. A discussion of the more common cycling injuries follows.

Head and Neck Injuries

If you cycle, you must wear a helmet to prevent head and neck injuries. Any improved, impact-resistant, hard-shell helmet that will provide maximum protection is suitable. Any fall from a bicycle that does result in an injury to the head and neck demands medical care.

One day, while waiting for a light to change, I saw a cyclist killed when a car threw him many feet from his bike. I hadn't realized what a very dangerous sport this is in today's traffic. Drivers often have difficulty seeing riders of bicycles or motorcycles—especially when the riders weave in and out of traffic lanes. It is a sort of one-vehicle game of "chicken."

Prior to any bicycling activity a rider who has had neck problems should perform neck exercises that strengthen and maintain neck movement up, down, and sideways (see Chapter 4). This activity prevents later problems with neck fatigue. A good rule is to rest any injured area until it is no longer symptomatic or until strength returns to preinjury level. Shoulder and upper-limb injuries are the most common injuries because of falls, which occur when the bicycle loses traction and the rider lands on his or her outstretched hand or the point of the shoulder. Any injury can be serious, and among the most common are injuries to the acromioclavicular joint at the top of the shoulder. Fractures of the clavicle (collarbone) and upper arm are also not uncommon. Any injury that causes pain, swelling, or loss of function requires medical attention. However, initially you can manage simple abrasions or sprains in the shoulder or upper extremity if you use ice, compression, and rest. When the pain and function loss remain after 24 to 48 hours, seek medical care. Another possible problem in the upper arm is compression of the nerves, which usually develops from wrong positioning of hands on the handlebars. The bicyclist may experience numbness or tingling, even loss of function in the hands. Any similar problem not soon resolved may be associated with nerve damage, and you should consult a physician immediately.

Back and Spine Pain

Although the back and spine are rarely afflicted with pain from cycling (because it is not a sport involving repetitive-loading and weight-bearing on the lower leg), some individuals may develop low-back strain after long hours of cycling. If lower-back pain does develop, you can rest and perform strengthening exercises for alleviation. Here, too, a key element is prevention (Table 14-6).

General overall conditioning is also effective if you are to prevent lower-back strain. Most hip problems result from the overuse syndrome and tend to develop into bursitis and tendinitis. Pain is a result of repetitive motion over the outer side of the hip joint and is often diagnosed as bursitis. When pain does develop in this area, rest, aspirin, and heat will usually solve the problem. However, occasionally the pain is persistent enough to prompt medical care. As in most cases, prevention is paramount. The bicycle seat should be appropriately tilted so that you will be in a comfortable position. Handlebars should be at the proper height, and the seat should be high enough so your lower leg can almost be extended. Wearing absorbent clothing will prevent other problems in the hip area and also skin problems.

Knee Problems

Knee problems are also the bane of cyclists but not the plague they are for runners. These problems involving the kneecap joint usually cause pain, which results from softening of the undersurface cartilage of the kneecap, a process known as *chondromalacia patellae*. Cyclists who experience pain and perhaps a feeling of swelling usually sense a tenderness when the patella is compressed. Rest, ice, and aspirin may help; however, prevention is, of course, better. Place the seat so that it prevents a flexed-knee position. Rather, try to stretch your knee out on the downward stroke. You should ascertain the appropriate position and perform exercises to strengthen both the quadriceps and hamstring muscles (Chapter 10). The development of a 2 to 1 relationship between the strength of the front thigh muscles and hamstrings is important.

Foot and Ankle Problems

Foot and ankle problems are very uncommon in a cyclist; however, some develop pain in the front of the foot from improperly placed tongue pads or an improper foot position. Using a relief pad in the shoe can help a great deal. Again, prevention is better still. Position the foot properly with the ball of the foot over the pedal axle; cleats on bicycle shoes and toe clips aid in this positioning. Make sure you are comfortable on the bicycle. Pain in the back of the ankle can result from Achilles tendinitis caused by overstrain. The same simple maneuvers previously described for runners are usually effective; but if pain persists, seek medical care. Being cautious and taking preventive measures will increase your enjoyment of bicycling immeasurably.

General Cautionary Measures

We can't stress enough that prevention is imperative. In athletes there is always the drive to push a little more, but this can prove harmful.

> Gradual *conditioning* and strengthening shouldn't be neglected. Gradually increase your mileage but never go beyond your capabilities. Caution will prevent most injuries.

> Choose standard *equipment,* matched to your ability. Take proper care of tires. Wear riding gloves to protect your palms from abrasions as well as to allow you to maintain stability. Padded handlebars will help prevent upper extremity problems.

> Proper riding *techniques* can eliminate many injuries. Tilting the bicycle seat slightly forward prevents nerve compression at the wrist by reducing arm and hand tension. Be sure to move your hands frequently during prolonged riding.

Conditioning, proper equipment, and technique all will work together to keep cycling free from injury.

Golf

Golf more than many other activities is less strenuous to the musculoskeletal system, but injuries do occur because of the demanding swing. Appropriate preseason conditioning, strengthening, and proper swing practice are important; using good equipment will usually protect you from most injuries. Common problems are wrist sprains and injuries—rather than lower back, hand, and shoulder problems. The swing accounts for most of these problems, but contact with objects other than the ball brings a few injuries! Not long ago we heard of a certain "fit-full" golfer here in Toledo who threw his club not at a tree but above his head. He was thinking even less when it descended, bonked him on the noggin, and sent him to the hospital.

Overuse- or impact-type problems in turn cause wrist sprains. You can employ the simple first-aid remedies we have outlined: rest, ice, compression, and elevation. Control of the club head, maintenance of wrist strength, and appropriate acceleration of the club prevent many injuries (Table 14-7).

Hand and shoulder problems occur from any part of the swing; namely, the first part, which is the take-away position; the second, impact; and the third, follow-through. Follow-through results in a hyperextension, or a C position, of your back, and puts a tremendous strain on it. Strengthening exercises and stretching can eliminate hand and shoulder problems. If you have problems with the wrist, an analysis of your swing by a competent professional can reveal which portion is your major handicap. Wrist problems more commonly result from improper take-away position or the impact of your swing rather than your follow-through. Sometimes your back pain and strain may result from both an improper take-away position and follow-through. But, primarily, back pain is a local problem associated with inadequate muscle strength. You need appropriate muscle strength and exercises to strengthen the abdominals, lower back, and forearms. These are critical if you wish to avoid injury and overuse syndromes. Gradual stretching also helps prevent back injuries.

If pain from overuse occurs in any one of these areas, use first-aid (the RICE program) and stretching. Resume activity when function and strength are fully returned. The local club professional can help you evaluate your swing and your positioning if you are having chronic problems.

However, here too prevention is the key element in any of these activities. Do strengthening exercises to develop muscles of the upper and lower extremities or visit a local gym or health club or have your physician refer you to a physical therapist, if you feel the need. The instructor or therapist will outline a program for strengthening the buttocks, lower back, quadriceps, hamstrings, shoulder, arm, and forearm muscles. Undertake the exercises gradually and only after receiving medical advice and evaluation. This goes a long way toward a problem-free golf game as well as most other activities.

Stretching activities also maintain appropriate mobility of the joints involved in all three parts of the swing. Remember cardiovascular exercise is important if you are to walk an 18-hole golf course. You can incorporate a home-exercise program to help in developing strength and endurance. The muscles mentioned are important in improving all three processes of the swing and the follow-through. Strengthening these muscles goes a long way toward decreasing injury possibilities.

Skiing

Skiing injuries are usually specific injuries but may also be the result of overuse. Most of them range from a minor bruise to major knee damage, with falls accounting for most. If a fall does bring a bruise, be sure to realize that any pain complex reduces your efficiency. Injuries such as contusions, with mild pain, should be treated aggressively with rest, ice, compression, and elevation. Alert skiers seek medical care if problems persist. Overuse syndromes are very common in skiing injuries, and prevention is paramount (Table 14-8).

It is critical that you train, including strengthening the muscles of the lower leg, especially the quadriceps (Table 10-6). Also undertake appropriate warm-up exercises that include stretching. At the beginning of the day, stay on the lower slopes. Lessons from an experienced instructor will improve technique and ability. Equipment that is fitted to the individual (not necessarily the most expensive) and is maintained in top condition over a prolonged period of time will add to your skill and prowess. Many participants ski beyond their endurance and ability, attempting too much. And they don't always stop skiing before fatigue or cold set in. Always use strap grips, but don't wrap them around your thumbs if you want to prevent many of the ski injuries to the upper extremities. Be especially careful when conditions are not perfect. Learn to fall with your body relaxed and your hands and arms tucked in. Roll forward to spread the impact throughout your entire body line. In general, skiing can be enjoyable sport. Don't ruin the fun of it.

A general conditioning program that includes strengthening all muscles and especially the quadriceps is invaluable. Many skiing injuries, other than simple bruises, require medical attention.

Although we have emphasized some general points in each section, here too, the best treatment is avoiding treatment. Prevention counts most. You must know your body and its capabilities. Because we all have a competitive spirit, it isn't always easy to determine just what you are capable of. Middle-aged athletes cannot hope to reach the level of younger individuals and should not become overly involved in competitive activities. Doing the general overall strengthening exercises, maintaining physical condition, using only appropriate equipment, and participating only at your capability usually prevent most overuse syndromes described here. You can enjoy these sports for many years to come.

Table 14-1
Warm-up Exercises

1. *Trunk stretch:* Sit on the floor, legs out straight, toes pointing up. Reach overhead, then bend forward from the waist and exhale as you move your trunk, head, and arms forward until your hands are touching the legs or feet. Now grasp your legs or feet as far forward as you can, and slowly breathe in. Bend your elbows and pull your chest and head toward your feet, stretching the hamstrings, calves, and back muscles. Hold for 10 to 20 seconds, then grasp further forward if you can, and relax. Repeat 3 to 6 times over 1 to 2 minutes before sports (Figure 9-20).
2. *Shoulder and trunk stretch:* Stand with your arms behind your head, hands on the opposite elbow; bend your trunk to the right side and pull the left elbow to the right, keeping your arms behind your head. Stretch the left side for 1 minute; repeat for the opposite side.
3. *Abdominal curls:* Lie on your back, draw up the knees, but still keep your feet on floor. Flatten your back and try to push into the floor by contracting the abdomen and rotating the pelvis so your waist contacts the floor. Now slowly raise your chest, neck, and head as a unit about 3 inches. Keep your chin tucked in, like a soldier at attention. Don't jut the head forward as you begin. Hold your chest up from the floor for 20 seconds, repeat 3 times (Figure 9-15).
4. *Hip flexors stretch:* Lie on your side. Push the uppermost thigh backward. Grasp your upper foot behind you and pull slowly. Hold 10 seconds; repeat for 1 minute (Figure 9-7).

(continued)

5. *Calf stretch:* Stand an arm's length from a wall and slowly reach upward on the wall overhead. Keep your heels to the floor. Now slowly push your body in toward the wall, stretching your heel cords. Hold 10 seconds; repeat for 1 minute. See Figure 11-4.

6. *General warm-up:* Increase circulation by riding a stationary bicycle. Do jumping jacks or jog in place a few minutes.

Table 14-2
Preventive Measures for Home-Exercise Equipment

1. Discuss your plan with your physician after a physical examination.
2. Test similar equipment before purchase.
3. Perform stretching movements before exercising to improve flexibility.
4. Wear loose-fitting clothing, free of hooks and buckles and that can't be caught in the equipment.
5. Wear well-fitting protective shoes.
6. Begin slowly and exercise regularly.
7. Build gradually.
8. Respect pain. Don't exceed your capability!

Table 14-3
Preventive Measures for Racket Sports

1. Discuss the proposed activity with your physician after your physical examination.
2. Use a racket that fits your grip.
3. Wear well-fitting shoes that provide good heel stability and shock absorption.
4. Have your racket strung at approximately 55-pound tension.
5. Stretch before play.
6. Perform general strengthening exercises between playing sessions.
7. Review your performance at regular intervals with a professional.
8. Respect pain. Quit before it becomes too severe.

Table 14-4
Preventive Measures for Joggers and Runners

1. Discuss this activity with your physician after your physical examination. Make certain the physician has checked for minor structural disorders of the lower limbs. If any exist, follow the advice for adaptive measures (e.g., soft shoe inlays, knee supports).
2. Women might consider pads beneath brassiere hooks.
3. Before running, perform warm-up exercises to stretch trunk and leg muscles.
4. Build up your mileage gradually.
5. Avoid hard surfaces, hills, and uneven terrain.
6. Examine shoe fit, support, and degree of wear.
7. Between running sessions perform exercises to strengthen and maintain muscles.
8. If you are over 40, limit your mileage to 20 miles per week and have your cardiovascular system checked periodically.
9. Do not run when you are tired or unduly stressed.
10. Respect pain. Quit before it becomes too severe.

Table 14-5
Preventive Measures for Swimmers

1. Discuss the activity with your physician after your physical examination.
2. Perform a warm-up with stretching exercises beforehand.
3. Discuss shoulder-strengthening exercises with a professional. Develop a gradual strengthening program and continue this program as long as you swim!
4. Keep duration and distance within your capacity.
5. Review your style with a professional at regular intervals.
6. Respect pain.

Table 14-6
Preventive Measures for Bicyclists

1. Discuss the activity with your physician after your physical examination.

(continued)

2. Wear appropriate shoes and gloves.
3. Position seat and handlebars for comfort and for relief of hand strain.
4. Observe grip position and the strength of grip while bicycling.
5. Wear protective equipment in traffic.
6. Build up mileage slowly.
7. Perform mobilizing as well as neck-, trunk-, and limb-strengthening exercises on a regular basis.
8. Wear clothes that absorb moisture and fit properly.
9. Respect pain.

Table 14-7
Preventive Measures for Golfers

1. Discuss the activity with your physician after your physical examination. Have regular cardiovascular-fitness examinations.
2. Review your technique with a professional at regular intervals.
3. Perform abdominal, low-back, thigh-, shoulder-, arm-, and forearm-strengthening exercises regularly.
4. Perform a gradual warm-up stretch before play.
5. Perform other aerobic exercises to keep your cardiovascular system fit.

Table 14-8
Preventive Measures for Skiers

1. Discuss skiing with your physician after your physical examination.
2. Learn how to fall with your body relaxed, arms tucked in. Roll forward to spread the impact throughout your body.
3. Begin with a slow warm-up on the lower slopes.
4. Consult an experienced instructor to improve technique. Learn conditioning exercises.
5. Perform conditioning exercises between sessions.
6. Wear properly fitted, well-maintained equipment.
7. Avoid skiing under risky conditions.

Chapter 15

Drugs, Diets, and Devices

We will talk about prescription and nonprescription drugs, rub-on medications, unproven remedies, diets, and other treatments for arthritis. We will also provide you with information, so you can sort out what is of value. The public today is more knowledgeable and informed than ever before, yet quackery continues to exist and find its way to new customers.

Drugs

Generic or Brand Name?

We are often asked to write generic prescriptions and are happy to do so if a generic drug is available, and if we have experienced satisfactory results with it. A generic product cannot be sold until the drug patent has expired. Therefore most NSAIDs are not yet available as generic drugs. The company that develops an arthritis drug must recover the costs of development and testing. This runs into the tens of millions of dollars! The longer the Food and Drug Administration takes to approve a drug, the higher your cost will be. Generic drugs are supposed to be "bioequivalent" (exact duplications). The generic drug chemical may be bioequivalent, yet the generic drug may have different effects than the brand-name drug. Why? Because the binders, solvent, fillers, coating, and other substances used in production may change absorption or effectiveness. Also, allergies to the fillers, coatings, or binders may occur. Ask your doctor and your pharmacist about their experience with a particular generic drug. Twenty years ago, an Air Force base had an epidemic of streptococcal infections. The antibiotics used were generic, produced outside the United States. They didn't work! And the base ran out of penicillin. We are skeptical of generic drugs until our own experience proves them safe and effective.

Steroids

When cortisone was discovered, it appeared to be a miraculous treatment for rheumatoid arthritis. The next decade, the 1950s, witnessed the most dramatic rise, and later fall, in the expectations of arthritis patients. Cortisone provided immediate relief of pain, swelling, stiffness, and misery. However, side effects of diabetes, cataracts, high blood pressure, stomach ulcers, and a "moon face" soon became apparent. Early in the 1960s, studies revealed that steroids resulted in three times more bone damage than that seen in similar patients not treated with steroids. Today, oral steroids (synthetic forms of cortisone) should be used only for certain specified arthritis diseases and their complications. Prednisone is the most widely prescribed oral steroid and is used in rheumatoid arthritis, particularly when complications occur. These include inflammation of the lung, heart sac, eye, or blood vessels (vasculitis). Other diseases for which we prescribe oral steroids include polymyalgia rheumatica, temporal (giant-cell) arteritis, polymyositis, dermatomyositis, systemic lupus erythematosus, mixed connective-tissue disease, and many forms of vasculitis. We always try for the lowest possible dose, sometimes using 1-milligram tablets. Sometimes prednisone can be used as infrequently as every other day, and this can further reduce side effects.

Steroid injections are used in several ways. Some rheumatic diseases that haven't responded to any form of treatment can be treated with "bolus steroids" (intravenous methylprednisolone). For example, when a huge dose of steroid is administered into the vein on 3 successive days and repeated every 6 to 12 weeks the disease may be reversed temporarily. This is thought to paralyze the immune system. Risks include serious infection, possible heart attack, and severe damage to the ends of bone—particularly in the hips and shoulders.

Some injectable steroids are manufactured as minute crystals. A vial of this form of medication has the appearance of milk and in this form is very helpful when injected directly into a swollen joint. Used in this manner, the steroid reduces the inflammation and may retard the bone damage. Studies at Case Western Reserve University and at the University of Indiana have shown that artificially induced arthritis damage in animals is slowed down when the joint is injected with a crystalline-type steroid. But steroid joint injections require care. If the physician is unskilled, the needle can penetrate and damage the soft cartilage. Or if the skin is not correctly prepared, the needle can carry germs into the joint and cause a joint abscess. Lastly, if the injections are performed too often, bone damage may result. We try to avoid frequent joint injections, and we try to limit injections of any one joint to not more than three a year. If the joint is swollen, as much fluid as possible should be removed. Arthritis joint fluid contains enzymes and acids that further harm the joint.

Steroid injections are of considerable help in soft-tissue rheumatism—bursitis, tendinitis, trigger finger, carpal-tunnel syndrome, and regional pain syndromes such as frozen shoulder, myofascial trigger points, back pain, some cases of sciatica, heel pain, tennis and golfer's elbow, and some cases of fibrositis. Here, too, careful technique, proper intervals between injections, and use of a crystalline form of steroid will avoid complications. We have used products such as methylprednisolone acetate (Depo-Medrol) and triamcinolone hexacetonide (Aristospan) because they are poorly absorbed and tend to avoid side effects.

In summary, steroids are used for specific diseases or disease complications. Great care must be taken because of long-term complications. Steroids can cause symptoms of arthritis (pseudorheumatism) as well as treat them! If you are on steroids, you must keep a close check on blood pressure and blood potassium and sugar levels. You should maintain a good intake of calcium, reduce your starchy food intake, avoid salt, and have your doctor use the lowest possible dose. You should wear a "cortisone alert" tag or bracelet. If you miss doses because of illness or injury, you might go into shock. Never stop oral steroids suddenly. The dosage must be reduced gradually.

Nonsteroidal Anti-inflammatory Drugs (NSAIDs)

Aspirin and salicylate drugs are the most widely used NSAIDs. More than 30 others are in use or being tested for use. They all can relieve pain, attack inflammation, and reduce fever.

Aspirin (acetylsalicylic acid) is widely known and widely used. What is not so widely known is that the amount needed to reduce inflammation is much greater than that needed to reduce pain. Buffered aspirin is easier on the stomach, and more rapidly absorbed; but it is a little more expensive. You can treat a headache with two tablets every 4 to 6 hours, but to treat arthritis you may need three or more per dose. Because arthritis treatment requires such a large dose, manufacturers now produce timed-release aspirin, arthritis-strength aspirin, and liquid forms of salicylate. Always take aspirin with food, milk, or an antacid. Crackers or a small glass of milk will do. We often have the patient begin with a total of 10 or 12 aspirins a day, and raise the dosage by two tablets every 3 or 4 days until either stiffness and swelling begin to subside or side effects occur.

Tinnitus, a ringing sensation in the ears, may be one of the side effects and may occur before an adequate dosage is achieved. If hearing and thinking are not impaired, we tell our younger patients who have persisting arthritis symptoms and who have mild ringing or buzzing noise to cautiously keep on increasing the dosage. The dosage can be increased unless hearing and thinking might be impaired. Older patients may already have impaired hearing; they may not hear the ringing, and therefore they are more likely to seriously overdose themselves. Therefore, we are more cautious with older patients. If side effects occur, the dosage is reduced or temporarily stopped and then resumed, but at two tablets less per day than the dosage that was toxic. For example, if 18 tablets a day was an excessive dosage, we would cut to 8 tablets, and then gradually raise the dosage to 16 per day. The key to using aspirin is to raise the dosage slowly and maintain a safe blood level by taking it regularly with food or milk (doses not longer than 8 hours apart nor closer together than 3 hours). Also, any missed doses should be made up by taking an extra dose in the middle of the night. *Aspirin sensitivity,* or allergy, can cause a stuffy nose, wheezing, skin rash (particularly on the front of the lower legs), polyps in the nose, hives, and swelling of the tongue and lips. Other rare reactions include liver irritation, kidney damage, and (in children) an increase in acidity of the blood, fever, and rapid breathing.

Enteric-coated aspirin is used if the patient has had stomach ulcers, a hiatus hernia, or other stomach sensitivity to aspirin. Sodium salicylate is also available, but blood levels are hard to maintain. We do not recommend sodium salicylate for patients with inflammatory types of arthritis.

Aspirin prolongs bleeding time by interfering with cells needed for blood clotting. Therefore, if you are going to have a tooth extracted or surgery, stop aspirin at least 10 days before the procedure. You can substitute a nonacetylated aspirin that still has the anti-inflammation benefit of aspirin without the bleeding tendency. Products such as choline salicylate (Arthropan) (1 teaspoon equals two regular aspirin tablets) can be used without risk of bleeding. Of course the cost of treatment is greater. Other nonacetylated salicylates are available by prescription.

Prescription salicylates include slow-release aspirin (ZORprin), enteric-coated salicylate (Easprin), and compounds in which the acetyl portion is replaced with some other molecule. The acetyl portion of aspirin is the cause of stomach-lining irritation and an increased tendency toward bleeding. The nonacetylated prescription salicylates include salsalate (Disalcid), magnesium salicylate (Magan), and choline and magnesium salicylate (Trilisate). These agents are much more easily tolerated by some patients, but they are more expensive than aspirin products.

Nonsalicylate NSAIDs

As mentioned, manufacturers are testing a great number of these products. Those available at the time this chapter is being written include:

Diflunisal (Dolobid)

Fenoprofen (Nalfon)

Ibuprofen (Advil, Haltran, Medipren, Motrin, Nuprin, Rufen)

Indomethecin (Indocin)

Ketoprofen (Orudis)

Meclofenamate sodium (Meclomen)

Naproxen (Naprosyn)

Piroxicam (Feldene)

Sulindac (Clinoril)

Tolmetin sodium (Tolectin)

Phenylbutazone (Butazolidin)

Similarities of these compounds include cost per day of treatment, effectiveness, potential for fluid retention, rash, gastrointestinal irritation, interaction with blood-thinner drugs, and potential liver irritation. Rare side effects include bone-marrow reactions, vision impairment, aggravation of asthma, headache, and insomnia. Sulindac has a longer duration of action, and renal toxicity may be slightly less common for sulindac. Special precautions are urged for patients taking diuretics, blood thinners, or diabetic agents. Some people show signs of liver toxicity and kidney problems. Blood and urine can be monitored to enhance safety when a patient requires one of these agents. Phenylbutazone is more toxic particularly for older patients, and generally this drug should not be used unless the others have all been tried unsuccessfully. Indomethecin is available as a suppository for nighttime use; at times it causes severe mental reactions. Meclofenamate sometimes causes severe symptoms of cramps and diarrhea. In general, however, these drugs have proved very safe; serious reactions occur about one time in 5000 patient years of use. Thus, 5000 people could take one of these drugs for a year with only one of them having a serious liver, bone-marrow, or kidney reaction. Risk of bone-marrow damage is higher with phenylbutazone.

These drugs and aspirin or salicylates are useful for osteoarthritis, rheumatoid arthritis, gout, pseudogout, ankylosing spondylitis, psoriatic arthritis, and lupus erythematosus, and also for the inflammation and pain of bursitis, tendinitis, and myofascial disorders.

Painkillers

If we ever had a drug that eradicated all pain, the person with arthritis would grind the involved joint to powder! Relief of pain is a goal of treatment, but not entirely. We do want to reduce pain when it is severe, when the cause is known, and when we know the patient will not abuse the body. Painkillers do nothing to inflammation nor do they slow damage; rather they may worsen the damage. Some of the nonnarcotic oral painkillers are:

Acetaminophen (more than 50 compounds available without prescription)

Salicylates and NSAIDs (discussed above)

Propoxyphene HCl (Darvon compounds, Wygesic)

The problem in using a painkiller is double-edged. It may lose effectiveness with time, and the disease causing the pain may be worsening. When used only as a temporary treatment, the three agents above are fine, safe, and reliable. Sometimes, though, pain pills can make you forgetful, and you may not remember when you took your last dose. Also, the medication may lose potency, and you might begin to overdose. Used in excess, certain painkillers can damage the liver. If you think you have overdosed, call your doctor and induce vomiting.

Pain-Modifying Drugs

Drugs that modify pain can also change your awareness or recognition of pain. Most were originally used to treat depression. Later, it was learned that in smaller doses they could alter pain perception. Whenever pain has persisted beyond 6 months and has no identifiable source (such as some cases of headache or backache), these drugs can prove helpful. They have been proved safe in most cases. These drugs include:

Amitriptyline HCl (Elavil, Endep)

Amoxapine (Asendin)

Desipramine HCl (Norpramin)

Doxepin HCl (Adapin, Sinequan)

Imipramine HCl (Tofranil)

Maprotiline HCl (Ludiomil)

Nortriptyline HCl (Pamelor)

Protriptyline HCl (Vivactil)

Trazodone HCl (Desyrel)

Trimipramine maleate (Surmontil)

All of these may take up to 3 weeks before results are noted. They can be given in small dosage with gradual increases and can be taken over several hours before retiring. They often cause a dry mouth and have a sedative effect; therefore, most physicians recommend their use before you retire. Patients with glaucoma, heart disease, or constipation should discuss these problems with their physician before obtaining a prescription. Some patients are stimulated by these drugs. Insomnia may be aggravated and a rapid or irregular heartbeat can occur. A patient should consider periodic tests for liver toxicity if long-term use is contemplated. Be careful about drinking alcohol and driving when taking one of these drugs. They can remain in the system for 10 or more days. One of our patients after taking amitriptyline and having one drink drove her car through a billboard!

Muscle Relaxants

No drug can relax a tight muscle in spasm, particularly if the muscle is repeatedly being injured by improper body mechanics. In addition, muscle spasm sometimes feeds on itself. Then a pain-spasm-pain cycle is suspected. In such cases a muscle relaxant used alone or in combination with a painkiller (or a pain-modifying drug) and stretching exercises can be remarkably helpful. Commonly prescribed muscle relaxants include:

> Carisoprodol (Soma)
> Chlorphenesin carbamate (Maolate)
> Chlorzoxazone (Paraflex)
> Cyclobenzaprine HCl (Flexeril)
> Diazepam (Valium)
> Methocarbamol (Robaxin)
> Orphenadrine citrate (Norflex)
> Quinine sulfate (Q-vel, Quinamm)

These drugs usually have to be taken on a continued basis for several days. Taking them can worsen glaucoma, heart diseases, and blockage of the bladder. Cyclobenzaprine is recommended only for brief use. Quinine can help stop leg cramp and can be taken more regularly, used in periodic courses. See Chapter 11.

Rub-ons

Rub-ons, and other topical (applied to the skin) products include counterirritants, pressurized coolant sprays, and topical anesthetic agents. Counterirritants relieve pain, perhaps by confusing the nervous system. They can provide temporary local pain relief for arthritis and soft-tissue injuries. They include:

Absorbine Jr.

Aspercreme

Banalg

Ben-Gay

Deep-Down

Doan's Backache Spray

Icy Hot

infraRUB

Mentholatum

Mobisyl Creme

Myoflex Creme

Sportscreme

Vaporub

Caution is required. Using a rub-on over a fracture or tumor may delay proper diagnosis and treatment! Also, we have seen a few bad rashes after a patient has used a rub-on.

DMSO (dimethyl sulfoxide) has enjoyed a wide press but is of little real therapeutic value. Because it is a solvent, it can carry poisonous material through the skin into the bloodstream. Patients who have tried it know it gets into the bloodstream and imparts a garliclike odor to their breath! In some patients who were also taking sulindac, a severe neuritis developed where they had applied DMSO.

Arnica has also been used in various liniments but has a distinctly unpleasant odor.

Pressurized coolant sprays, available by prescription, require detailed professional instruction. They are helpful when used in conjunction with stretching exercises. Ethyl chloride is widely available, but it is flammable. Fluorimethane is preferred for home use. The procedure is to slowly spray from the trigger point into the pain zone. Two slow sweeps can be applied, followed by a hot pack. The spray should precede the stretching action.

Remittive Drugs for Specific Diseases

In some rheumatic diseases, when the immune system has gone berserk, remittive drugs seem to correct the system, at least partly.

Remittive agents are slow-acting drugs. They must be given in addition to NSAIDs. They include chloroquine, hydroxychloroquine sulfate, penicillamine, and the following gold salts: aurothioglucose (Solganal), gold sodium thiomalate (Myochrysine), and auranofin (Ridaura). They can improve a resistant case of *rheumatoid arthritis* but may take up to 6 months to produce results. Each agent works in about two-thirds of cases. These agents have potentially toxic effects on the eye, liver, kidney, and bone marrow. Gold is the safest; although side effects are common, they are not permanent. (Remember, the crippling effect of rheumatoid arthritis is very permanent!) Chloroquine and hydroxychloroquine can impair vision; periodic eye examinations are required. If you have systemic disease with nerve damage or vasculitis, the doctor may use immunosuppressive chemotherapy. Immunosuppressive drugs include azathioprine (Imuran), cyclophosphamide (Cytoxan), methotrexate, chlorambucil (Leukeran), mechlorethamine HCl (Mustargen HCl), triethylenethiophosphoramide (Thiotepa), and 6-mercaptopurine. Others are also under investigation. These agents can damage normal blood cells; therefore frequent laboratory tests to monitor the blood counts are essential when these drugs are used. Cyclophosphamide can induce scarring and bleeding of the bladder, and urine tests should be checked regularly. The drugs can also cause inflammation of the lung. Theoretically, they may induce cancer. These are cancer-treatment drugs used in smaller dosage. Only experts who have had experience and training should administer them.

Some cases of *systemic lupus erythematosus* respond to hydroxychloroquine, and steroids can be avoided or reduced. Like rheumatoid arthritis, if systemic illness is severe or if more than 20 mg of steroid a day is needed, then many patients are advised to try immunosuppressive treatment.

No treatment for *scleroderma (progressive systemic sclerosis)* has proved remittive, but we have been testing penicillamine for the past 5 years. Some striking remissions have occurred after 1 or 2 years of treatment. Colchicine may be helpful also.

Gouty arthritis can occur by way of a number of pathways. Uric acid overproduction or uric acid retained by the kidney may result. Drugs that increase the elimination of uric acid such as probenecid or that block the liver from producing uric acid, such as allopurinol, are helpful long-term. But these agents must be added while colchicine or an NSAID is being used. If probenecid or allopurinol is used alone, gouty arthritis can worsen. Never take aspirin regularly while you are on probenecid. Aspirin counteracts probenecid.

Diet

If a food or an ingredient in a food were the cause of any form of arthritis, the association would have been recognized years ago. When vitamins were first discovered there was great interest in the study of the effects of diets and vitamins on arthritis. That was 40 years ago! Special hospital studies were carried out in which volunteer patients with arthritis were hospitalized for up to 6 months and fed various diets deficient in some nutrients or excessive in other foods. No relationship could be determined. Recently, studies have shown that rheumatoid arthritis did flare up occasionally in patients if milk products were introduced into their diet. To prove the association, all of the foods were put into capsules so the patients did not know what they were eating. Thus many food substances could be tested by elimination. The tests produced no significant findings.

However, many people claim bad attacks after eating certain foods. One patient claims a different food every 2 years! Obviously, her attacks coincide with eating the same food this year, another food next year; but the association is coincidental. A well-balanced diet providing protein, minerals, and vitamins is essential to the healing process. Eat sensibly and moderately. Patients with arthritis can't burn off calories easily. If you are obese, then less medication gets to your joint tissues. You should lose weight, and this is a struggle that requires thinking before eating.

Many books urge the use of special diets or megadoses of vitamins and minerals, fish oils, seaweed, and other substances. They offer testimonials, anecdotes, and uncontrolled studies to back their claim. They never mention the carefully performed studies that fail to support such treatments.

Assistive Devices

When you are in pain you should look for ways to alleviate the pain, ways to save those joints that cause your discomfort. Pain tells you to modify use of the involved joint or muscle, and often you will have to find a permanent way to reduce joint work. There are many assistive devices on the market. But you must choose very carefully because some of them may actually worsen your problem. For example, using a hydraulic-lift chair seat will result in further loss of the quadriceps muscles that brace the knees. This can lead to further loss of knee-joint stability. Using a walker may damage the shoulder. Forearm canes might be less troublesome.

There are also many good books in print that can help you:

> *Aids and Adaptations,* compiled by the Occupational Therapy Department, Canadian Arthritis and Rheumatism Society, British Columbia Division, Vancouver, Canada. (Contains designs and instructions for fabrication. Available from CARS, 45 Charles Street E, Toronto, Ontario, Canada. Cost, $2.50.)

> Arthritis Foundation, *Understanding Arthritis. What It Is, How It's Treated, How to Cope with It,* Scribner, New York, 1985.

> Irene Crawford, *Aids to Independence; A Guide to Products for the Disabled and Elderly,* TAB Books, Summit, N.J., 1985. ($11.95)

> James F. Fries, *Arthritis, A Comprehensive Guide* (2d ed), Addison-Wesley, Reading, Mass., 1986.

> K. Lorig and J. F. Fries, *The Arthritis Helpbook: What You Can Do for Your Arthritis* (2d ed), Addison-Wesley, Reading Mass., 1986.

> Anita L. Mayer, *Clothing for the Handicapped, the Aged, and Other People with Special Needs,* Interweave, 1984. (Interweave, 306 N. Washington Avenue, Loveland, CO 80537.)

The Arthritis Foundation sends its monthly newsletter to those who join the organization. They also have many excellent pamphlets on arthritis and related disorders. Write to The Arthritis Foundation, 1314 Spring Street, Atlanta, GA 30309, or call your local chapter.

And here are a few of the items on the market:

Eating: Long, built-up handles for forks, knives, and other utensils; suction cups for plates or serving trays; two-handled cups and pots; potholder mit; jar opener; and scouring brush with long handle.

Dressing: Long-handled shoehorn; sock aid; button hook; zipper pull; Velcro fasteners; elastic shoe laces; and front-fastening clothing.

Personal care: Long-handled comb, brush, and sponge; shower hose; bathroom grab bars; shower stool; bathtub transfer bench; raised toilet seat; portable commode to locate on the first floor to avoid the use of stairs; special toothbrushes.

Miscellaneous: Book holder; doorknob extension; key holder; pencil holder; felt-tip pen; car-door opener; wrist, thumb, knee braces, or supports; back support for bed or automobile; adjustable desk chair; bar stool; padded gloves for gardening; pipe insulation for hand tools; electric screwdriver; long-handle extenders for changing lightbulbs; hospital bed; pull-rope for assistance in getting out of bed; "egg-crate" foam mattress pad; elbow and heel pads; foot cradle to keep covers off the feet at night; long-handed "grabber" tongs.

Here are addresses for catalogs that feature assistive devices:

Attainment Company, Inc.
P.O. Box 103
Oregon, WI 53575
(For the professional)

Cleo, Inc.
3957 Mayfield Road
Cleveland, OH 44121

Comfortably Yours
Aids for Easier Living
52 W. Hunter Avenue
Maywood, NJ 07607

Crow River Industries, Inc.
7550 Washington Avenue South
Eden Prairie, MN 55344

Danmar Products, Inc.
2390 Winewood
Ann Arbor, MI 48105

Dr. Leonard's Health Care Catalog
74 20th Street
Brooklyn, NY 11232
(This is an excellent resource.)

Enrichments, Inc.
P.O. Box 579
Hinsdale, IL 60521
1-800-343-9742
(This is an excellent resource.)

Equipment Shop, Inc.
P.O. Box 33
Bedford, MA 01730
(For the professional)

Exceptionally Yours, Inc.
22 Prescott Street
Newtonville, MA 02160
(Clothing)

Fashion Able
5 Crescent Avenue
Box 5
Rocky Hill, NJ 08553
(Hard-to-find items)

Fashion Ease
Division of M & M
Health Care Apparel Co.
1541 60th Street
Brooklyn, NY 11219
(Clothing)

Fleetwood Furniture
25 E. Washington Street
Zeeland, MI 49464
(For the professional)

Gunnell, Inc.
221 N. Water Street
Vassar, MI 48768
(For the professional)

Handicapped Children's
   Technological Services
Box 7
Foster, RI 02825
(For the professional)

Luxury Liners
18929 Norwalk Blvd.
Suite 105
Artesia, CA 90701

Maddak, Inc.
6 Industrial Road
Pequannock, NJ 07440
(This is an excellent resource)

Mobility Plus, Inc.
P.O. Box 391
215 N. 12th Street
Santa Paula, CA 93060

Be OK!
Fred Sammons, Inc.
Box 32
Brookfield, IL 60513
1-800-323-7305
(This is an excellent resource.)

Rifton Equipment for the
   Handicapped
Route 213
Rifton, NY 12471
(For the professional)

Rolyan Medical Products
N93 W14475 Whittaker Way
Menomonee Falls, WI 53051
(For the professional)

Therafin Corporation
3800 S. Union Avenue
Steger, IL 60475
(For the professional)

Ways & Means
28001 Citrin Drive
Romulus, MI 48174
(Catalog, $2.50)
(This is an excellent resource.)

WFR/Aquaplast Corp.
P.O. Box 327
Ramsey, NJ 07446
(For the professional)

Unproven Treatment

We are sure you are aware of many things that some people recommend as sure cures for arthritis that are not worth a penny or even

thinking about (Table 15-1). But where do you draw the line between what is downright quackery and what is helpful but unproved? One simple way is to examine the claims of the promoter. If the claim is for an arthritis cure, forget it! There are no cures! If the claim covers a multitude of diseases, forget it! There are no universal treatment measures. Aspirin is the closest drug to a universal agent, but you know that aspirin is far from being a cure-all. Mexican-border clinics that claim their pills contain DMSO are run by quacks. Can you imagine getting turpentine to turn to a solid? Then how do you get a similar agent, DMSO, into a pill?

Table 15-1
Status of Unproven Treatments

Seaweed; immune milk; snake venom; red-ant serum; Certo; honey and vinegar; alfalfa; "arthritis diets"	To our knowledge, valid scientific (double-blind) studies where the investigator and patient can't tell whether the treatment is real or placebo have not been performed.
Nitroimidazoles: antibiotics used to treat amoeba infections have been claimed to help rheumatoid arthritis.	Perhaps of use someday, but to date studies show little more benefit than with standard drugs. Also, there are many more side effects.
Lasers are used in many fields of surgery with striking benefit. Some of our patients have bought units intended for use in veterinary medicine, and tried them on their back, feet, hands, and other joints badly afflicted by injury or osteoarthritis; they claimed benefit.	One controlled study did not show any benefit when compared with placebo laser treatment. But laser technology is in its infancy. It may yet prove useful.
Cod-liver oil	It can be dangerous. It contains large doses of vitamin A and D, which can be toxic. The idea that an oil, taken by mouth, can lubricate the joints is unsound. The body cannot absorb it

(continued)

	undigested. Oils are broken down before absorption into the bloodstream.
Vitamins; zinc and copper	No valid (double-blind) studies support their value. Doses recommended may cause significant side effects.

Special diets published for the treatment of arthritis can be harmful to your health. One of them caused two preventable deaths, as a result of severe depletion of vitamin C (scurvy). This can cause you to bleed to death.

Should You Be a Guinea Pig?

Why not? If you have rheumatoid arthritis, every treatment in one way or another is an experiment! We don't know the cause of most types of arthritis, so our treatment is based on empirical experience. When a drug manufacturer wants to test a drug, and your doctor is satisfied that the earlier research has shown that the safety margin is satisfactory, what can you lose? You can lose this potentially better drug because the manufacturers must prove it is both safe and effective. If you don't volunteer, who will? We have been doing research on arthritis drugs for 20 years. We have never seen a permanent injury from a research drug. Today, the rigorous monitoring of research patients probably allows better overall management of the patient who volunteers to test a drug. And you save money. The company pays for most of your care. However, beware of research advertisements. Some good research is done that way; but often if a research center has to advertise to get patients into the program, the study isn't well designed. Their results may not be accurate.

Glossary

This glossary will help you understand the terms used in your discussions with health professionals, though we have tried to avoid the use of technical terms in this book. The list is far from complete, but we hope you will find the definitions and terms helpful.

Acetominophen   A commonly used painkiller; not an anti-inflammatory drug.

Achilles Tendon   The heel cord.

Acromioclavicular Joint   The joint between the collarbone and the shoulder blade protrusion. The joint is the nob on top of the shoulder.

Acromion   The part of the shoulder blade bone that protrudes forward and lies above the top of the arm bone.

Activities of Daily Living (ADL)   An assessment technique for tasks and movements necessary in independent living.

Acupuncture   A Chinese technique for pain relief. Needles are inserted at specific points on the body. It is not widely accepted in western cultures.

Acute   Having sudden or very recent onset of symptoms or disease.

Adhesive Capsulitis   The scarring down of the membrane surrounding the joint. Sites include the shoulder, hip, and ankle. It may follow injury, infection, or adjacent tendinitis.

ADL   See *Activities of Daily Living.*

Allergy   See *Hypersensitivity.*

Allied Health Professions Association (AHPA)   Members include physical therapists, occupational therapists, nurses, and researchers interested in arthritis and affiliated with the American Rheumatism Association.

American Rheumatism Association (ARA)   Members include physicians and researchers interested in arthritis and immunity.

ANA   See *Antinuclear Antibodies (ANA).*

Ankylosing Spondylitis   A widespread disease that results in a gluing together of the spine and sacroiliac joints. It can also result in inflammation of the eye, heart, and lower limb joints. Inheritance factors are involved.

Anserine Bursitis   Inflammation of a bursa on the inner aspect of the knee.

Antibodies   Proteins that stick to foreign invaders of the body and, after attachment, cause inflammation. This is how we fight off germs. (See *Autoantibodies.*)

Antigens   Protein substances and organisms that stimulate the production of antibodies.

Antimalarials   Antibiotics that fight malaria and are often used to treat connective-tissue diseases such as rheumatoid arthritis and lupus erythematosus.

Antinuclear Antibodies (ANA)   A group of autoantibodies directed against proteins in the nucleus (command center) of cells.

Apatite   A calcium salt that forms very small crystals in tissues and can be seen only with an electron microscope.

ARA   See *American Rheumatism Association (ARA).*

Arthralgia   Joint pain without swelling; may precede swelling.

Arthritis   Inflammation within the joint. Features of warmth, redness, and swelling may not be evident, but pain, tenderness, and stiffness are common.

Arthritis Foundation   The only national agency with the mission of finding the cause and cure for all forms of arthritis and rheumatism. There are chapters in all 50 states, and it is affiliated with other similar organizations worldwide. Headquarters: 1314 Spring Street NW, Atlanta, GA 30309.

Arthrocentesis   Removal and examination of joint fluid.

Arthrography   Injection of air or substance into a joint to outline the interior of the joint on an x-ray.

Arthropathy   A general term for joint disease.

Articular   Pertaining to a joint.

Aspirin   Acetylsalicylic acid. Discovered a century ago, it is helpful in both relieving pain and combating inflammation.

Autoantibodies   Antibodies directed against the body's own tissues. They are usually the result of a faulty immune system and are likely to be involved in tissue destruction in rheumatoid arthritis, systemic lupus erythematosus, rheumatic fever, and other diseases.

Autoimmune   Pertaining to the reactions that follow the production of autoantibodies.

Baker's Cyst   A swelling behind the knee. It usually results from knee arthritis and excessive joint fluid that is pushed back out of the knee joint (similar to the formation of a hernia).

Bicipital Tendinitis   Swelling and inflammation of the covering of the biceps tendon (upper end of the biceps muscle) in front of the shoulder.

Biofeedback   A technique of controlling body functions that are usually not under our control; useful in treatment of headache, high blood pressure, abnormal nerve functions, pain, etc.

Bone Scan   Following injection of a harmless radioactive isotope into the arm, a special sensor generates a picture on x-ray film; measures bone and joint irritation or damage.

Bouchard Nodes   Bony enlargement of the middle finger joints; usually due to osteoarthritis.

Bursa (pl. bursas)   A saclike structure that protects soft tissue from the underlying bony parts of a joint.

Bursitis   Inflammation of a bursa as a result of infection or irritation.

Calcaneal   Pertaining to the heel bone.

Calcific Tendinitis   A pastelike deposit of calcium salts within a tendon sheath. It may spill over into a bursa and result in bursitis or tendinitis or both.

Callus   A thickening of the skin over a bony prominence usually on the foot.

Capsule   Covering tissue that surrounds the joint into which muscles and tendons attach.

Carcinoma   A malignancy (cancer).

Carpal-Tunnel Syndrome   Disease within the wrist canal that results in pressure on the nerve to the palm and to the thumb, index, and long finger.

Cartilage   The spongy tissue on the end of a bone that acts as a cushion. This is the tissue that is the first to be damaged by arthritis.

Cellulitis   Infection of the deep-skin tissues.

Cervical   Referring to the neck area.

Cervical-Disc Disease   Diseased pad between the neck bones (vertebrae), often in association with arthritis of the neck.

Chondrocalcinosis   Deposition of calcium salts in the cartilage of joints. It is common in elderly persons and may be symptom-free or associated with pseudogout.

Chronic   Pertaining to longstanding symptoms or disease.

Chrysotherapy   Treatment with gold salts for rheumatoid arthritis; rarely used in other types of arthritis.

Coccygodynia   A condition that causes pain surrounding the tailbone.

Coccyx   The tailbone. Last segment of the sacrum that lies below the lumbar spine.

Cockup Toe   See *Hammertoe*.

Collagen   A microscopic weblike series of protein strands in connecting tissues.

Computed Tomography (CT) Scan   After a series of x-rays are taken, a computer rearranges the information to form a new image.

Congenital   Pertaining to a disease process that begins before birth and is not an inherited abnormality.

Connective Tissue   Fibrous tissue that provides support to other body tissues.

Corticosteroids A family of drugs derived from cortisone. Effects on the body include reduction of inflammation, a rise in blood pressure, a rise in blood sugar, and depletion of bone calcium. Prolonged use can cause diabetes, high blood pressure, cataracts, and stomach ulcers. Crystalline suspensions of corticosteroids can be used with less risk for local injections to combat inflammation.

Cortisone A hormone secreted by the adrenal gland; it is essential for sustaining circulation and other body functions.

CREST Syndrome A form of systemic sclerosis (scleroderma) with features of tight skin, red spots on the skin, calcium deposits in the skin, abnormal swallowing, and Raynaud's phenomenon.

C Reactive Protein (CRP) A test that measures inflammation.

CRP See *C Reactive Protein (CRP)*.

Cryoglobulin A protein complex of antigens and antibody that solidify in the cold and then can be measured.

Crystal Arthritis Gout, pseudogout, and some other rare types of arthritis that result when chemicals in the body crystallize.

CT See *Computed Tomography (CT) Scan*.

Cutaneous Pertaining to or involving the skin.

Cytotoxic Drug Drugs that kill rapidly growing cells; often combined with other drugs and collectively are a form of chemotherapy used in cancer and leukemia. Much smaller doses are used to treat arthritis. Drugs include cyclophosphamide (Cytoxan), chlorambucil (Leukeran), methotrexate, and azathioprine (Imuran).

Degenerative Arthritis See *Osteoarthritis*.

De Quervain's Tenosynovitis Washerwoman's tendinitis. Swelling of the tendons that draw the thumb outward from the palm.

Dermatomyositis A connective-tissue disease that kills muscle cells. The main feature is weakness about the neck, shoulders, and hips.

Diffuse Generalized, all over.

Disc A steel wool–like mesh pad between vertebrae; a cartilage plate between bones in some joints.

D Penicillamine Drug used to break down rheumatoid chemicals in rheumatoid arthritis; also under investigation in the treatment of systemic sclerosis (scleroderma).

Dupuytren's Contracture A nodular scarring of the tissue beneath the skin of the palm.

Edema Accumulation of fluid in the tissues under the skin as a result of noninflammatory processes.

Enthesis Site of attachment of tendons to bones.

Enthesopathy Inflammation or deterioration of the site of tendon attachment to bone.

Entrapment Neuropathy Squeezing of a nerve by surrounding tissue. Common at the wrist (carpal-tunnel syndrome), ankle (tarsal-tunnel syndrome, and in the spine (spinal stenosis).

Eosinophilic Fasciitis An unusual disease that inflames the deep-skin tissues of the legs and arms. May be related to localized forms of scleroderma.

Epicondylitis Tennis elbow.

Erosion A pitting (usually seen on x-ray) at the ends of bones as a result of inflammation or infection.

Erythema Nodosum A reddish, painful crop of nodules on the legs due to infections and other diseases or allergy.

Erythrocyte Sedimentation Rate (ESR) See *Sedimentation Rate*.

ESR See *Sedimentation Rate*.

Exercise Therapy A system of exercise that strengthens specific muscles.

Familial Pertaining to a condition that occurs in family members more often than would happen by chance alone.

Fascia Lata A fibrous band on the side of the thigh that separates the front thigh muscles from the back thigh muscles.

Fasciitis Irritation of the fibrous membranes that are between the muscles and line the palm or sole of the foot.

Fibromyalgia See *Fibrositis*.

Fibrositis A condition with features of widespread pain and aching, worse in the morning. It involves the neck, shoulder, and hip areas; has characteristic tender points; and may result from specific sleep disorders.

Flatfeet   Congenital disorder in which, upon standing, the inner foot flattens and the heel inclines outward; the feet may point outward.

Forefoot   Portion of the foot containing the metatarsal joints (the ball of the foot).

Frozen Shoulder (Painful-Arc Syndrome)   Shoulder condition with pain and loss of motion, particularly outward, upward, and backward.

Functional   (1) Affecting a tissue's action. (2) Affecting a psychologic function. Not affecting organic structure. Migraine headaches and fibrositis are functional disorders in that no definite tissue alteration is seen.

Gait   Manner of walking that is determined by the spine, hips, knees, feet, and supportive tissues.

Ganglion   Cystic swelling derived from a joint or tendon.

GC Arthritis   Gonorrhea-related arthritis.

Giant-Cell Arteritis   Disease of larger blood vessels with a characteristic microscopic picture. Occurs after age 55 and can cause swollen joints, severe stiffness, headaches, and jaw pain and fatigue. A serious disease that can lead to stroke, heart attack, or blindness.

Glucocorticoids   See *Steroids*.

Gold Treatment   Gold, originally tried as an antibiotic, is used to induce a "turn off" of the immune system in rheumatoid arthritis. Can be given by injection (shot) or in capsule form.

Gout   A backing up or overproduction of uric acid with acute, severely painful attacks of arthritis in joints of the lower or upper limbs.

Grip Strength   A measurement performed for comparing rates of progress in arthritis.

Hallux   Of or relating to the big toe.

Hallux Valgus   Outwardly deviated big toe that creates a bunion.

Hammertoe   Upward deviation of a toe joint from birth defects or tight shoes, often with a painful thickening on top.

Hamstrings   The muscles behind the thigh.

Heberden Nodes   Nobby enlargement of the end joints of the fingers, usually due to osteoarthritis.

Herniated Disc   Rupture of the nucleus pulposus (gelatinous material) from the disc into the spinal canal against the nerve root.

HLA B27, HLA DW4, etc.   Sites of genes along the sixth chromosome in cell nuclei that direct the immune system. May affect the manner of rheumatic involvement; also may be the reason only certain people respond to a specific medicine.

Holistic   Pertaining to the whole person. A practice that encompasses multiple treatment regimens. Many are unproven.

Housemaid's Knee (Prepatellar Bursitis)   Painful swelling over the kneecap. Comes from kneeling, or other activities performed while on hands and knees.

Hydroxyapatite   Accumulation of a calcium salt around tendons and joints as a result of a defect in metabolism. Causes sudden attacks of tendinitis in the shoulder, hip, wrist, or ankle areas.

Hyperlipidemia   Excessive accumulation of fats in the blood. Can lead to hardening of arteries and also arthritis.

Hypermobility   A condition in which joint motion exceeds normal range, for example, the ability to draw the thumb downward until it touches the forearm or to lay the palms on the floor with knees straight. Other joints can be similarly involved.

Hypersensitivity   Overactivity of the immune system caused by foods, chemicals, dust or mold, or drugs.

Ibuprofen   Chemical (generic) name for a nonsteroidal anti-inflammatory drug contained in Motrin, Rufen, Advil, Medipren, and Nuprin.

Idiopathic   Pertaining to a disease process of uncertain cause.

Immune-Complex Disease   Diseases that result when the immune system produces antibodies against the body's own proteins. The antibodies then attach to these proteins and form complex proteins. These in turn trigger further chemical reactions that lead to tissue damage. Examples include rheumatoid arthritis and systemic lupus erythematosus.

Immunity   Response of the blood system to protect the body against disease, usually against germs.

Indomethacin (Indocin)   One of the first nonsteroidal anti-inflammatory drugs. Still widely used to stop acute attacks of joint swelling.

Inflammation   A process of walling off an injury that progresses to redness, warmth, swelling, and pain. Helps to get rid of a germ or other noxious agent.

Inflammatory-Joint Disease   Arthritis that is just part of a bodywide reaction. Examples include rheumatoid arthritis, ankylosing spondylitis, rheumatic fever, and systemic lupus erythematosus.

Joint   Where two bones are attached. In the skull, the bones are fused, whereas in the remainder of the body the bones may form a ball-and-socket joint or hinge-type joint.

Joint Fluid   A naturally occurring, thick, clear amber fluid that cleanses and carries nutrients to the joint and then carries wastes away from the joint. Secreted by the synovial membrane.

Joint Protection   A technique of performing tasks by less strainful means.

Kyphosis   Abnormal backward curvature of the spine; humpback.

Leg Length   Measured from the front of the pelvis bone to the inner ankle bone. Up to 1/2-inch discrepancy between the two legs can be normal.

Ligament   A thick fibrous-tissue hinge between two bones.

Limitation of Motion (LOM)   The amount of lost motion determined by measurement with a compasslike device called a goniometer.

Locking   Joint movement is suddenly temporarily halted, usually by a free-floating fragment of bone or cartilage within the joint.

LOM   See *Limitation of Motion (LOM)*.

Lumbar   The segment of the spine between the waist (below the last rib) and the pelvic bone (sacrum).

Lupus Erythematosus   Literally "red wolf." A disease so named because of the bright red mask across the cheeks and bridge of the nose. The disease inflames many organs and tissues, and there is damage to many internal organs.

Magnetic Resonance Imaging (MRD)   A diagnostic test that uses magnetism rather than x-rays.

Malignancy   A cancerous disease.

Mixed Connective-Tissue Disease   An uncommon disease with features of lupus erythematosus, rheumatoidlike arthritis, myositis, and systemic sclerosis. Thought to be less severe than any of the other individual diseases.

Morning Stiffness   A gelling of the joints when you first arise after sleep. Only significant if it lasts longer than 30 minutes. A cardinal sign of an inflammatory arthritis.

MRI   See *Magnetic Resonance Imaging (MRI)*.

Musculoskeletal   Refers to the tissues that provide movement.

Myalgia   Pain or aching of muscle origin.

Myofascial Pain   Pain in a body region that results from a trigger point located in an injured muscle.

Myositis   Inflammation within muscle tissue, usually part of a body-wide disease process (such as polymyositis or dermatomyositis).

Necrotizing Vasculitis   A disease that destroys tissue by attacking the walls of blood vessels. (See *Vasculitis*.)

Neoplasm   A new growth, a tumor. May be benign or malignant.

Neuropathy   Disease that harms nerve tissue.

Nonarticular Rheumatism   Diseases of the supporting joint tissues rather than the bony parts of the joint or the membrane within the joint.

Nonsteroidal Anti-inflammatory Drug (NSAID)   Drugs without corticosteroid properties but with properties that do fight inflammation and reduce fever, pain, and inflammatory swelling.

NSAID   See *Nonsteroidal Anti-inflammatory Drug*.

Nucleus Pulposus   A ball-like structure within the center of a vertebra. Contains a gelatinous center, which often ruptures into the spinal canal.

Obesity   The condition in which body weight exceeds normal weight by 20 percent or more.

Occupational Therapist (OT)   A specialist in the mechanical stresses that add to joint deformity; knowledgeable in techniques of joint protection, energy conservation, and rehabilitation. Fashioning braces and splints are also the specialized services of the occupational therapist.

Olecranon Pertaining to the point of the elbow.

Oral Of the mouth; given through the mouth.

Orthopedic Pertaining to corrective measures for skeletal deformity or crippling.

Osteoarthritis Arthritis that results from loss of the cartilaginous protective layer within a joint. It results from inherited factors (particularly when the fingers and great toe are involved) or from congenital mild structural changes in the shape of a bone (particularly in the hip and knee).

Osteomyelitis An infection of bone.

Osteoporosis Porous bones as a result of decreased protein and calcium in bone tissue. Causes include heredity, early menopause, decreased calcium intake or increased calcium loss, and hormonal imbalance in the regulation of calcium. In many cases the causes are not well understood.

OT See *Occupational Therapist (OT)*.

Painful-Arc Syndrome See *Frozen Shoulder*.

Patella The kneecap.

Patellofemoral Joint The joint between the kneecap and the femur.

Periarthritis Inflammation or irritation of the capsule and other supportive tissues surrounding a joint.

Physical Therapy Treatment with mechanical, thermal, or soundwave methods of transferring energy. Includes exercises to strengthen, realign, or improve joints or the spine.

Piriformis Syndrome Irritation of the piriformis muscle deep in the buttock. Can cause sciatica without impairment of the sciatic nerve.

Plantar Refers to the bottom of the foot.

Plica A fold of synovium (joint membrane) that can interfere with smooth joint motion.

Podagra Acute and very painful arthritis of the big toe joint, usually due to gout.

Polyarteritis Many inflamed vessels; a type of vasculitis.

Polyarthritis Many inflamed joints. A term often used when classical features of rheumatoid arthritis or other types of arthritis are lacking for diagnosis.

Polymyalgia Rheumatica   Aching and stiffness in many muscle areas, usually about the shoulders and hips. Often, it is a condition that stops as suddenly as it begins.

Polymyositis   A disease that inflames and damages many muscles in the neck, trunk, shoulders, and upper leg areas.

Popliteal   Refers to the area behind the knee.

Prednisone   The most commonly prescribed artificial (manufactured) corticosteroid. About four times more potent than cortisone.

Prepatellar Bursitis   See *Housemaid's Knee.*

Pseudogout   A condition that mimics gout but is due to a calcium salt (calcium pyrophosphate).

PSS   See *Systemic Sclerosis.*

Psychogenic Rheumatism   Musculoskeletal pain and disability due primarily to psychologic stress.

Psychosocial   Refers to conditions that relate to stress from emotional and situational events.

Radiographic   Pertaining to features seen on x-ray images.

Raynaud's Phenomenon   Cold sensitivity of distal parts (hands and feet) that turn blue, white, or red after exposure to cold. (Two or all three colors may be present.)

Referred Pain   When pain has traveled from an internal structure outward, upward, or downward. (The gallbladder, for example, can refer pain into the right shoulder blade.)

Reflex Sympathetic Dystrophy   A reaction in one or more limbs with burning and throbbing pain, edema, paleness, and sweaty limb that ultimately becomes waxy pale, with limited motion. Thought to result from a short-circuiting of the sympathetic nervous system.

Rheumatic   Pertaining to disease of the musculoskeletal system.

Rheumatic Fever   Arthritis that moves from joint to joint following a strep infection. Can cause inflammation within the walls of the heart or brain.

Rheumatism   An ailment of the musculoskeletal system.

Rheumatoid Arthritis A chronic illness with profound morning stiffness in joints, swelling of joints, painful joint motion; it may involve deep tissues in the skin, lungs, heart, nerves, and joints.

Rheumatoid Factor An antibody to the body's own gamma globulin and other proteins of the circulating blood.

Rheumatoid Spondylitis A term that is no longer used. See *Ankylosing Spondylitis*.

Schober Test A measurement for spinal flexibility.

Sciatica Pain that travels down the leg from the lower fold of the buttock.

Scleroderma See *Systemic Sclerosis*.

Scoliosis A side-to-side curvature of the spine.

Sedimentation Rate (Sed Rate) A screening test for body-wide inflammation.

Sed Rate See *Sedimentation Rate*.

Seronegative Test result indicating that the blood does not reveal an arthritis factor.

Shin Splints Cramp and pain in the inner foreleg that is relieved by rest.

Shoulder-Hand Syndrome Related to reflex sympathetic dystrophy but with a painful, stiff shoulder and a swollen hand.

Sjogren's Syndrome Condition with dryness of the eyes, mouth, and vagina.

SLE See *Lupus Erythematosus*.

Slipped Disc Improper term for ruptured disc.

Soft Tissue The nonbony parts of the musculoskeletal tissues.

Spondylitis Inflammatory disease of the sacroiliac and spinal joints.

Spondyloarthropathy Arthritis disorders that share features of eye inflammation and sacroiliac joint inflammation and are genetically linked.

Spondylolisthesis Condition when one vertebra can slide forward on another; usually a result of a congenital break in the small bones behind the involved vertebra.

Sprain A violent injury to a joint with injury to the ligaments.

Stenosing Tenosynovitis   Swelling and thickening of the sheath that surrounds a tendon, resulting in compression of the tendon. Can cause trigger finger.

Steroids   Natural or synthetic hormones derived from glands; usually refers to those produced by the adrenal gland.

Strain   Injury from overuse, overstretching, or squeezing.

Synovial Membrane   A lining within the cavity of a joint. The site of inflammation in many forms of arthritis.

Synovitis   Inflammation of the synovial membrane.

Systemic   Pertaining to a condition that involves most or all of the body.

Systemic Lupus Erythematosus (SLE)   See *Lupus Erythematosus*.

Systemic Sclerosis   A connective-tissue disease that hardens the lining of the skin, intestine, and lung. Raynaud's phenomenon may precede onset of this disease.

Tarsal   Refers to the ankle.

Tarsal-Tunnel Syndrome   Compression of the nerves that serve the bottom of the foot within a tunnel at the inner aspect of the ankle.

Temporal Arteritis   See *Giant-Cell Arteritis*.

Temporomandibular Joint   The jaw joint.

Temporomandibular Joint (TMJ) Syndrome   Painful disorder of the neck and face, often with headache. Usually due to or aggravated by unconscious jaw-clenching.

Tender Points   A series of painful points located within the musculoskeletal system that when persistent suggests a diagnosis of fibrositis.

Tendinitis   An inflammation or degeneration of the tissues constituting and covering a tendon.

Tendon   A fibrous cord that attaches a muscle to another body part.

Tennis Elbow   Irritation of the forearm tissues that causes pain along the outer or inner aspect of the elbow.

Tenosynovitis   Inflammation or degeneration of the sheath that covers a tendon.

TENS   See *Transcutaneous Electric Nerve Stimulator (TENS)*.

Thoracic   Refers to the upper trunk or chest.

Thoracic-Outlet Syndrome   Compression of the nerves and vessels of the arm within one of three tunnels at the top of the chest on each side.

TMJ Syndrome   See *Temporomandibular Joint Syndrome*.

Transcutaneous Electric Nerve Stimulator (TENS)   A device that transmits a small charge of electricity into the skin and can dull pain.

Traumatic Arthritis   Arthritis that results directly from trauma, usually in association with a fracture into the bony joint.

Trigger Finger   A momentarily locked state of finger movement. Can result from many problems within the finger or palm region.

Trigger Point   A spot within a muscle that causes pain at a distant point in the body, usually as a result of injury to the muscle.

Unproved   Lacking scientific proof. Requires standard research methods such as double-blind comparison against placebo.

Vascular   Refers to the system of blood vessels.

Vasculitis   A group of diseases with predominant injury to the blood vessels.

Vertebra   One of the back bones.

Xiphoidalgia   Pain in the lowest part of the breastbone.

Appendix

Products and Manufacturers

Products and manufacturers are listed here for your convenience.

Absorbine Jr.	W. F. Young, Inc. Springfield, MA 01103
ACE Bandage	Becton Dickinson Consumer Products 365 W. Passaic Street Rochelle Park, NJ 07662
Adapin	Pennwalt Pharmaceutical Corporation 755 Jefferson Road Rochester, NY 14623
Advil	Whitehall Laboratories Inc. 685 Third Avenue New York, NY 10017
Aristocort	Lederle Laboratories One Cyanamid Plaza Wayne, NJ 07470
Aristospan	Lederle Laboratories One Cyanamid Plaza Wayne, NJ 07470

Arthropan	The Purdue Frederick Co. 100 Connecticut Avenue Norwalk, CT 06854
Asendin	Lederle Laboratories One Cyanamid Plaza Wayne, NJ 07470
Aspercreme	Thompson Medical Company 919 Third Avenue New York, NY 10022
Atromid-S	Ayerst Laboratories 685 Third Avenue New York, NY 10017
Banalg	Thompson Medical Company 919 Third Avenue New York, NY 10022
Benemid	Merck Sharp & Dohme West Point, PA 19486
Ben-Gay	Leeming Division Pfizer Inc. 100 Jefferson Road Parsippany, NJ 07054
Butazolidin	Geigy Pharmaceuticals Ardsley, NY 10502
Cervipillo	TRU-EZE Mfg. Company 27635 Diaz Temecula, CA 92390
Clinoril	Merck Sharp & Dohme West Point, PA 19486
Cupramine	Merck Sharp & Dohme West Point, PA 19486
Cytoxan	Bristol-Myers Products 345 Park Avenue New York, NY 10154
Darvon	Eli Lilly and Co. Lilly Corporate Center Indianapolis, IN 46285
Deep-Down	J. B. Williams Co., Inc. 767 Fifth Avenue New York, NY 10022

DePen	Wallace Laboratories P.O. Box 1 Cranbury, NJ 08512
Depo-Medrol	The Upjohn Company 7000 Portage Road Kalamazoo, MI 49001
Desyrel	Mead Johnson & Company 2404 W. Pennsylvania Street Evansville, IN 47721
Disalcid	Riker Laboratories, Inc. 225-1S-07 3M Center St. Paul, MN 55144
Doan's Backache Spray	Jeffrey Martin Co. Union, NJ 07083
Dolobid	Merck Sharp & Dohme West Point, PA 19486
Easprin	Parke-Davis 201 Tabor Road Morris Plains, NJ 07950
Elavil	Merck Sharp & Dohme West Point, PA 19486
Endep	Roche Laboratories Manati, Puerto Rico 00701
Feldene	Pfizer Laboratories Division Pfizer Inc. 235 E. 42d Street New York, NY 10017
Flexeril	Merck Sharp & Dohme West Point, PA 19486
Fluori-Methane	Gebauer Chemical Co. 9410 St. Catherine Avenue Cleveland, OH 44104
Haltran	The Upjohn Company 7000 Portage Road Kalamazoo, MI 49001
Icy Hot	Searle Consumer Products Box 5110 Chicago, IL 60680

Imuran	Burroughs Wellcome Co. 3030 Cornwallis Road Research Triangle Park, NC 27709
Indocin	Merck Sharp & Dohme West Point, PA 19486
infraRUB	Whitehall Laboratories Inc. 685 Third Avenue New York, NY 10017
Isotoner gloves	Artis Isotoner Inc. 417 5th Avenue A 166 New York, NY 10016
Leukeran	Burroughs Wellcome Co. 3030 Cornwallis Road Research Triangle Park, NC 27709
Librium	Roche Laboratories Manati, Puerto Rico 00701
Ludiomil	Ciba Pharmaceutical Company 556 Morris Avenue Summitt, NJ 07901
Magan	Adria Laboratories P.O. Box 16529 Columbus, OH 43216
Maolate	The Upjohn Company 7000 Portage Road Kalamazoo, MI 49001
Meclomen	Parke-Davis 201 Tabor Road Morris Plains, NJ 07950
Medipren	McNeil Consumer Products Co. Fort Washington, PA 19034
Mentholatum	Mentholatum Company Buffalo, NY 14213
Methotrexate	Lederle Laboratories One Cyanamid Plaza Wayne, NJ 07470
Mobisyl Creme	B. F. Ascher & Company, Inc. 15501 W. 109th Street Lenexa, KS 66219

Motrin

The Upjohn Company
7000 Portage Road
Kalamazoo, MI 49001

Mustargen

Merck Sharp & Dohme
West Point, PA 19486

Myochrysine

Merck Sharp & Dohme
West Point, PA 19486

Myoflex Creme

Adria Laboratories
P.O. Box 16529
Columbus, OH 43216

Nalfon

Dista Products Company
Lilly Corporate Center
Indianapolis, IN 46285

Naprosyn

Syntex Laboratories, Inc.
3401 Hillview Avenue
P.O. Box 10950
Palo Alto, CA 94303

Norflex

Riker Laboratories, Inc.
225-1S-07 3M Center
St. Paul, MN 55144

Norpramin

Merrell Dow Pharmaceuticals Inc.
Cincinnati, OH 45242-9553

Nuprin

Bristol-Myers Products
345 Park Avenue
New York, NY 10154

Orudis

Wyeth Laboratories
P.O. Box 8299
Philadelphia, PA 19101

Pamelor

Sandoz, Inc.
Route 10
East Hanover, NJ 07936

Paraflex

McNeil Consumer Products Co.
Fort Washington, PA 19034

Plastizote

Spectrum Sports
Twinsburg, OH 44087

Quinamm

Merrell Dow Pharmaceuticals Inc.
Cincinnati, OH 45242-9553

Q-vel

Bio Products, Inc.
Westport, CT 06880

Ridaura	Smith Kline & French Laboratories 1500 Spring Garden Street P.O. Box 7929 Philadelphia, PA 19101
Robaxin	A. H. Robins Company 1407 Cummings Drive Richmond, VA 23220
Rufen	Boots Pharmaceuticals, Inc. 6540 Line Avenue Shreveport, LA 71106
Sinequan	Roerig Division Pfizer Pharmaceuticals 235 E. 42d St. New York, NY 10017
Solganal	Schering Corporation Galloping Hill Road Kenilworth, NJ 07033
Soma	Wallace Laboratories P.O. Box 1 Cranbury, NJ 08512
Spandex	E. I. du Pont deNemours & Co, Inc. Wilmington, DE 19898
Spenco	Spenco Medical Products P.O. Box 2501 Waco, TX 76702
Sportscreme	Thompson Medical Company 919 Third Avenue New York, NY 10022
Surmontil	Wyeth Laboratories P.O. Box 8299 Philadelphia, PA 19101
Tagamet	Smith Kline & French Laboratories 1500 Spring Garden Street P.O. Box 7929 Philadelphia, PA 19101
Thiotepa	Lederle Laboratories One Cyanamid Plaza Wayne, NJ 07470

Titralac	Riker Laboratories, Inc. 225-1S-07 3M Center St. Paul, MN 55144
Tofranil	Geigy Pharmaceuticals Ardsley, NY 10502
Tolectin	McNeil Consumer Products Co. Fort Washington, PA 19034
Trilisate	The Purdue Frederick Co. 100 Connecticut Avenue Norwalk, CT 06854
Valium	Roche Laboratories Manati, Puerto Rico 00701
Vaporub	Richardson Vicks Wilton, CT 06897
Vivactil	Merck Sharp & Dohme West Point, PA 19486
Wal-Pil-o	RoLoke Co. Box 24DD3 West Los Angeles, CA 90024
Wygesic	Wyeth Laboratories P.O. Box 8299 Philadelphia, PA 19101
Zantac	Glaxo Inc. Five Moore Drive Research Triangle Park, NC 27709
ZORprin	Boots Pharmaceuticals, Inc. 6540 Line Avenue Shreveport, LA 71106
Zyloprim	Burroughs Wellcome Co. 3030 Cornwallis Road Research Triangle Park, NC 27709

Index